Rapid On-Site Evaluation (ROSE)
in Diagnostic Interventional Pulmonology

Jing Feng · Wen Ning
Dianhua Jiang · Jingyu Chen · Bo Wu
Editors

Rapid On-Site Evaluation (ROSE) in Diagnostic Interventional Pulmonology

Volume 2: Interstitial Lung Diseases

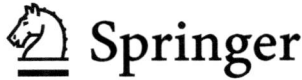 Springer

Editors
Jing Feng
Pulmonary and Critical Care Medicine
Tianjin Medical University General
Hospital
Tianjin
China

Dianhua Jiang
Cedars-Sinai Medical Center
Los Angeles
USA

Bo Wu
Lung Transplantation Group
Nanjing Medical University
Wuxi
China

Wen Ning
College of Life Sciences
Nankai University
Tianjin
China

Jingyu Chen
Lung Transplantation Group
Nanjing Medical University
Wuxi
China

ISBN 978-981-15-0938-4   ISBN 978-981-15-0939-1   (eBook)
https://doi.org/10.1007/978-981-15-0939-1

This Springer imprint is published by the registered company Springer Nature Singapore Pte Ltd. The registered company address is: 152 Beach Road, #21-01/04 Gateway East, Singapore 189721, Singapore

Contents

Rapid On-Site Evaluation (ROSE) in Diagnostic Interventional Pulmonology: Introduction and Detailed Methods

Jing Feng, Qiang Li, Yi Shi, and Ke Wang

In recent years, the use of diagnostic interventional pulmonology has been booming due to the increased prevalence of lung cancer, more drug-

The content of the Chapter 1 has been published in "Rapid On-Site Evaluation (ROSE) in Diagnostic Interventional Pulmonology Volume 1: Infectious Diseases"
Print ISBN 978-981-13-3455-9
Online ISBN 978-981-13-3456-6
Chapter 1 Rapid On-Site Evaluation (ROSE) in Diagnostic Interventional Pulmonology: Introduction and Detailed Methods
Jing Feng, Qiang Li, Yi Shi, Ke Wang
Pages 1–9
https://link.springer.com/chapter/10.1007/978-981-13-3456-6_1

J. Feng (✉)
Pulmonary and Critical Care Medicine, Tianjin Medical University General Hospital, Tianjin, China
e-mail: zyyhxkfj@126.com

Q. Li
Department of Respiratory and Critical Care Medicine, Shanghai East Hospital, Tongji University School of Medicine, Shanghai, China
e-mail: liqressh@hotmail.com

Y. Shi
Department of Respiratory and Critical Care Medicine, Jinling Hospital of Nanjing University, Nanjing, Jiangsu, China
e-mail: shiyi56@163.com

K. Wang
Department of Respiratory Medicine, The 1st Affiliated Hospital of Guangxi Medical University, Nanning, China
e-mail: 497256113@qq.com

resistant pathogen infections of lower respiratory tract, and urgent request for diagnosis of baffling and critical respiratory diseases. The efficiency of interventional diagnostics has become one of the most important references for rating pulmonology or cancer center, which promote the clinical application of numerous advanced technologies and facilities. As a "real-time accompany technique" for diagnostic interventional pulmonology, rapid on-site evaluation (ROSE) has also been paid an unprecedented attention and develops promptly.

1.1 Definition and Work Content of Diagnostic Interventional Pulmonology ROSE

The diagnostic interventional pulmonology ROSE is a real-time cytological examination technique which accompanies sequential sampling. The process of ROSE is as follows: A small part of every tissue specimen sampled from target lesion is smeared on a slide without losing tissue material significantly. Then the cytological slide is stained as soon as possible. Finally, the stained slide is interpreted immediately under specialized microscope integrating with all the available clinical information. The cytological content to be interpreted includes cellular morphology, differential cell counts, constituent ratio, cellular array, mutual relation, cytological background, and analysis of exotic substance.

J. Feng et al. (eds.), *Rapid On-Site Evaluation (ROSE) in Diagnostic Interventional Pulmonology*,
https://doi.org/10.1007/978-981-15-0939-1_1

As a carrier of cells, ROSE slide plays the following roles: evaluation of adequate sampling, real-time guidance for interventional methods and modalities, approaching a preliminary diagnosis or narrowing differential diagnosis spectrum, optimizing processing scheme for target lesion specimen, analyzing patients' disease status, and prognosis in combination with all available clinical and cytological information. It is still controversial about whether ROSE can increase the rate of successful diagnosis in diagnostic interventional pulmonology.

1.2 Historic Evolution and Prospect Forecast of ROSE Clinical Practice

"Modern" ROSE was first applied in interventional pulmonology in 1981. Pak et al. [1] used a quick staining and rapid interpretation technique in the procedure of percutaneous transthoracic fine needle aspiration biopsy under fluoroscopic guidance. Staining could be accomplished within 5 min, and interpretation was available less than 15 min after sampling target lesions. Successful diagnosis was achieved in 36 of 37 patients (97%). An improved rate of successful diagnosis following the "bedside" rapid stain was then proposed, which reflected the advantage of being able to determine the adequacy of specimens before releasing patients from the procedure room.

The use of "modern" ROSE in interventional operation with flexible bronchoscopy began from 1990. Davenport [2] suggested that ROSE might significantly improve the diagnostic yield of transbronchial aspirates.

Around 2005, "minimally invasive internal medicine" techniques with favorable sensitivity and specificity, including transbronchial needle aspiration (TBNA), began to spread widely. These techniques were not only applied to the diagnosis of lung/mediastinal malignancies but also benign diseases such as sarcoidosis, tuberculosis, etc.

If operators are satisfied with the specimen got through these procedures, it is not necessary to perform more invasive surgeries such as mediastinoscopy, video-assisted thoracoscopic surgery (VATS), and open lung biopsy. Meanwhile, inter-

ventional pulmonologists have to answer questions regarding the following: Whether the target specimen is obtained and sufficient? How to deal with target specimen appropriately? Can a preliminary diagnosis be achieved or a wide differential diagnosis spectrum be narrowed? Can patients' disease status and prognosis be analyzed comprehensively in combination with all available clinical and cytological information? Obviously, this "real-time feedback" ROSE information is invaluable.

During interventional procedures, if target specimen is satisfactory, the procedure stops where it should stop, which can not only save time and medical resources but also reduce pain, trauma, and complications. On the contrary, the procedure should be continued, and interventional methods and modalities may have to be changed appropriately. If a preliminary diagnosis is made, differential diagnosis spectrum is narrowed, or disease status is integrated, an important reference may be provided for clinicians to establish a thorough diagnostic protocol and treatment regimen. And it can also help to select processing scheme for target lesion specimen including oncological examinations such as immunohistochemistry, polymerase chain reaction (PCR), chromosome fluorescence in situ hybridization (FISH), electron microscopy, and microbiological examinations such as special staining, grinded tissue culture, etc. And it can also assist in the selection of further means of procedures. In a case for which ROSE in TBNA has provided a relatively definite diagnosis of malignant tumor and obtained satisfactory specimens for follow-up oncology-related examination, the transbronchial lung biopsy (TBLB) with higher risks of complications is then not necessary [3]. The entire interventional diagnostic operation is thus considered optimized. Therefore, ROSE has been widely accepted and utilized during this period [4] and is matured in about 2010 [5, 6].

Since 2010, high-tech equipment represented by virtual bronchoscopy navigation (VBN), ultrathin bronchoscopy, endobronchial ultrasound (EBUS), electromagnetic navigation (EMN) bronchoscopy, etc. was widely used in interventional pulmonary diagnosis and treatment [7, 8]. Due to the high cost of such technical equipment, relatively complicated manipulating process, and expensive consumable items, an extremely high success rate of intervention diagnosis is required; with the addition of the urgent needs of microbial etiology in critical respiratory disease, ROSE has almost become a "standard configuration" in interventional lung disease diagnosis and treatment center.

In 1997, the birth of clone sheep shocked the world, and it showed that single somatic cell could contain almost all the life information. Recently, rapid development and extensive application of molecular diagnostics have brought cytological technology to rejuvenate. At present, the ability to diagnose of cytology is almost comparable to that of histology [9] and is distinctly advantageous in many aspects [10, 11]. ROSE glass slide, as a cell carrier, can not only be used to make cytological interpretation but also can be a "treasure trove" for preserving and studying cells. All cell-based molecular biology and gene technology can be carried out using the ROSE glass slides, including PCR, FISH, immunocytochemistry, second-generation gene sequencing, etc. [11, 12]. The development of biotechnology is at a tremendous pace, especially that the progress of molecular biology and genetic technology is beyond imagination. In this scenario, the future of ROSE is anticipated.

1.3   Basic Working Conditions and Equipment Requirements of ROSE

1.3.1   ROSE Cytological Microscope

The main equipment of ROSE is a dedicated cytological microscope, and the ocular lens are usually ×10 (10 times), while the wide-field objective lens are ×10 (10 times) and ×40 (40 times). "Oil-free" ×100 objective lens (100 times) is recommended, which is not only necessary for observing characteristics of microorganisms but also an easy access to get high-quality graphic information.

1.3.2   Graphic Imaging and Photographic System

It should be equipped with high-resolution graphic imaging and photographic system for

report making, data summary, case review, academic exchange, clinical education, etc. A high-resolution camera with autofocus function is recommended to integrate on a microscope as its graphic system.

1.3.3   ROSE for Infectious Diseases

In principle, the preparing of infection-related ROSE slides should be carried out in Class II biosafety cabinet. The slides and staining liquor should be specially treated after interpretation. After all, the operators must get biosafety-related training and have the required qualifications.

1.3.4   Location Requirements

ROSE must be positioned at the procedure room, providing primary cytological interpretation and exchanging real-time impression. The advanced interventional pulmonary center may be equipped with a professional ROSE room, which should connect to the procedure site or can show microscope graphic information directly to operators in real time through electronic systems.

1.3.5   Preparation for ROSE

Sterile cytological slides with cell adhesion, absorbent paper, powder-free latex gloves, and disposable 2.5/5 mL syringe needles should be prepared before procedure, and a full set of Diff-Quik (DQ) staining liquor can be poured into sealed glass dyeing cylinders for convenience.

1.3.6   Conservation of Stained Slides

Stained slides and dyeing liquor for infectious diseases should be treated after use following Class II biosafety protocols. It is recommended to place stained cytological slides in a cool and dry place directly for long-term preservation and not to use neutral gum for slide sealing to avoid missing cytological information.

1.4 The Detailed Work Process for ROSE

ROSE is to proceed with the three steps of preparing, staining, and interpreting continuously. As ROSE needs to "guide interventional pulmonary procedures" real time, in clinical practice, preparing, staining, and interpreting of ROSE slides should be accomplished in succession promptly.

1.4.1 The Preparation of Cytological Slides for ROSE

1.4.1.1 Imprinting (Rolling)

It is the most commonly used method, suitable for transbronchial lung biopsy (TBLB), conventional transbronchial needle aspiration (TBNA) with tissue-incising needles (such as Wang's MW-319 needle), mucosa biopsy under direct bronchoscopic vision, medical thoracoscopy biopsy under direct scopic vision, and percutaneous tissue-incising needle lung biopsy.

After target site sampled, the tissue pellets are picked up with a disposable 2.5/5 mL syringe needle from biopsy forceps cup or percutaneous tissue-incising needle groove or are pushed out from tissue-incising needle (such as Wang's MW-319 needle). Then the specimens are smeared roundly on the one-third dyeing side of cytological slide, which should have a strong cell adhesion, with a diameter of about 1 cm and a proper thickness without losing materials for histopathological exam as its premise. After that, the tissue pellets are processed conventionally step-by-step including pathologic or microbiological exams, and the target specimen flow direction is optimized according to the results of ROSE interpretation, thus adjusting further process means.

1.4.1.2 Brushing

It is applicable to specimens brushed with ordinary cell brush, protected specimen brush, or ultrafine cell brush, as well as semiliquid speci-

mens including sputum, viscous body fluid, etc. After target site is drawn, the brush tip is pushed out, and the specimens are smeared on the one-third dyeing side of cytological slide, which should have a strong cell adhesion, forming a rectangle of about 1×2 cm. Slides in other processes such as regular slides sent to pathology department and microbiology laboratory should be still prepared according to the conventional methods.

1.4.1.3 Spraying

It is applicable for fine needle aspiration (FNA) and conventional transbronchial needle aspiration (TBNA) with cytological needle such as SW-121, SW-122, SW-521, and SW-522 type of Wang's needle and so on. After target site sampled, the needle tip is pressed against the one-third dyeing side of cytological slide, which should have a strong cell adhesion. As air pressurizing at needle tail, the specimens are smeared roundly with a diameter of about 1 cm and a proper thickness without losing materials for histopathological exam as its premise. Slides in other processes such as regular slides sent to pathology department and microbiology laboratory should be still prepared according to conventional methods.

1.4.1.4 Leaving

It is appropriate to endobronchial ultrasonography (EBUS)-induced transbronchial needle aspiration (TBNA), so-called EBUS-TBNA. After target site sampled, the needle tip is pressed against the one-third dyeing side of cytological slide, which should have a strong cell adhesion, and the tissue paste is pushed out with the inner needle. After most of the tissue specimens are taken away with filter paper hold by pointed tweezers, the cytological material will be left on the slide to become a ROSE film. Then the tissue paste sent to pathology department and microbiology laboratory should be still prepared according to conventional methods. Or ROSE cytological slides in EBUS-TBNA can also be prepared using the aforementioned "spraying" method.

1.4.2 Rapid Staining of ROSE Cytological Slides (Staining)

The World Health Organization (WHO) recommends the use of Diff-Quik (DQ) staining liquor to rapidly stain ROSE cytological slides. DQ staining has been modified from Romanowsky stain technology, which has the similar interpreting results to Wright's staining. DQ staining liquor contains acid dye (eosin) and alkaline dye (methylene blue). DQ staining's rationale is the constituents to be dyed have different affinities to staining liquor and show different colors for identifying the morphological characteristics. It consumes very short time (only about 30–70 s) for cytological slides to be stained after the target site is sampled. Thus, the interpreting process of ROSE forms a "real-time" feedback to interventional procedure because of time-saving preparing and staining.

It is recommended to use "dip" staining rather than "drop" staining to improve quality and efficiency. DQ A solution, DQ B solution, phosphate-buffered saline (PBS), and water are poured, respectively, in glass vials with lids. Individual ROSE slide is dipped in DQ A solution for 10–30 s and transferred to PBS vial washing DQ A solution. Then the slide is soaked in DQ B solution for 20–40 s and washed in water tank. Finally, residual liquid is removed from slide with bibulous paper. Glass vials holding DQ A solution, DQ B solution, and PBS should be sealed after use because these solutions are volatilizable.

1.4.3 To Interpret ROSE Cytological Slides Promptly and Comprehensively

The stained ROSE slide should be delivered immediately to the assistant and interpreted real timely with specialized cytological microscope. Cytological interpreting impression is indispensable part of the information needed for analyzing disease status comprehensively. In practice, ROSE interpretation should be based on all the available knowledge and clinical information, which should include the following:

1. Multidisciplinary knowledge about respiratory diseases, interventional pulmonology, pathology, clinical microbiology, infectious diseases, oncology, etc.
2. Detailed medical history and physical examination.
3. All the diagnosis and treatment process and development of the disease.
4. Imaging manifestations, especially comparison of imaging data before and after treatment.
5. Laboratory tests and comparison of laboratory data before and after treatment.
6. Manifestations of endoscopic vision and physical properties of the specimens obtained during the interventional procedure.
7. "Real-time" ROSE impression of the cytological interpretation after target site is confirmed and sampled precisely.

1.5 ROSE Implications for Disease/Disease Status

In general, ROSE is significative and putative in the diagnosis and differential diagnosis of lung disease/disease status as listed below:

1. Most common types of solid malignancies and histological typing of tumor.
2. Tuberculosis and its different development stages.
3. Sarcoidosis.
4. Mycoplasma pneumonia.
5. Viral pneumonia.
6. Some kinds of mycotic pneumonia (such as aspergillus, cryptococcus, or candida).
7. Organizing pneumonia or organizing status (i.e., organization) or fibrosis.
8. Pyogenic infection.
9. Necrotic infection or necrotic changes (necrosis).
10. Some kinds of allergic diseases or allergic changes.
11. Some kinds of rheumatic diseases, immune diseases (such as certain types of vasculitis), or immune changes.
12. Others, such as post-chemotherapy immune reconstitution or related changes after lung transplantation.

1.6 Consensus and Controversy in Clinical Practice of ROSE

1.6.1 ROSE and Histopathology/ Laboratory Medicine Are Mutual Complementation Rather than Mutual Repulsion

ROSE is a carrier of cytological information, and it is independent and interrelated among cytology, histopathology, and ecsomatics. ROSE will not compromise the status of histopathology or ecsomatics in clinical diagnosis. On the contrary, high-quality specimens can be obtained and delivered to the department of pathology and laboratory with the help of ROSE. Thus, the target specimen quality can be controlled, and the use of specimens can be optimized, when it will provide focus of attention to the auxiliary departments without delay. Similarly, the evaluation of ROSE cytological significance should not depend absolutely on whether the histopathology/laboratory examination has "positive results" or not. Cytological interpretation of ROSE is based on its own analysis index. ROSE impressions should be considered as a key component of diagnosis basis and integrated with all the available clinical information. It is not appropriate to excessively limit the flow of specimens according to ROSE impressions unless ROSE diagnosis is definite or the specimen amount is insufficient and further sampling is impossible. It is recommended to add nonstandard specimen inspection process not designed originally, such as special pathogen staining on tissue sections, according to ROSE results, thereby increasing the diagnostic efficiency.

1.6.2 Obtaining Target Lesion Is the Basis of ROSE Interpretation

The interpreting and comprehensive analyzing of ROSE should not be carried out until the specimen is obtained precisely from target lesions. Otherwise, the ROSE interpretation is worthless or even misleading clinical decision. If target lesion is not obtained, interventional modes and modalities should be modified to attempt repeatedly with the help of ROSE.

1.6.3 ROSE Is Not Exactly "Observe the Pathogenic Microorganism Itself"

In some kinds of mycotic pneumonia pathogens (such as aspergillus, cryptococcus, or candida), ROSE can interpret the pathogen directly according to microbial morphology. In case of other infectious diseases like tuberculosis, interpreting ROSE should be based more on cytological background integrated with available clinical information. ROSE is not only a "real-time" state analysis of illnesses but also an auxiliary beforehand anticipation for progression of disease.

1.6.4 It Is Still Controversial Whether ROSE Can Increase the Yield Rate of Diagnostic Interventional Pulmonology

In the 1980s, emergence of ROSE was aimed at improving the yield rate of diagnostic interventional pulmonology [1, 2]. As a carrier of cytological information, ROSE clinical value is continuously explored, and it is utilized further with the development of biotechnology. In recent years, there have been researches to question ROSE's "original intention" in improving diagnostic yield rate.

The controversy is mainly reflected in TBNA for lymph nodes, regardless of conventional lymph node TBNA or EBUS-lymph node TBNA. In cases of conventional lymph node TBNA, some researchers argue that ROSE can improve the positive rate [13, 14], while others thought that it cannot [5]. Similar arguments have been put forward for EBUS-lymph node TBNA. Some argue ROSE's positive value [15–17], especially for lymph node malignancy genotyping [18] or benign diseases [19], when others deem there is no difference [20–22]. However, from the perspective of reducing complications and improving the "exact diagnosis" efficiency, using ROSE is not only recommended in conventional lymph node TBNA [5] but also suggested in EBUS-lymph node TBNA [3], which was demonstrated by a large multicenter study.

In other diagnostic interventional procedures in applications of "high-tech equipment" except of lymph node TBNA, such as pulmonary peripheral lesion TBNA [23], positioning biopsy with peripheral lung radial EBUS (R-EBUS) [24, 25], peripheral lung precise bronchoscopic brushings [26], and positioning biopsy with peripheral pulmonary EMN [27–29], ROSE is proven to increase the positive rate of diagnostic interventional procedures in majority of current studies. More prospective randomized controlled studies are warranted for further conclusions.

1.6.5 Applying ROSE May Benefit More to the Following Interventional Procedures

1. Procedures applying "high-tech equipment" such as EMN and R-EBUS.
2. Target lesions difficult to sample, such as lesions that cannot directly be viewed through endoscope, very small target lesions, or lesions difficult to access.
3. Procedures with high risk of complications, to minimize the sampled material and stop where it should stop.
4. Short of sampled material may optimize the use of specimens with the help of ROSE preliminary impression.
5. Diagnosis and treatment that should be completed at the same time, such as EMN positioning thermal ablation for pulmonary peripheral nodules.
6. Urgent target lesion assessment for critical respiratory diseases requires timely differential diagnosis and treatment plan.
7. To narrow the spectrum of differential diagnosis or analyze patients' disease status and prognosis in combination with all available clinical and cytological information.
8. "Exact diagnosis" or "immediate diagnosis" must be made in a single procedure or the

obvious existence of psychological and objective pressure.
9. Operation demo, academic exchange, technical training, or clinical teaching.

1.6.6 Who Will Interpret ROSE Slides?

ROSE should be completed under the predominance of a clinical (interventional) physician, and so is a comprehensive evaluating process rather than just a histopathology/laboratory process. Staffs involved in ROSE interpretation should be cytopathologists, cytopathological technicians, laboratorians and trained clinical/interventional physicians, nurses, common technicians, interns, etc. [30]. If ROSE report is needed for medical records or charges, it can be issued by a qualified cytopathology physician or laboratorian.

References

1. Pak HY, Yokota S, Teplitz RL, Shaw SL, Werner JL. Rapid staining techniques employed in fine needle aspirations of the lung. Acta Cytol. 1981;25(2):178–84.
2. Davenport RD. Rapid on-site evaluation of transbronchial aspirates. Chest. 1990;98(1):59–61.
3. Eapen GA, Shah AM, Lei X, Jimenez CA, Morice RC, Yarmus L, Filner J, Ray C, Michaud G, Greenhill SR, Sarkiss M, Casal R, Rice D, Ost DE. American College of Chest Physicians Quality Improvement Registry, Education. Complications, consequences, and practice patterns of endobronchial ultrasound-guided transbronchial needle aspiration: results of the AQuIRE registry. Chest. 2013;143(4):1044–53.
4. Gasparini S. It is time for this 'ROSE' to flower. Respiration. 2005;72(2):129–31.
5. Trisolini R, Cancellieri A, Tinelli C, Paioli D, Scudeller L, Casadei GP, Parri SF, Livi V, Bondi A, Boaron M, Patelli M. Rapid on-site evaluation of transbronchial aspirates in the diagnosis of hilar and mediastinal adenopathy: a randomized trial. Chest. 2011;139(2):395–401. https://doi.org/10.1378/chest.10-1521.
6. Diacon AH, Koegelenberg CF, Schubert P, Brundyn K, Louw M, Wright CA, Bolliger CT. Rapid on-site evaluation of transbronchial aspirates: randomised comparison of two methods. Eur Respir J. 2010;35(6):1216–20. https://doi.org/10.1183/09031936.00050809.
7. Asano F, Eberhardt R, Herth FJ. Virtual bronchoscopic navigation for peripheral pulmonary

lesions. Respiration. 2014;88(5):430–40. https://doi.org/10.1159/000367900.

8. Zaric B, Stojsic V, Sarcev T, Stojanovic G, Carapic V, Perin B, Zarogoulidis P, Darwiche K, Tsakiridis K, Karapantzos I, Kesisis G, Kougioumtzi I, Katsikogiannis N, Machairiotis N, Stylianaki A, Foroulis CN, Zarogoulidis K. Advanced broncho-scopic techniques in diagnosis and staging of lung cancer. J Thorac Dis. 2013;5(Suppl 4):S359–70. https://doi.org/10.3978/j.issn.2072-1439.2013.05.15.

9. Travis WD, Brambilla E, Noguchi M, Nicholson AG, Geisinger K, Yatabe Y, Ishikawa Y, Wistuba I, Flieder DB, Franklin W, Gazdar A, Hasleton PS, Henderson DW, Kerr KM, Petersen I, Roggli V, Thunnissen E, Tsao M. Diagnosis of lung cancer in small biopsies and cytology: implications of the 2011 International Association for the Study of Lung Cancer/American Thoracic Society/European Respiratory Society clas-sification. Arch Pathol Lab Med. 2013;137(5):668–84. https://doi.org/10.5858/arpa.2012-0263-RA.

10. Fischer AH, Cibas ES, Howell LP, Kurian EM, Laucirica R, Moriarty AT, Renshaw AA, Zakowski MF, Young NA. Role of cytology in the manage-ment of non-small-cell lung cancer. J Clin Oncol. 2011;29(24):3331–2; author reply 3332–3. https://doi.org/10.1200/JCO.2011.35.2534.

11. Chandra S, Chandra H, Sindhwani G. Role of rapid on-site evaluation with cyto-histopathological correlation in diagnosis of lung lesion. J Cytol. 2014;31(4):189–93. https://doi.org/10.4103/0970-9371.151128.

12. Rekhtman N, Brandt SM, Sigel CS, Friedlander MA, Riely GJ, Travis WD, Zakowski MF, Moreira AL. Suitability of thoracic cytology for new thera-peutic paradigms in non-small cell lung carcinoma: high accuracy of tumor subtyping and feasibility of EGFR and KRAS molecular testing. J Thorac Oncol. 2011;6(3):451–8. https://doi.org/10.1097/JTO.0b013e31820517a3.

13. Bruno P, Ricci A, Esposito MC, Scozzi D, Tabbì L, Sposato B, Falasca C, Giarnieri E, Giovagnoli MR, Mariotta S. Efficacy and cost effectiveness of rapid on site examination (ROSE) in management of patients with mediastinal lymphadenopathies. Eur Rev Med Pharmacol Sci. 2013;17(11):1517–22.

14. Madan K, Dhungana A, Mohan A, Hadda V, Jain D, Arava S, Pandey RM, Khilnani GC, Guleria R. Conventional transbronchial needle aspiration versus endobronchial ultrasound-guided transbron-chial needle aspiration, with or without rapid on-site evaluation, for the diagnosis of sarcoidosis: a random-ized controlled trial. J Bronchol Interv Pulmonol. 2017;24(1):48–58.

15. Nakajima T, Yasufuku K, Saegusa F, Fujiwara T, Sakairi Y, Hiroshima K, Nakatani Y, Yoshino I. Rapid on-site cytologic evaluation during endobronchial ultrasound-guided transbronchial needle aspira-tion for nodal staging in patients with lung cancer. Ann Thorac Surg. 2013;95(5):1695–9. https://doi.org/10.1016/j.athoracsur.2012.09.074.

16. Cardoso AV, Neves I, Magalhães A, Sucena M, Barroca H, Fernandes G. The value of rapid on-site evaluation during EBUS-TBNA. Rev Port Pneumol (2006). 2015;21(5):253–8. https://doi.org/10.1016/j.rppnen.2015.02.003.

17. Guo H, Liu S, Guo J, Li B, Li W, Lu Z, Sun J, Zhang B, Yu J. Rapid on-site evaluation during endobron-chial ultrasound-guided transbronchial needle aspi-ration for the diagnosis of hilar and mediastinal lymphadenopathy in patients with lung cancer. Cancer Lett. 2016;371(2):182–6. https://doi.org/10.1016/j.canlet.2015.11.038.

18. Trisolini R, Cancellieri A, Tinelli C, de Biase D, Valentini I, Casadei G, Paioli D, Ferrari F, Gordini G, Patelli M, Tallini G. Randomized trial of endobron-chial ultrasound-guided transbronchial needle aspi-ration with and without rapid on-site evaluation for lung cancer genotyping. Chest. 2015;148(6):1430–7. https://doi.org/10.1378/chest.15-0583.

19. Plit ML, Havryk AP, Hodgson A, James D, Field A, Carbone S, Glanville AR, Bashirzadeh F, Chay AM, Hundloe J, Pearson R, Fielding D. Rapid cytological analysis of endobronchial ultrasound-guided aspi-rates in sarcoidosis. Eur Respir J. 2013;42(5):1302–8. https://doi.org/10.1183/09031936.00128312.

20. Joseph M, Jones T, Lutterbie Y, Maygarden SJ, Feins RH, Haithcock BE, Veeramachaneni NK. Rapid on-site pathologic evaluation does not increase the efficacy of endobronchial ultrasonographic biopsy for mediastinal staging. Ann Thorac Surg. 2013;96(2):403–10. https://doi.org/10.1016/j.athoracsur.2013.04.003.

21. Griffin AC, Schwartz LE, Baloch ZW. Utility of on-site evaluation of endobronchial ultra-sound-guided transbronchial needle aspiration specimens. Cytojournal. 2011;8:20. https://doi.org/10.4103/1742-6413.90081.

22. Oki M, Saka H, Kitagawa C, Kogure Y, Murata N, Adachi T, Ando M. Rapid on-site cytologic evaluation during endobronchial ultrasound-guided transbron-chial needle aspiration for diagnosing lung cancer: a randomized study. Respiration. 2013;85(6):486–92. https://doi.org/10.1159/000346987.

23. Mondoni M, Sotgiu G, Bonifazi M, Dore S, Parazzini EM, Carlucci P, Gasparini S, Centanni S. Transbronchial needle aspiration in peripheral pulmonary lesions: a systematic review and meta-analysis. Eur Respir J. 2016;48(1):196–204. https://doi.org/10.1183/13993003.00051-2016.

24. Chen CH, Cheng WC, Wu BR, Chen CY, Chen WC, Hsia TC, Liao WC, Tu CY, Shih CM, Hsu WH, Wang KP. Improved diagnostic yield of bronchoscopy in peripheral pulmonary lesions: combination of radial probe endobronchial ultrasound and rapid on-site evaluation. J Thorac Dis. 2015;7(Suppl 4):S418–25. https://doi.org/10.3978/j.issn.2072-1439.2015.12.13.

25. Zaric B, Eberhardt R, Herth F, Stojsic V, Carapic V, Popovic ZP, Perin B. Linear and radial endobronchial ultrasound in diagnosis and staging of lung cancer.

Expert Rev Med Devices. 2013;10(5):685–95. https://doi.org/10.1586/17434440.2013.827512.

26. Steinfort DP, Leong TL, Laska IF, Beaty A, Tsui A, Irving LB. Diagnostic utility and accuracy of rapid on-site evaluation of bronchoscopic brushings. Eur Respir J. 2015;45(6):1653–60. https://doi.org/10.1183/09031936.00111314.

27. Loo FL, Halligan AM, Port JL, Hoda RS. The emerging technique of electromagnetic navigation bronchoscopy-guided fine-needle aspiration of peripheral lung lesions: promising results in 50 lesions. Cancer Cytopathol. 2014;122(3):191–9. https://doi.org/10.1002/cncy.21373.

28. Balbo PE, Bodini BD, Patrucco F, Della Corte F, Zanaboni S, Bagnati P, Andorno S, Magnani C. Electromagnetic navigation bronchoscopy and rapid on site evaluation added to fluoroscopy-guided assisted bronchoscopy and rapid on site evaluation: improved yield in pulmonary nodules. Minerva Chir. 2013;68(6):579–85.

29. Karnak D, Ciledağ A, Ceyhan K, Atasoy C, Akyar S, Kayacan O. Rapid on-site evaluation and low registration error enhance the success of electromagnetic navigation bronchoscopy. Ann Thorac Med. 2013;8(1):28–32. https://doi.org/10.4103/1817-1737.105716.

30. Bonifazi M, Sediari M, Ferretti M, Poidomani G, Tramacere I, Mei F, Zuccatosta L, Gasparini S. The role of the pulmonologist in rapid on-site cytologic evaluation of transbronchial needle aspiration: a prospective study. Chest. 2014;145(1):60–5. https://doi.org/10.1378/chest.13-0756.

Anatomic Distribution and Morphology of Common Tracheal/Bronchial/Pulmonary Cells

2

Jing Feng, Pei Li, Xin Li, and Hongmei Zhou

2.1 Native Tracheal/Bronchial/Pulmonary Cells

2.1.1 Cell Components of Proximal Airways

Ciliary columnar epithelial cells (ciliated cells), goblet cells, brush cells, basal cells, and neuroendocrine cells.

2.1.2 Cell Components of Terminal Airways (Bronchioli)

These include ciliary columnar epithelial cells (ciliated cells) and glabrous cells.

The content of the Chapter 2 has been published in "Rapid On-Site Evaluation (ROSE) in Diagnostic Interventional Pulmonology Volume 1: Infectious Diseases"
Print ISBN 978-981-13-3455-9
Online ISBN 978-981-13-3456-6
Chapter 2 Anatomic Distribution and Morphology of Common Tracheal/Bronchial/Pulmonary Cells
Jing Feng, Pei Li, Xin Li, Hongmei Zhou
Pages 11–15
https://link.springer.com/chapter/10.1007/978-981-13-3456-6_2

Glabrous cells: Glabrous cells are mainly Clara cells. Others are bronchiolar neuroendocrine cells (labeled as K, very few) and various types of bronchiolo-epithelial cells (e.g., occasional distal airway basal cells). These cells can be collectively referred to as distal/terminal bronchiolar epithelial cells, or distal airway epithelial cells, or Feng's cells, labeled as F.

2.1.3 Cell Components of Gas Exchange Areas

Type II pneumocytes and Type I pneumocytes.

2.1.4 Other Native Cell Components

Fibroblasts and fibrocytes, glandular cells, myocytes, basement (membrane) cells of blood vessel (difficult to differentiate from airway basal cells), and others.

J. Feng (✉)
Pulmonary and Critical Care Medicine, Tianjin Medical University General Hospital, Tianjin, China
e-mail: zyyhxkfj@126.com

P. Li
Department of Respiratory Medicine, Taikang Xianlin Gulou Hospital, Nanjing University School of Medicine, Nanjing, China
e-mail: 13913881589@163.com

X. Li
Department of Pathology, Tianjin Haihe Hospital, Tianjin Institute of Respiratory Diseases, Tianjin, China
e-mail: x_li2012@hotmail.com

H. Zhou
grid.410560.6 0000 0004 1760 3078, Department of Respiratory and Critical Care Medicine, Affiliated Zhongshan Hospital of Guangdong Medical University, Guangzhou, China
e-mail: zhouhongmei2011e@163.com

2.2 Common Nonnative Tracheal/Bronchial/ Pulmonary Cells

Erythrocytes, neutrophils, eosinophils, basophils, lymphocytes, monocytes, macrophages, histiocytes, epithelioid cells, multinuclear giant cells, and others.

Morphology of Common Tracheal/Bronchial/ Pulmonary Cells (DQ Staining).

2.3 Native Tracheal/Bronchial/ Pulmonary Cell Morphology

2.3.1 Cell Morphology of Proximal Airways

Ciliary columnar epithelial cells (ciliated cells): The cells are roughly cylindrical, with the nucleus located in the middle. The end of the cell body is gradually tapered, the other end has a flat terminal bar, and the terminal bar is attached by pink-stained cilia.

Goblet cells: The cells are polar, the long axis of the nucleus is perpendicular to the long axis of the cell, the nucleus is located at one side which is narrow relatively, and the top of the other side expands, mostly empty vacuoles in cytoplasm, like a stemmed goblet.

Brush cells: Cells are roughly cylindrical and the nucleus is located in the middle. The cell body at one end is tapered, the other end has a flat terminal bar, and the terminal bar is lined with well-arranged microvilli. Another type of brush cells is hairless small fusiform (i.e., tapering at both ends) epithelial cells embedded in pseudostratified ciliated columnar epithelial structure.

Basal cells (reserve cells): The cells are small in size; the nucleus is similar in size to erythrocytes, conical or cuboidal in shape, and progressively smaller in nuclear-to-plasma ratio from deep to superficial; and cytoplasm is gradually increasing and eosinophilic, but nucleoplasm ratio is larger as a whole. These cells form a structure, appearing as a sheet. They are multidirectional stem cells and can differentiate and supplement other types of epithelial cells.

Neuroendocrine cells: The cells are rare and cylindrical or cubic, cytoplasm is abundant, and the overall nuclear-to-plasma ratio is small. Thick neurosecretory granules can be seen in the cytoplasm.

2.3.2 Cell Morphology of Terminal Airways (Bronchioli)

Clara cells: The nucleus size is about 1.2–1.5 times larger than that of erythrocyte. Nucleus size of these cells is further increased under disease conditions, but the overall nuclear-to-plasma ratio and morphology still suggest nonmalignant cells. The nuclear chromatin is delicate, overall lightly stained, and occasionally deeply stained under disease conditions.

The chromatin is slightly thick. The cell membrane is thin, incomplete, or even invisible, and there is a clear cytoplasm, but not much, which is grayish blue or gray in color. The nucleus located in the cytoplasm without cell membrane is an important feature of the cell, and there is no polarity. There are also Clara cells without cytoplasm, and they must be differentiated from reactive lymphocytes.

2.3.3 Cell Morphology of Gas Exchange Areas

Type II pneumocytes: Nuclear-to-plasma ratio is relatively small, nuclear is circular or quasi-circular, cytoplasmic staining is deeper compared with lung macrophages and histiocytes, and vacuoles are in the cytoplasm but have no phagocytosis like macrophages.

Type I pneumocytes: These cells can be seen only in the destruction of large amounts of lung tissue; the nucleus is oval-shaped with thin cytomembrane.

2.3.4 Other Native Cell Morphology

Fibroblasts and fibrocytes: Fibroblasts are large and round, abundant in cytoplasm, darkly stained, cyanophilic, with larger nuclei, and often more than two times the diameter of erythrocytes. Nuclear membrane is thick and cyanophilic and also has deep staining. The nuclei and the whole size of fibrocytes are smaller than those of the fibroblasts. Fibrocytes are elongated or spindle-shaped, often appearing in an aggregated manner and arranged in series.

Glandular cells: These cells are often sheet structure arranged, with abundant cytoplasm and vacuoles, lightly stained, and neutrophile, nuclear-to-plasma ratio is relatively small, and most of the eosinophilic nuclei are eccentric.

2.4 Common Nonnative Tracheal/Bronchial/ Pulmonary Cell Morphology

Erythrocytes: Erythrocytes have a diameter of 6–9 μm and average 7.2 μm and are light red or gray in DQ staining and often used as a cell size ruler.

Neutrophils: Neutrophils have a diameter of 10–12 μm. Cytoplasm in the DQ staining is colorless, the nuclei are darkly stained like curved rods (horseshoes) or lobulated, and the lobulated nuclei have usually two to five leaves, which are connected by filaments.

In the transbronchial lung biopsy (TBLB), neutrophils are in a very low magnitude. When there are no obvious infection and bleeding, it is extremely difficult to see neutrophils. Generally, when obvious distribution of neutrophils is seen, you can confirm that the relevant infection exists. When the density of neutrophils is relatively high, it can be confirmed that the relevant infection exists and is severe. It should be noted that the density of neutrophil distribution in the mucus/secretory substance is relatively high, so it must be considered comprehensively when making the interpretation.

In the activated phase, neutrophils are mainly composed of rod-shaped nuclei and two-lobule nuclei. The cytomembrane is relatively intact, and the cytoplasm is plump, showing "poisoning changes." In the necrosis phase, the neutrophils are mainly composed of three to five nuclei and

have often no membrane and no cytoplasm, showing neutrophil "debris and fragmentation."

In most cases of bacterial infections, "neutrophil phagocytosis of bacteria" is visible, which is of further significance for the interpretation of infections. According to cytology pertinent theory, neutrophils seldom phagocytize "colonized bacteria" but tend to phagocytize "pathogenic bacteria." Neutrophils are found in bacterial and fungal infections, that is, suppurative infections, partial rheumatism, and destructive damages to some lung lesions.

Eosinophils: Eosinophils have a diameter of 13–15 μm, their nuclear shape is similar to neutrophil, and they can have two to three leaves, generally two leaves like glasses, and are dark purple stained. Cytoplasm may have splintery eosinophilic particles. Eosinophilic cytoplasm is pale red. Eosinophils are easy to crumble, and particles can be distributed around the cells. When a large number of eosinophils disintegrate, diamond-shaped "Charcot-Leyden" crystals can be formed, and eosinophils are seen in tuberculosis, parasitic diseases, tumors, allergies, etc.

Basophils: They are 10–14 μm in diameter and round, and their cytoplasm contains coarse, different-sized, unevenly distributed, and blue-violet-dyed basophilic granules. Granules cover the nuclei, so nuclei of the basophils are often unclear, though their shape looks like the nuclei of the neutrophils with two to three leaves, usually two leaves, and increased basophils can also be seen in allergic diseases.

Lymphocytes: Lymphocytes are classified into three types, large (11–18 μm), medium (7–11 μm), and small (4–7 μm), according to diameter. Medium and small lymphocytes can be seen in TBLB. Large lymphocytes can be seen at the time of transbronchial needle aspiration (TBNA). And in TBLB, the nuclear-to-plasma ratio of lymphocytes is more and the cytoplasm is less. In the mature and stable lymphocytes, nuclei are of round type, with more chromatin and deeper staining, and the cytoplasm is blue.

The nuclei of reactive lymphocytes, often appearing in TBLB, are larger. The chromatin is even and loose, and the staining is more light than that in mature and stable lymphocytes. The cytoplasm is very little or no cytoplasm. In TBNA, the large lymphocytes are round, and the cytoplasm is more and light blue. Nuclei types are round and can have notch. Nuclear chromatin is concentrated, and nucleoli remnants are visible. The small lymphocytes are circular or quasi-circular and pale blue and have little or no cytoplasm and no particles. The nuclei are round, with visible notches and pits. Nuclear chromatin clumps, is purple, and has no nucleoli.

Plasmocytes: These cells, also known as effector B lymphocytes, are derived from the B lymphocytes by the stimulation of CD4+ lymphocytes, so they are consistent with the morphology of some B lymphocytes. Plasmocyte diameter is 10–20 μm. Nucleus is located on one side, and double nuclei are seen occasionally. The chromatin is thick and dense, and it is dyed into uneven lilac. There is often a half-moon, lightly stained area near the nucleus, and there may be vacuoles in the cytoplasm.

Plentiful of lymphocytes are likely to represent the acute phase of the lesion, seen in various types of inflammatory reactions, viral infections, tuberculosis (especially obvious), some rheumatism, some allergic reactions, and immune responses such as graft versus host. When plasmocytes appear, it is suggested that a chronic phase begins (but does not negate the acute phase).

2.4.1 Mononuclear Cell-Derived Non-epithelial Cells

2.4.1.1 Monocyte-Macrophage
Monocytes have a diameter of 12–20 μm and are round or irregular in shape. Occasionally, pseudopodia are visible. Nucleus morphology is irregular and can be kidney-shaped, horseshoe-shaped, and lobulated, often accompanied by notches, pittings, and obvious twisting and folding. The nuclear chromatin is more delicate, loose and silky, or cord-like. Generally, there is no nucleolus. The cytoplasm is more and grayish blue or pink in color. Fine purple-red particles are seen in the cytoplasm. Once the

monocytes migrate into the lungs, they become pulmonary macrophages; therefore, the lung is dominated by its macrophage subtype, and typical monocytes are rare.

Pulmonary macrophages differentiate from monocytes and are widely distributed in the stroma, with more in airways and alveolar septa below the bronchioles. Some migrate to the alveoli, so are called alveolar macrophages. Macrophages are 9–40 μm in diameter, their nuclei are circular or quasi-circular, and they are rich in cytoplasm and characterized by phagocytosis or being foamy. Early-phase lung macrophages are relatively small, with less cytoplasm and phagocytosis.

Histiocytes: These cells are differentiated from monocytes or transformed from alveolar macrophages (also monocyte origin) after phagocytosis for pathogens (such as tubercle bacillus). Cells are of different sizes, generally more than 7 μm, and round, oval, or irregular in shape. The cytoplasm is abundant and lightly stained, with thin or even incomplete cell membrane, and can undergo "cytoplasm shedding" to form naked nuclei. Nuclei contain fine vacuoles and show irregular round, oval, long, or kidney shapes, often sidely located. Sometimes, nucleoli are visible.

Epithelioid cells: Their morphology is similar to epithelial cells, so it is called. Epithelioid cells are the main cellular components of granuloma. They can be directly differentiated from monocytes or from histiocytes or pulmonary macrophages (all of which are monocyte in origin) after phagocytosis and digestion of pathogens (such as the tubercle bacilli containing waxy membrane). They are fusiform or polygonal, rich in cytoplasm, and lightly stained and have thin or even incomplete cell membrane. A considerable part of epithelioid cells can be "cytoplasm shedding" to form naked nuclei. Nuclei have fine vacuoles and are kidney-shaped, crescent-shaped, shoe-like, narrow, rod-shaped, or cucumber-shaped, with both ends blunt round.

Lots of histiocytes suggest a chronic phase and the appearance of hyperplasia and reparation (but not negate acute phase).

It can be considered that monocyte-macrophage, histiocyte, and epithelioid cells are different stages of the differentiation and evolution of the same monocyte cell line. During this evolution, the cells gradually become irregular. The cytoplasm gradually increases. The cytomembrane gradually becomes thin and gradually undergoes "cytoplasm shedding" to form naked nuclei. The nuclei gradually change from a round shape into an irregular shape and then become a kidney shape, a long shape, and a cucumber shape, which are growing longer and longer. These cells can array circularly together with lymphocytes to become multinucleated giant cells or become granuloma directly with more of these cells.

The multinucleated giant cells: More than three or even up to hundreds of epithelioid cells protrude out of cytoplasm, and then the cell bodies approach each other. Finally, the fusion of cytoplasmic protrusion causes the epithelioid cells to align circularly with lymphocytes and fuse together to form the multinucleated giant cells, so the giant cells are abundant in the cytoplasm. The nuclei of epithelioid cells scatter in the cytoplasm of giant cells. Multinucleated giant cells in tuberculosis are also called Langhans giant cells.

Mastocytes: Basophils are called mastocytes when they are in connective tissue or in mucosal epithelium. So their structure and functions are similar to those of basophils. Like blood basophils, they have basophilic granules. In DQ staining, they are characterized by the presence of toluidine blue-positive rose-red particles in the cytoplasm.

2.5 The Labeling of Cell Types and Cell States in this Book

In this book, we use two letters, in which the initial one is capitalized, of the cell name as the abbreviation of the cell type for legend and use the italic form of the two letters, also in which the initial one is capitalized, as the abbreviation of the cell state for legend.

- Ciliated cell, labeled as Ci.
- Glabrous cells: Glabrous cells are mainly Clara cells. Others are bronchiolar neuroen-docrine cells (labeled as K, very few) and various types of bronchiolo-epithelial cells (e.g., occasional distal airway basal cells). These cells can be collectively referred to as distal/terminal bronchiolar epithelial cells, or distal airway epithelial cells, or Feng's cells, labeled as F.
- Goblet cell, labeled as Go.
- Brush cell (including the glabrous spindle epithelial cell), labeled as Br.
- Basal cell (also known as reserve cell), labeled as Ba.
- Neuroendocrine cell (also known as small granulosa cell), labeled as K.
- Type II alveolar epithelial cells (Type II pneumocytes), labeled as Al2.
- Type I alveolar epithelial cells (Type I pneumocytes), labeled as Al1.
- Fibrocyte, labeled as Fi.
- Fibroblast, labeled as Fb.
- Glandular cell, labeled as Gl.
- Myocyte, labeled as My.
- Erythrocyte, labeled as Er.
- Neutrophil, labeled as Ne.
- Eosinophil, labeled as Eo.
- Basophil, labeled as Bp.
- Lymphocyte, labeled as Ly.
- Plasmocyte, labeled as Pl.
- Mononuclear-macrophage system.
- Migratory macrophage, or monocyte, collectively known as mononuclear cell, labeled as Mo.
- Macrophage, labeled as Ma.
- Histiocyte, labeled as Hi.
- Epithelioid cell, labeled as Ei.
- Multinucleated giant cell, labeled as Gi.
- Mastocyte, labeled as Mc.
- Mucus, labeled as Mu.
- Mesothelial cell, labeled as Me.
- Gomphosis, labeled as Gp.
- Keratinization, labeled as Ke.
- Cytoplasm, labeled as Cp.
- Cell state (italic).
- Hyperplasia, labeled as Hy.
- Necrosis, labeled as Nr.
- Aggregate, labeled as Ag.
- Giant cell reaction (cytomegalic), labeled as Gc (Cm).

- Some external objects.
- Hypha, labeled as Hp.
- Septum, labeled as Se.
- Spore, labeled as Sp.
- Bifurcate, labeled as Bi.

- Inclusion body, labeled as Ib.
- Amorphous material, labeled as Am.
- Tumor cell, labeled as Tc.
- All the others not mentioned here need to be specially marked.

Clustering (Categorizing) Analysis in ROSE Interpretation of Common Nonneoplastic Disease States of Lung/Mediastinum

3

Jing Feng, Pei Chen, Wei Chen, and Yao Li

For nonneoplastic diseases, ROSE is often the "cytologic version" of histopathology, that is, the manifestation of the cell shedding of correspond-

The content of the Chapter 3 has been published in "Rapid On-Site Evaluation (ROSE) in Diagnostic Interventional Pulmonology Volume 1: Infectious Diseases"
Print ISBN 978-981-13-3455-9
Online ISBN 978-981-13-3456-6
Chapter 3 Clustering (Categorizing) Analysis in ROSE Interpretation of Common Nonneoplastic Disease States of Lung/Mediastinum
Jing Feng, Pei Chen, Wei Chen, Yao Li
Pages 17–19
https://link.springer.com/chapter/10.1007/978-981-13-3456-6_3

J. Feng (✉)
Pulmonary and Critical Care Medicine, Tianjin Medical University General Hospital, Tianjin, China
e-mail: zyyhxkfj@126.com

P. Chen
Department of Respiratory Medicine, Xijing Hospital, Air Force Military Medical University, Xi'an, China
e-mail: 562892051@qq.com

W. Chen
Department of Respiratory Medicine, The Affiliated Huaian No.1 People's Hospital of Nanjing Medical University, Huai'an, China
e-mail: chenweijs@live.cn

Y. Li
Department of Respiratory Medicine, Shanghai Ninth People's Hospital, Shanghai Jiaotong University School of Medicine, Shanghai, China
e-mail: liyao_sjtu@163.com

ing tissue content, so the interpreter should have a deep understanding of the histopathology of corresponding diseases.

It should be noted that ROSE clustering (categorizing) analysis is the most common method we use in ROSE interpretation. This method is used throughout this book.

In general, nonneoplastic disease states of the lung/mediastinum can be classified into the following categories in ROSE interpretation (the detailed classification (clusters) of clustering analysis). Some of these categories can be classified as mild, moderate, and severe according to the specific situations.

3.1 Poorly Prepared ROSE Slides May Result in Meaningless Interpretations

At this point, the interpreter can be prompted to suggest that a bad slide preparation was gotten so as to make corresponding corrections in subsequent process.

3.2 "Inflammatory Changes"

The "inflammatory changes" are lacking in specificity, and there are differences in the degree.

The cells of tissue specimen drawn from target anatomic site/lesion (especially airway epithelial cells) are found to have hyperplasia, degeneration, necrosis, and denaturation; occasionally, a small number of inflammatory cells, such as scattered neutrophils, reactive lymphocytes or plasma cells, and excessive alveolar macrophages, are seen.

3.3 Approximately Normal/Mild Nonspecific Inflammatory Response

Scattered clear macrophages/clear macrophages are abundant, with mild "inflammatory changes."

3.4 Suppurative Infections (With or Without Visible Pathogens)

A variety of inflammatory cells mainly neutrophils, including lots of reactive lymphocytes and macrophages, are seen. Necrosis is obvious. Epithelial cell proliferation, degeneration, necrosis, and denaturation are visible.

3.5 May Conform to Viral Infections; May Conform to Mycoplasma Infections

In viral pneumonia, a variety of inflammatory cells mainly reactive lymphocytes, including scattered neutrophils and macrophages, and varying degrees of "inflammatory changes" are presented; type II pneumocyte hyperplasia is obvious. It may have "cytomegaly and karyomegaly," viral inclusions, "ciliocytophthoria," and some other features.

In mycoplasma pneumonia, a variety of inflammatory cells mainly mononuclear cells (early migratory macrophages), including scattered neutrophils, are presented. "Inflammatory changes" are obvious.

3.6 Granulomatous Inflammation

In inflammation phase, the key feature of "epithelioid cell subpopulation among reactive lymphocytes" is presented, namely, histiocytes and/or epithelioid cells are among lots of reactive lymphocytes.

In proliferation phase, many inflammatory cells mainly composed of histiocytes and/or epithelioid cells are found; multinucleated giant cells are visible.

3.7 May Conform to Organization

Organization is found secondary to infection or immune reasons. Abundant foamy macrophages aggregate, and scattered reactive lymphocytes and fibroblasts, with or without basophilic necrosis, can be seen.

3.8 May Conform to Fibrosis (Fibroblast Dominant/ Fibrocyte Dominant)

There are abundant fibroblasts and some of them have evolved to fibrocytes.

3.9 Lymphocyte-Based Immune Inflammatory Response

Abundant reactive lymphocytes are presented, and there are varying degrees of "inflammatory changes."

3.10 Eosinophil-Based Immune Inflammatory Response

Abundant eosinophils are presented, and there are varying degrees of "inflammatory changes."

3.11 Proliferative/Reparative Inflammatory Response

Histiocytes are dominating, and occasionally multinucleated giant cells and atypical granulomas are seen, with or without different numbers of reactive lymphocytes and plasma cells; varying degrees of "inflammatory changes" may be seen.

3.12 There Are Visible Pathogens, Characteristic Manifestations, or Foreign Objects

It may have hyphae, spores, cysts, bacteria, parasites, and other visible pathogens in the background, and some pathogens may be associated with eosinophils.

3.13 Necrotic "Inflammatory Changes"

Necrosis is evident. Most cells break up and disintegrate in the mucus background, and it is difficult to classify and count these cells.

3.14 Inconclusive Interpretation May Be Reached or the Interpretation Is Inconsistent with Clinical Information

At this point, the interpreter may be prompted to suggest that an invalid specimen was gotten or suggest that the clinical value of this interventional procedure is insufficient, and further clinical evidence should be sought.

ROSE Cytopathology Cases of Sarcoidosis

4

Jing Feng, Wen Ning, and Dianhua Jiang

4.1 Sarcoidosis Case 1

Brief history: Female, 58 years old, persistent coughing with mild shortness of breath, clinically diagnosed as sarcoidosis.

Technology to obtain the target lesions: Transbronchial needle aspiration (TBNA).

The preparation of cytological slides for ROSE: Imprinting (rolling).

Clustering (categorizing) analysis in ROSE interpretation:

- "Inflammatory changes".
- Granulomatous inflammation.
- Lymphocyte-based immune inflammatory response.

J. Feng (✉)
Pulmonary and Critical Care Medicine, Tianjin Medical University General Hospital, Tianjin, China
e-mail: zyyhxkfj@126.com

W. Ning
College of Life Sciences, Nankai University, Tianjin, China
e-mail: ningwen108@nankai.edu.cn

D. Jiang
Cedars-Sinai Medical Center, Los Angeles, USA
e-mail: Dianhua.Jiang@csmc.edu

Fig. 4.1 (a, b) Enlargement of subcarina and both pulmonary hilar lymph nodes

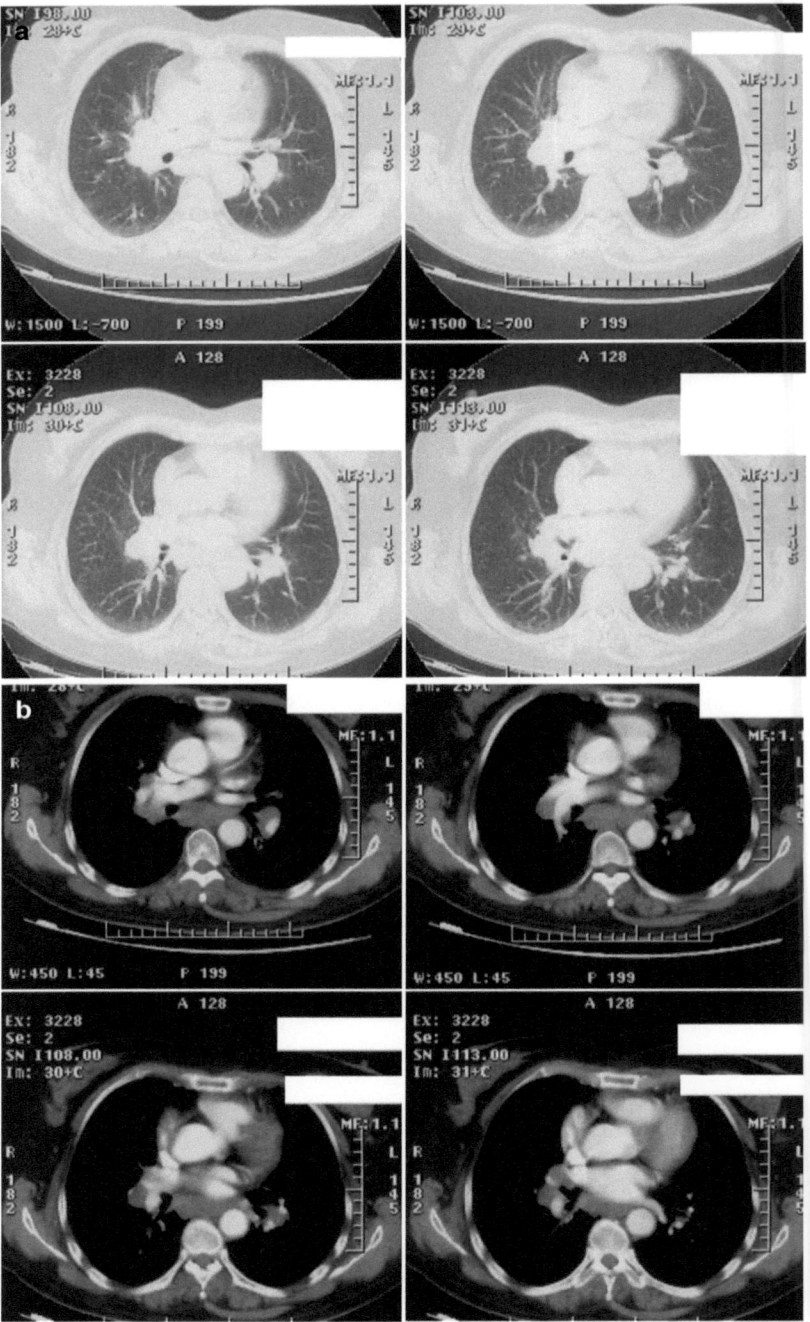

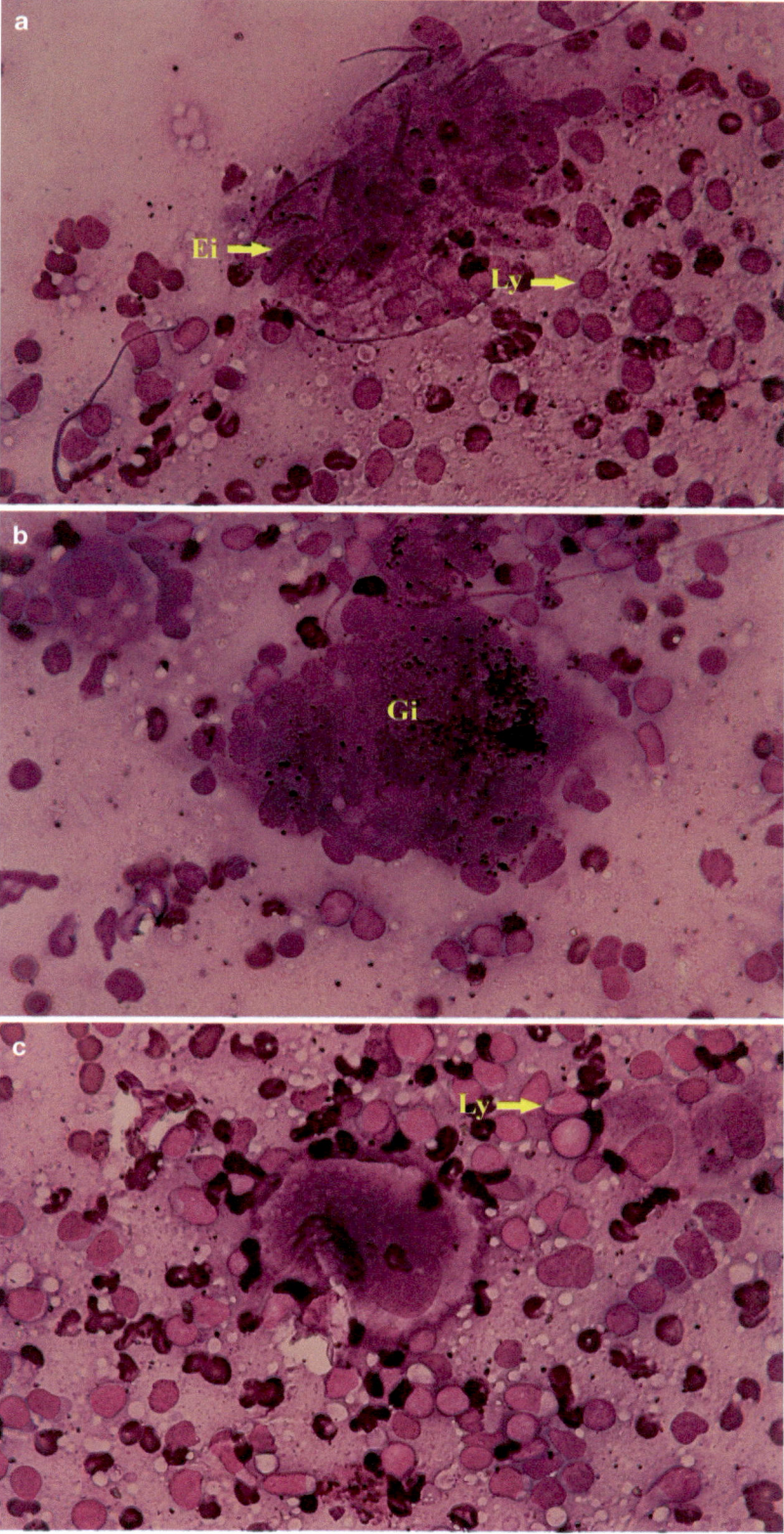

Fig. 4.2 (continued)

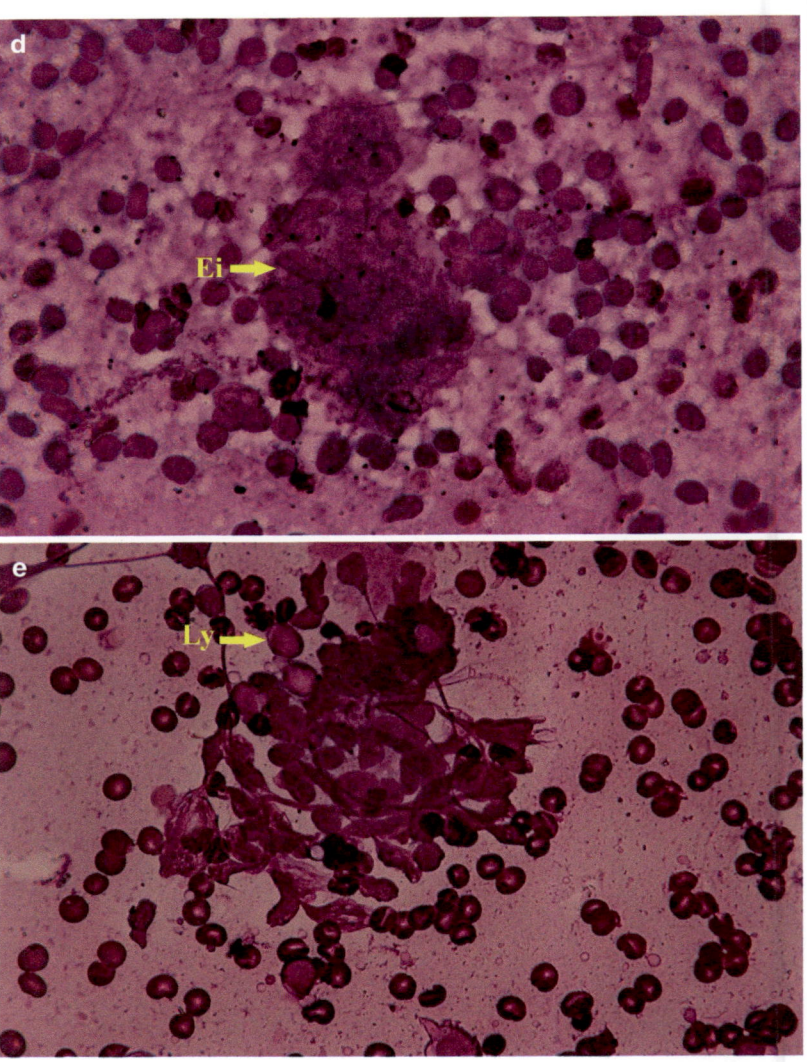

4.2   Sarcoidosis Case 2

Brief history: Female, 58 years old, persistent coughing with mild shortness of breath, clinically diagnosed as sarcoidosis.

Technology to obtain the target lesions: Transbronchial needle aspiration (TBNA).

The preparation of cytological slides for ROSE: Imprinting (rolling).

Clustering (categorizing) analysis in ROSE interpretation:

- "Inflammatory changes".
- Granulomatous inflammation.
- Lymphocyte-based immune inflammatory response.

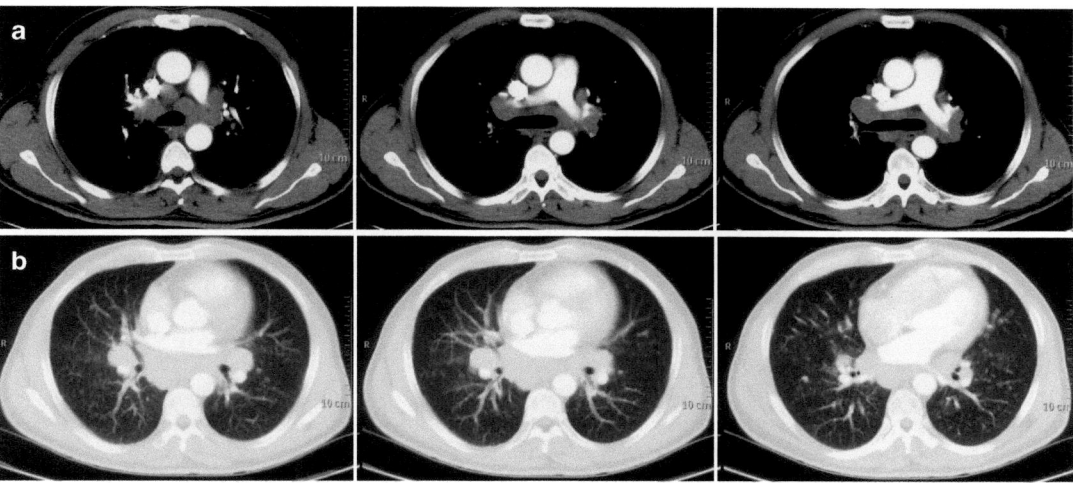

Fig. 4.3 (**a, b**) Enlargement of subcarina and both pulmonary hilar lymph nodes

Fig. 4.4 (a–e)
Annotated at the figure
(yellow arrow)

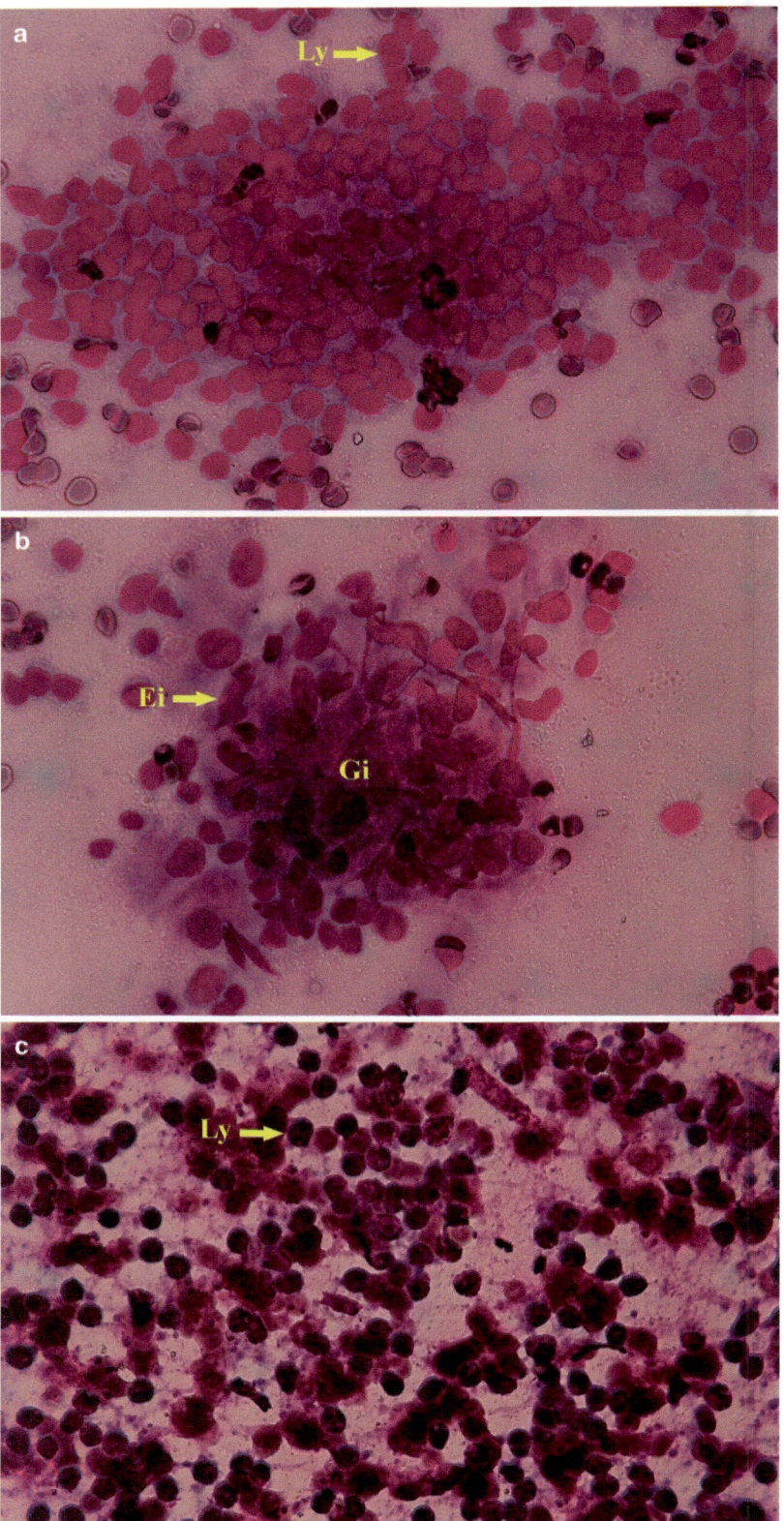

Fig. 4.4   (continued)

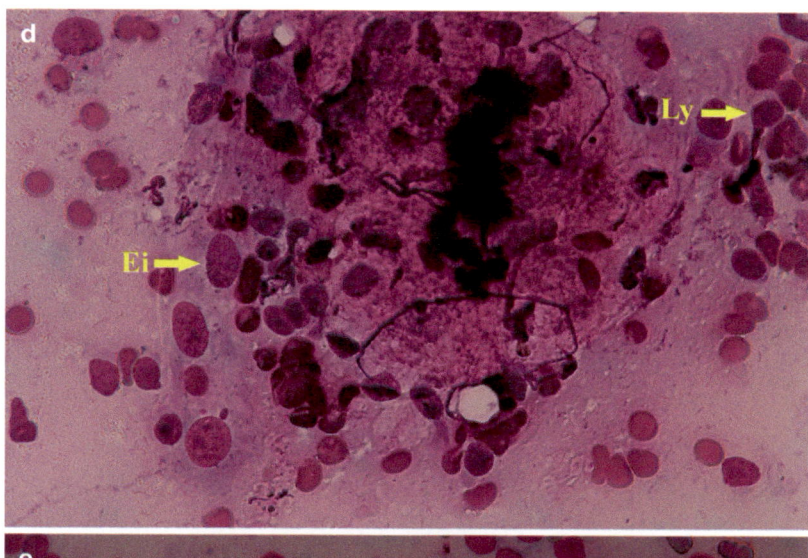

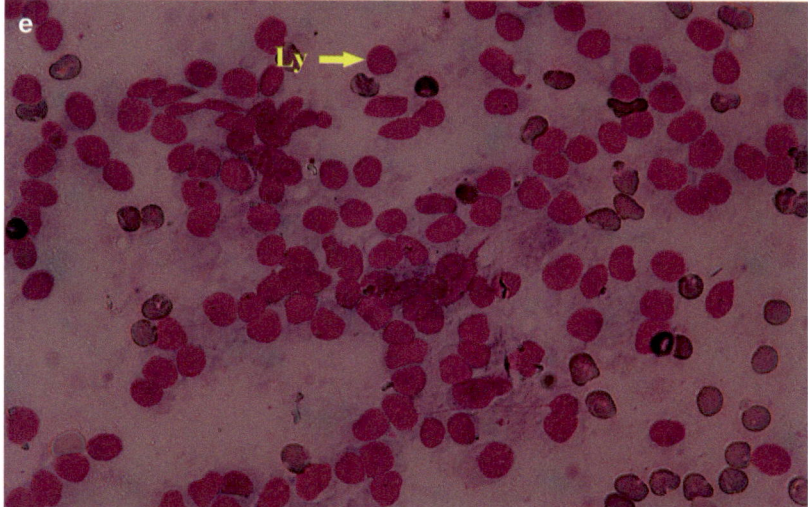

4.3   Sarcoidosis Case 3

Brief history: Male, 36 years old, persistent coughing with mild shortness of breath, clinically diagnosed as sarcoidosis.

Technology to obtain the target lesions: Transbronchial lung biopsy (TBLB).

The preparation of cytological slides for ROSE: Imprinting (rolling).

Clustering (categorizing) analysis in ROSE interpretation:

- "Inflammatory changes".
- Granulomatous inflammation.
- Lymphocyte-based immune inflammatory response.

Fig. 4.5 (a–d)
Enlargement of hilar and
mediastinal lymph nodes
and associated
reticulonodular
abnormalities involving
both lungs, resulting
from thickening of
interlobular septa and
intralobular irregular
lines, distributed along
the bronchovascular
bundles

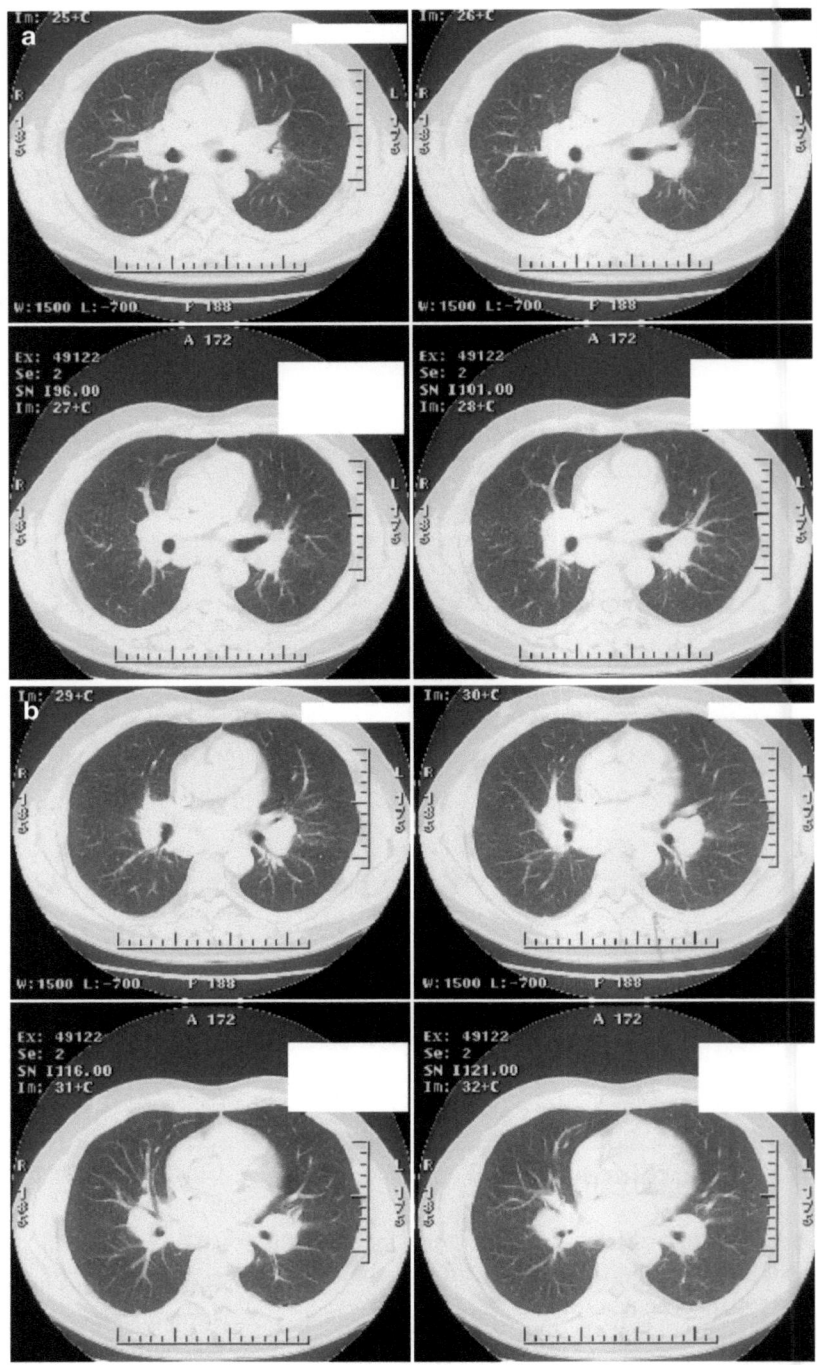

Fig. 4.5 (continued)

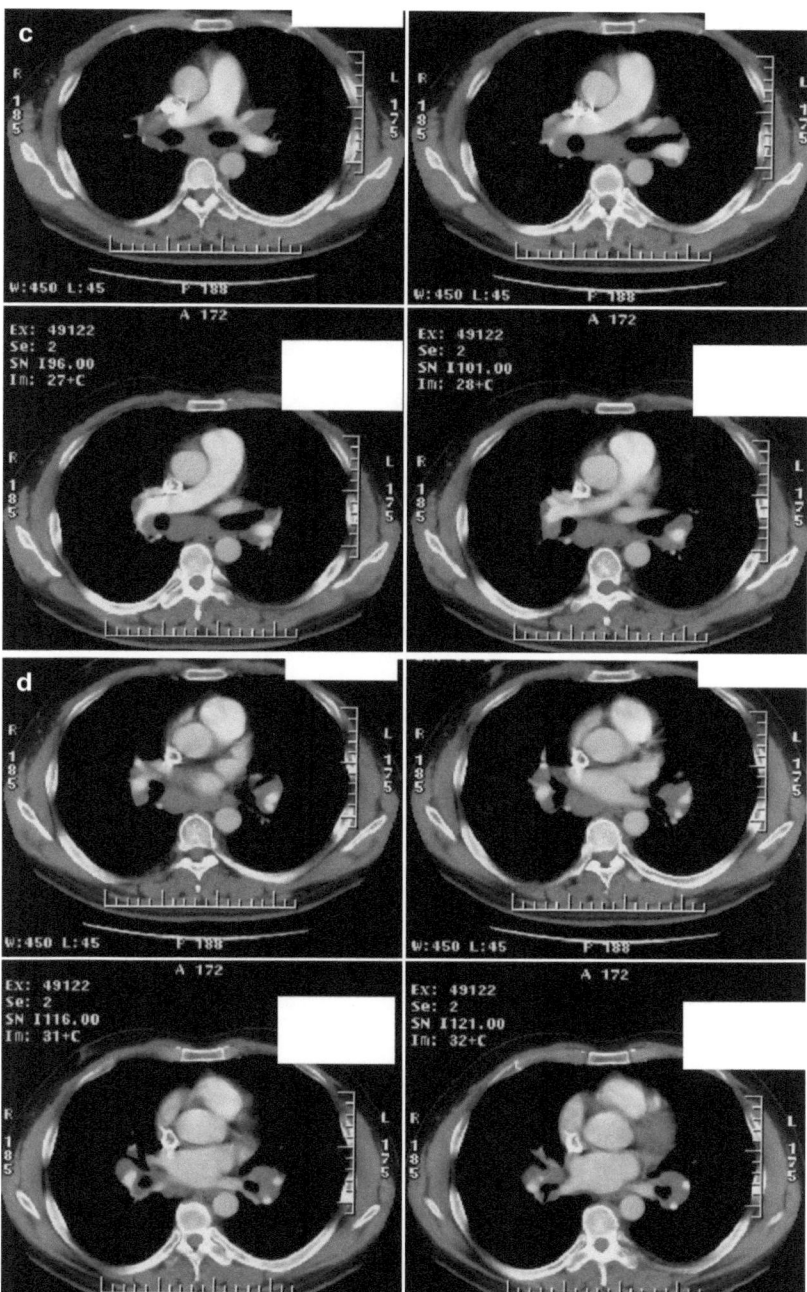

Fig. 4.6 (a–e)
Annotated at the figure
(yellow arrow)

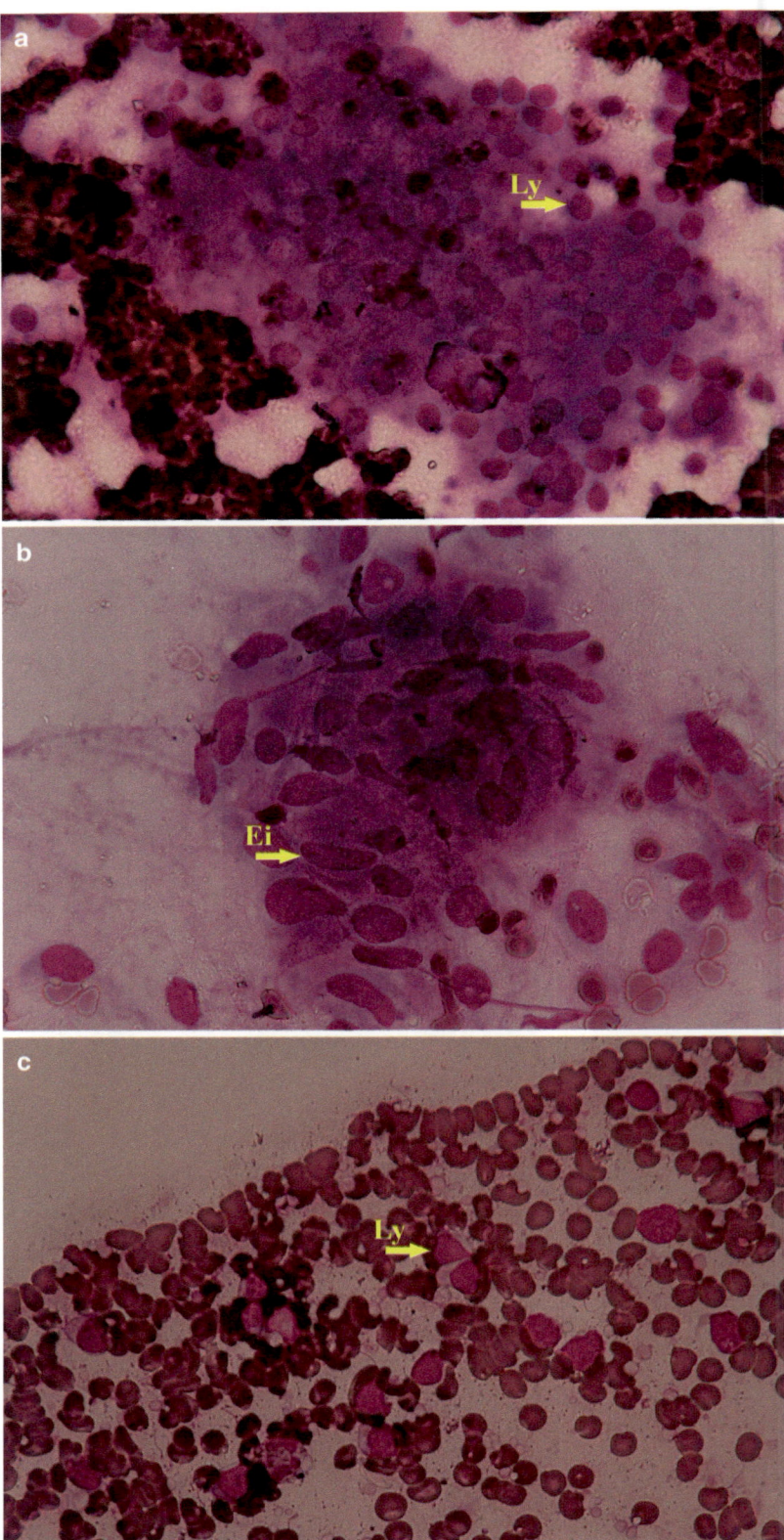

Fig. 4.6 (continued)

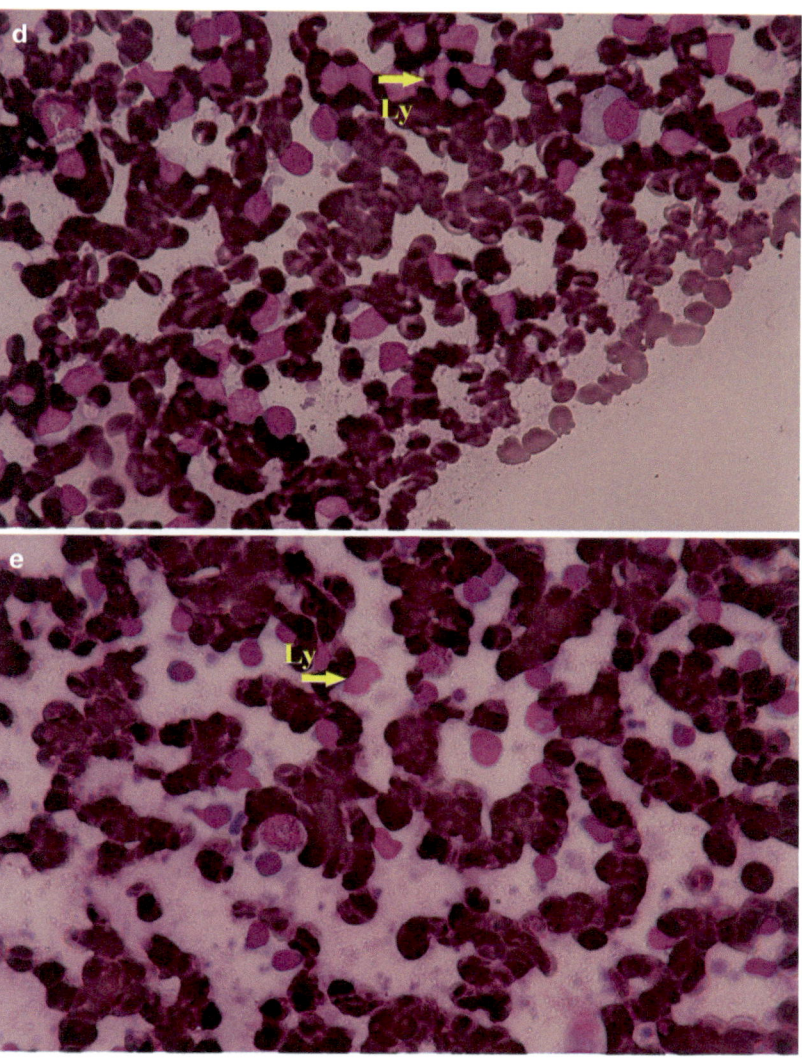

4.4   Sarcoidosis Case 4

Brief history: Female, 61 years old, persistent coughing with mild shortness of breath, clinically diagnosed as sarcoidosis.

Technology to obtain the target lesions: Transbronchial lung biopsy (TBLB).

The preparation of cytological slides for ROSE: Imprinting (rolling).

Clustering (categorizing) analysis in ROSE interpretation:

- "Inflammatory changes".
- Granulomatous inflammation.
- Lymphocyte-based immune inflammatory response.

Fig. 4.7 (a, b) Enlargement of hilar and mediastinal lymph nodes and associated reticulonodular abnormalities involving both lungs, resulting from thickening of interlobular septa and intralobular irregular lines, distributed along the bronchovascular bundles

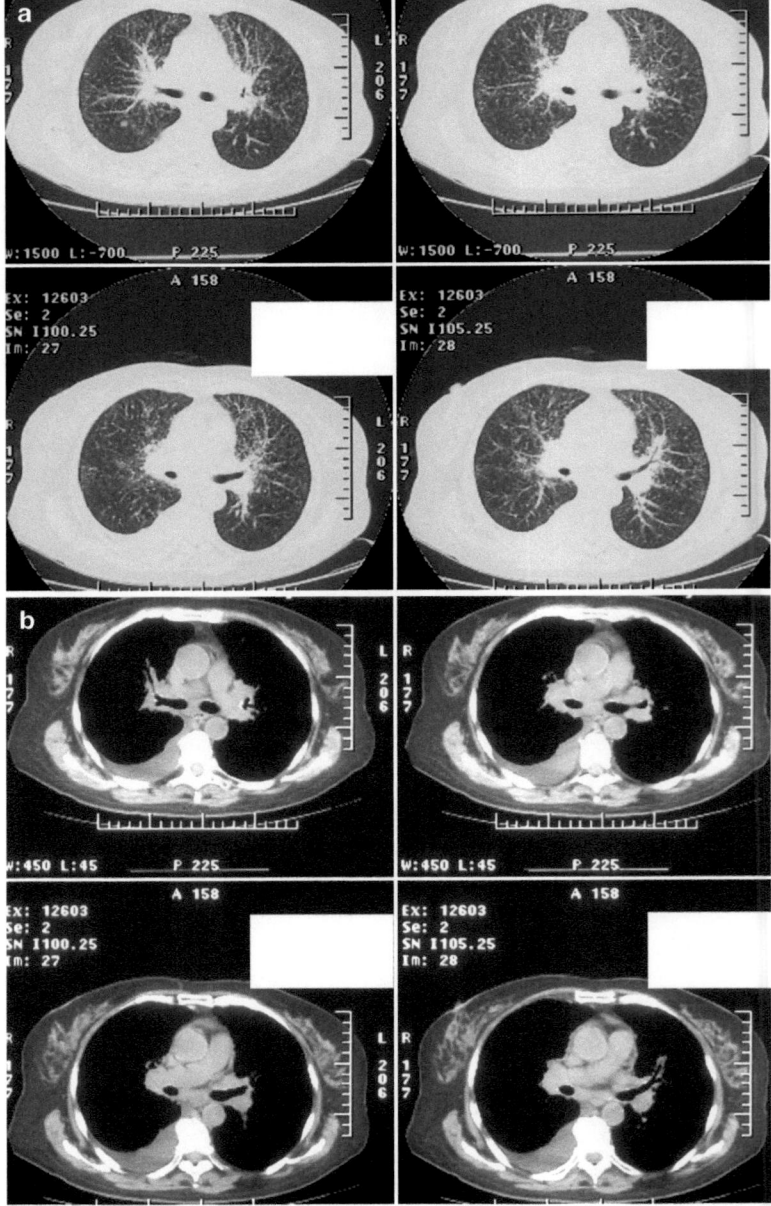

Fig. 4.8 (a–e)
Annotated at the figure
(yellow arrow)

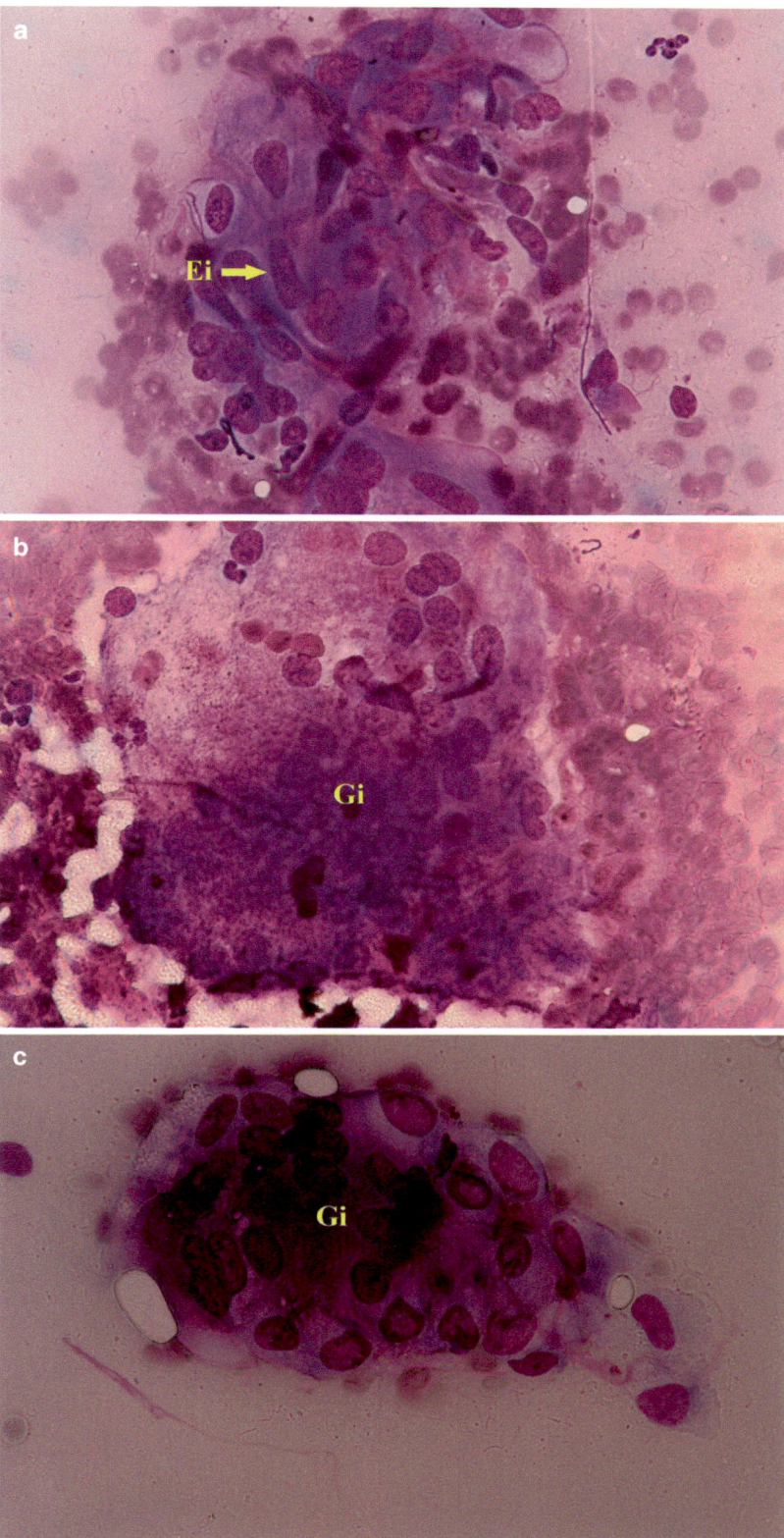

Fig. 4.8 (continued)

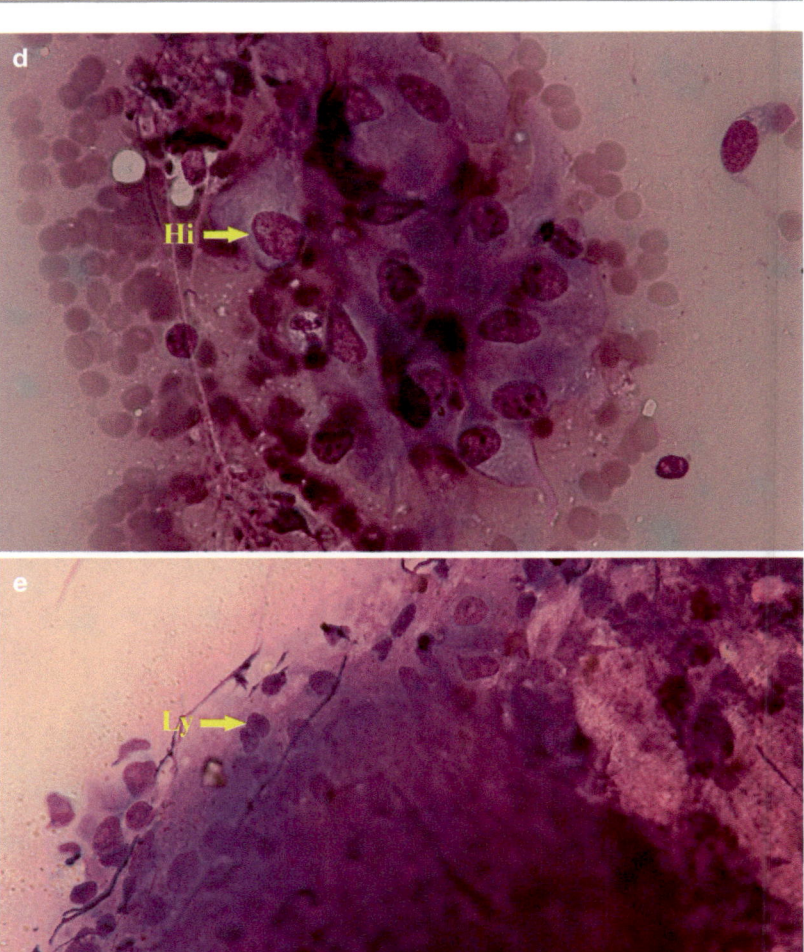

4.5   Sarcoidosis Case 5

Brief history: Male, 29 years old, persistent coughing with mild shortness of breath, clinically diagnosed as sarcoidosis.

Technology to obtain the target lesions: Transbronchial needle aspiration (TBNA).

The preparation of cytological slides for ROSE: Imprinting (rolling).

Clustering (categorizing) analysis in ROSE interpretation:

- "Inflammatory changes".
- Granulomatous inflammation.
- Lymphocyte-based immune inflammatory response.

Fig. 4.9 (**a, b**) Enlargement of hilar and mediastinal lymph nodes

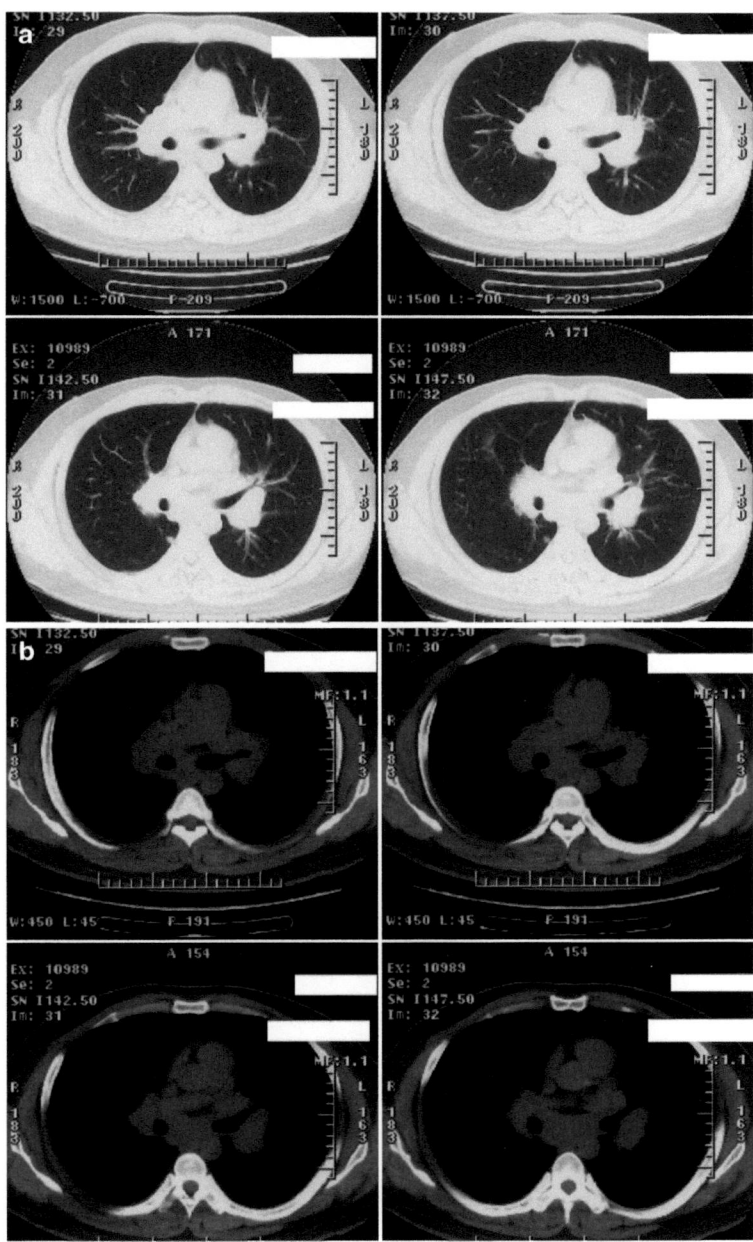

Fig. 4.10 (a–e)
Annotated at the figure
(yellow arrow)

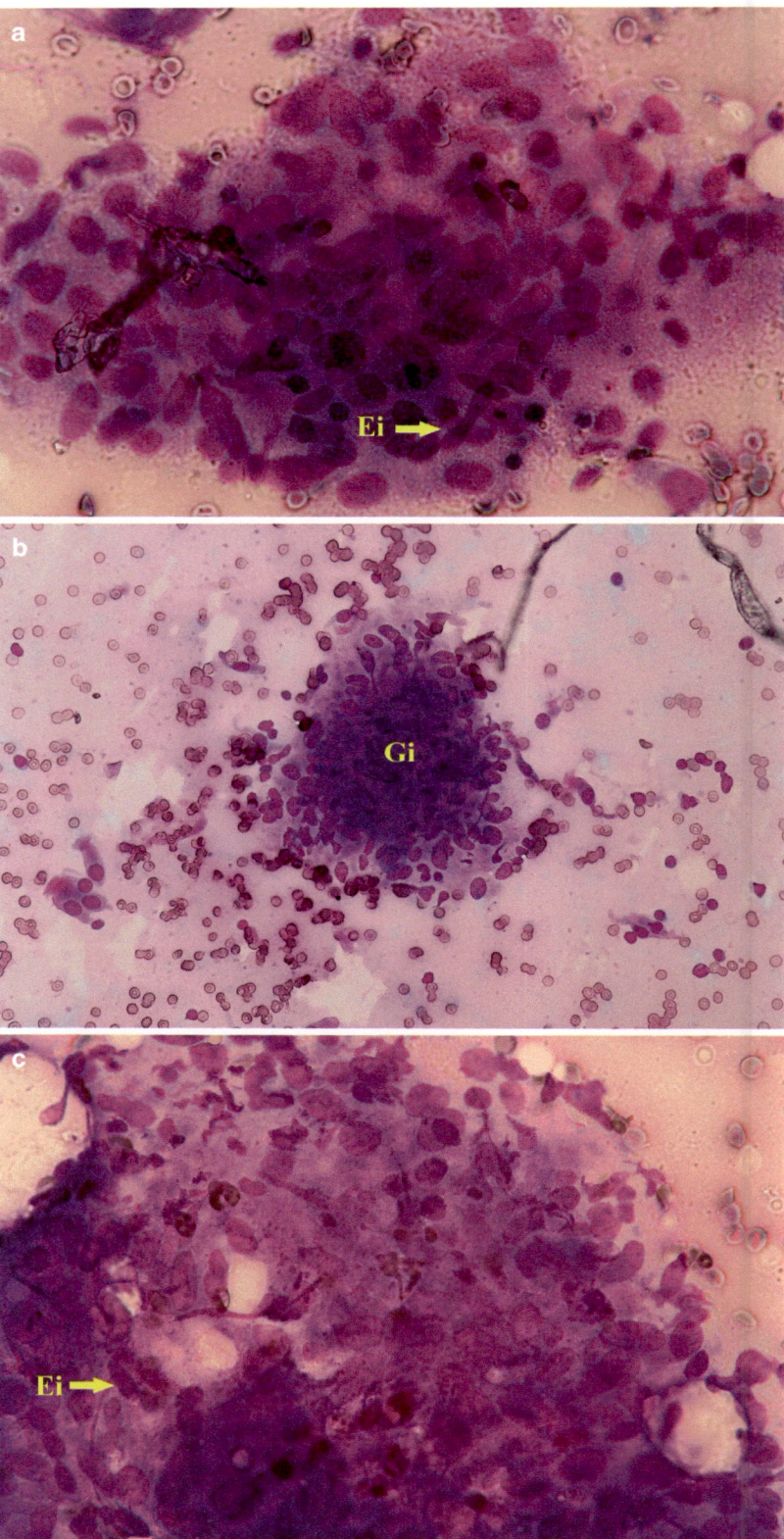

Fig. 4.10   (continued)

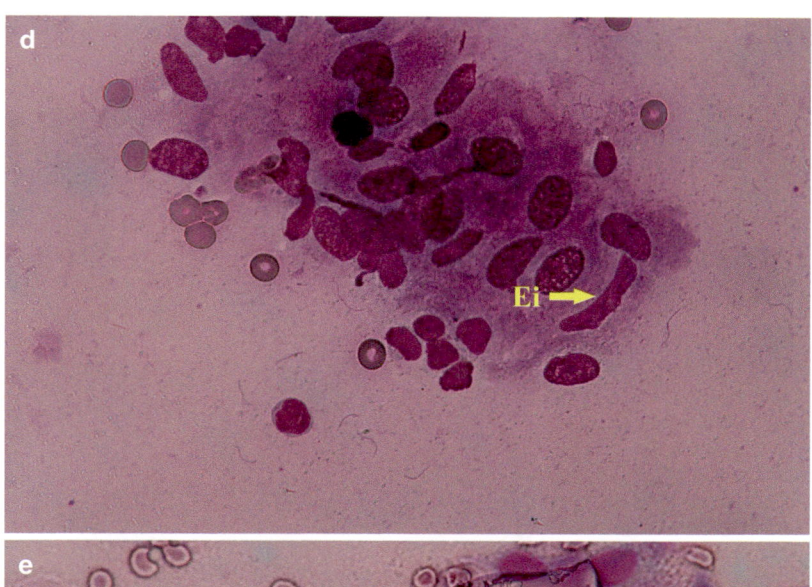

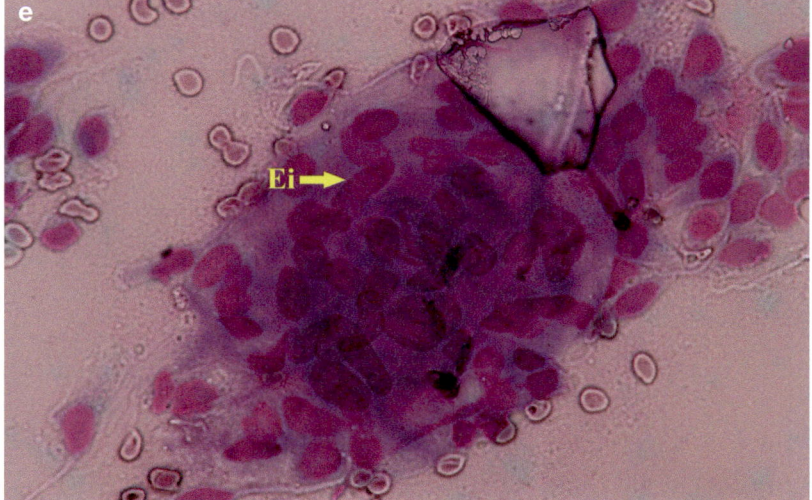

4.6   Sarcoidosis Case 6

Brief history: Female, 65 years old, persistent coughing with mild shortness of breath, clinically diagnosed as sarcoidosis.

Technology to obtain the target lesions: Transbronchial lung biopsy (TBLB).

The preparation of cytological slides for ROSE: Imprinting (rolling).

Clustering (categorizing) analysis in ROSE interpretation:

- "Inflammatory changes".
- Granulomatous inflammation.
- Lymphocyte-based immune inflammatory response.

Fig. 4.11 (a–d) Enlargement of hilar and mediastinal lymph nodes and associated reticulonodular abnormalities involving both lungs, resulting from thickening of interlobular septa and intralobular irregular lines, distributed along the bronchovascular bundles

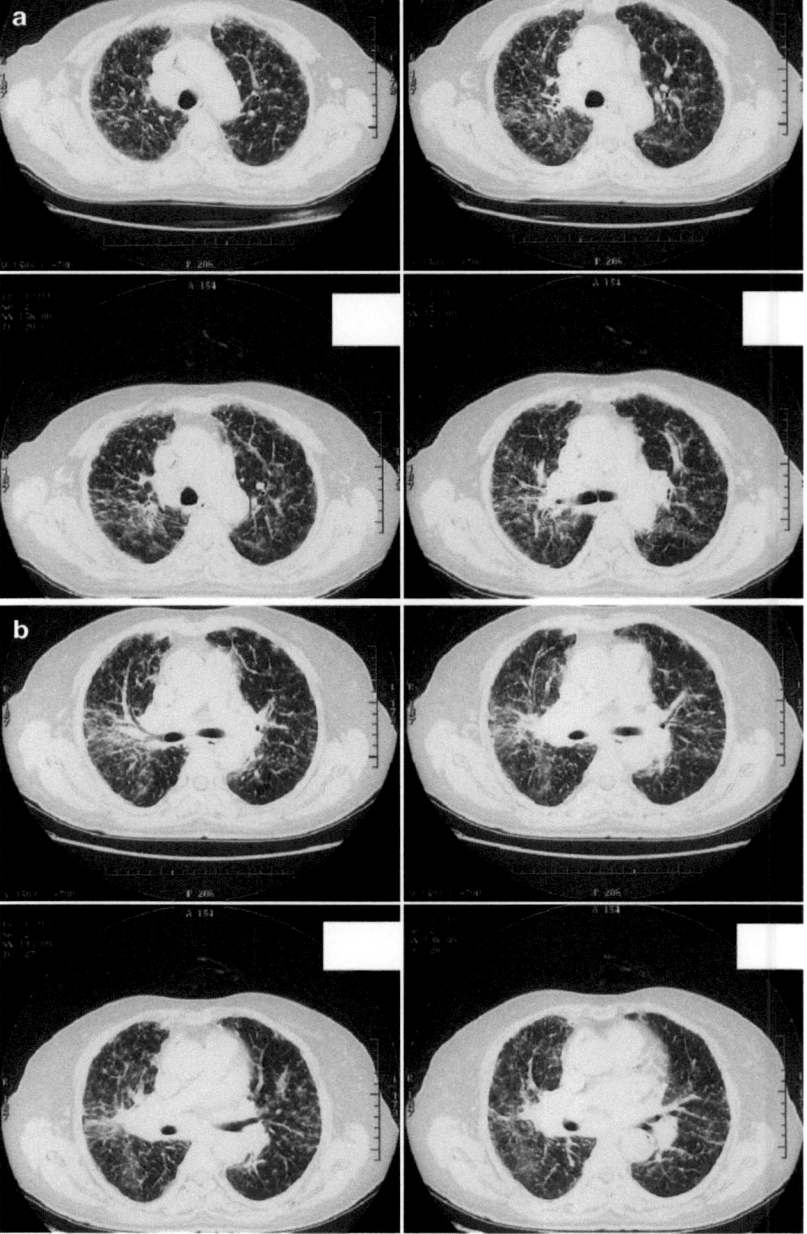

Fig. 4.11 (continued)

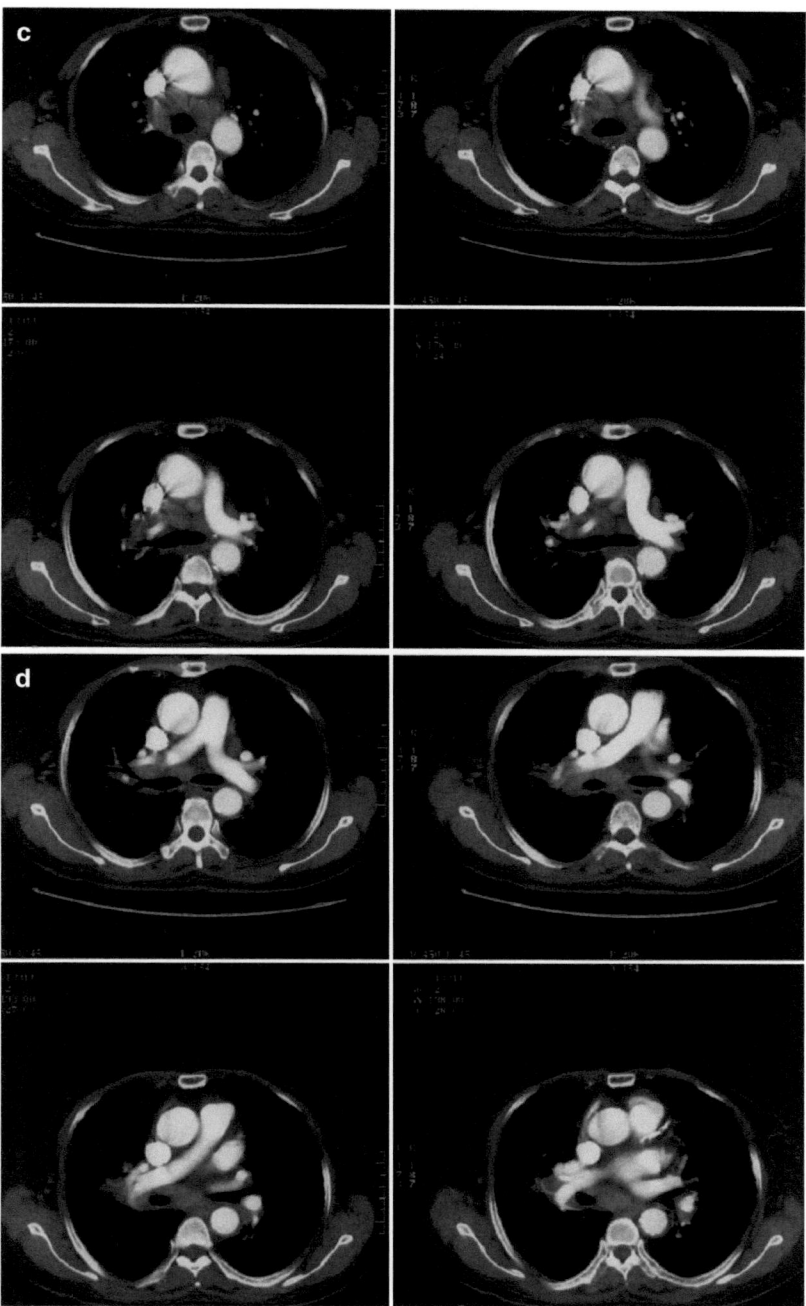

Fig. 4.12 (a–e)
Annotated at the figure
(yellow arrow)

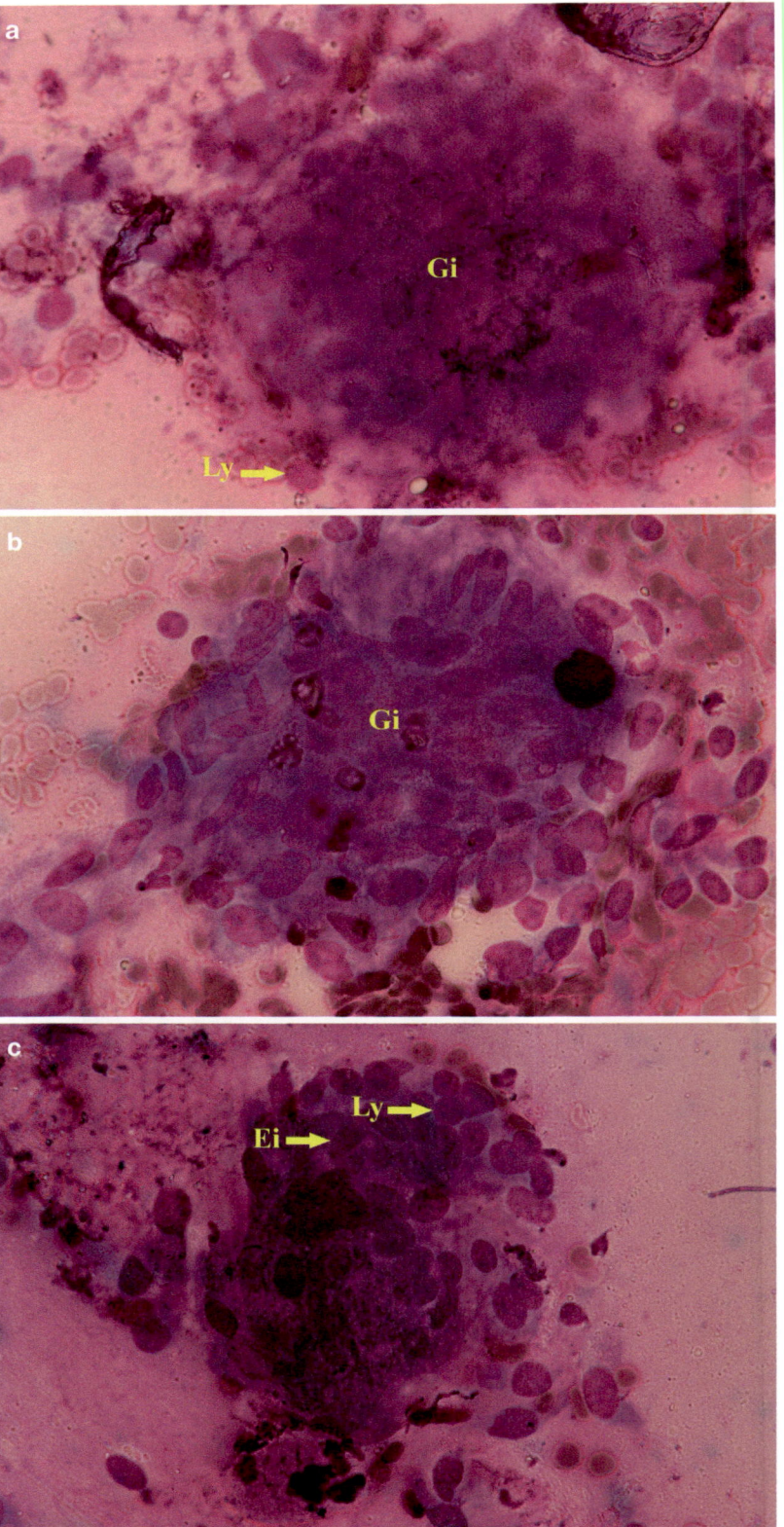

Fig. 4.12 (continued)

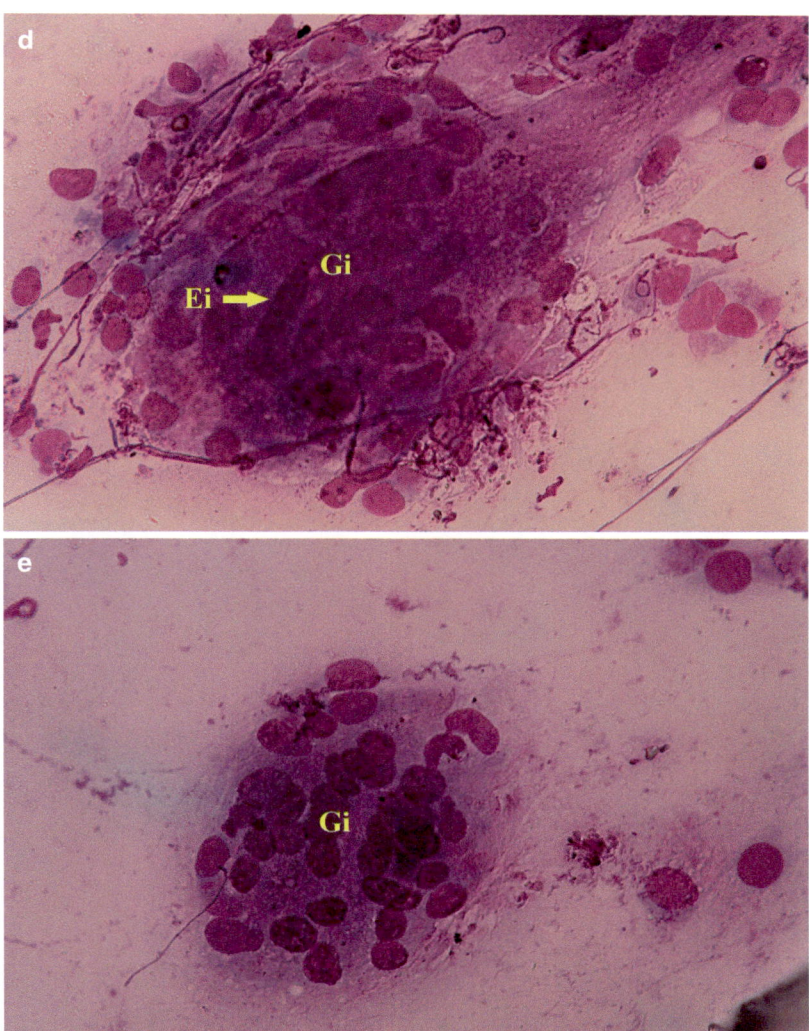

4.7   Sarcoidosis Case 7

Brief history: Female, 56 years old, persistent coughing with mild shortness of breath, clinically diagnosed as sarcoidosis.

Technology to obtain the target lesions: Transbronchial lung biopsy (TBLB).

The preparation of cytological slides for ROSE: Imprinting (rolling).

Clustering (categorizing) analysis in ROSE interpretation:

- "Inflammatory changes".
- Granulomatous inflammation.
- Lymphocyte-based immune inflammatory response.

Fig. 4.13 (a, b) Enlargement of hilar and mediastinal lymph nodes

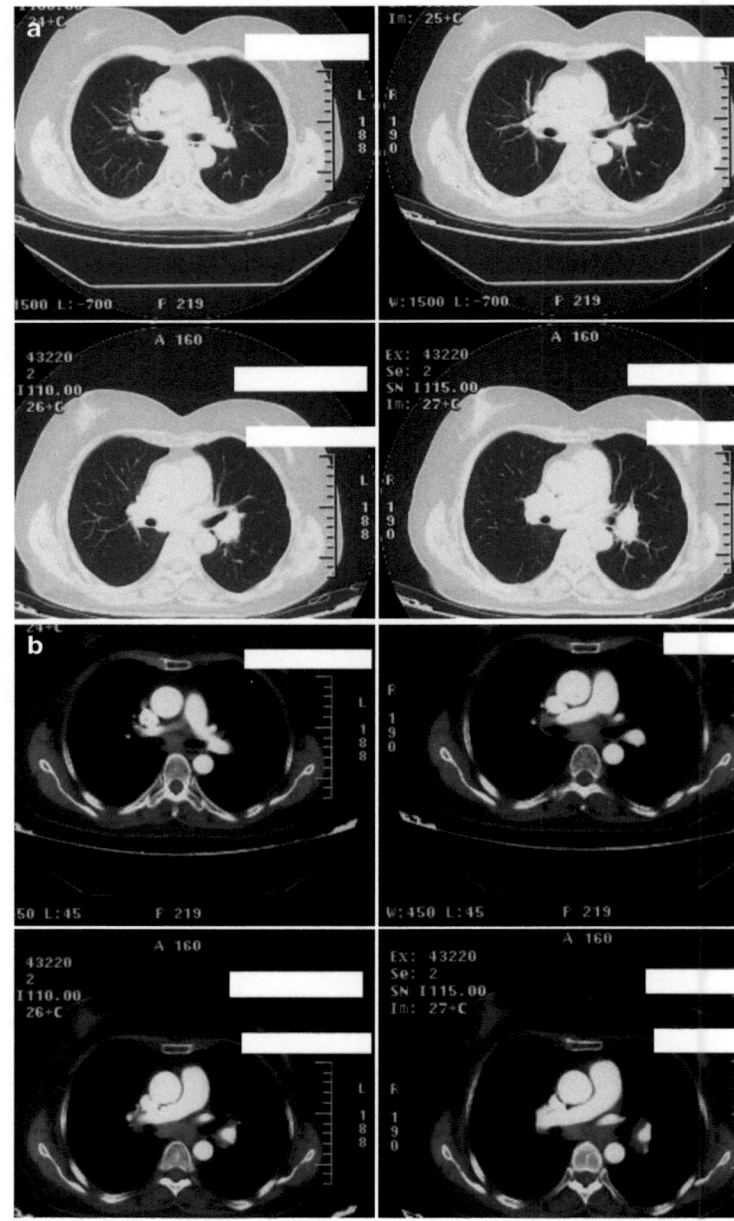

Fig. 4.14 (a–e)
Annotated at the figure
(yellow arrow)

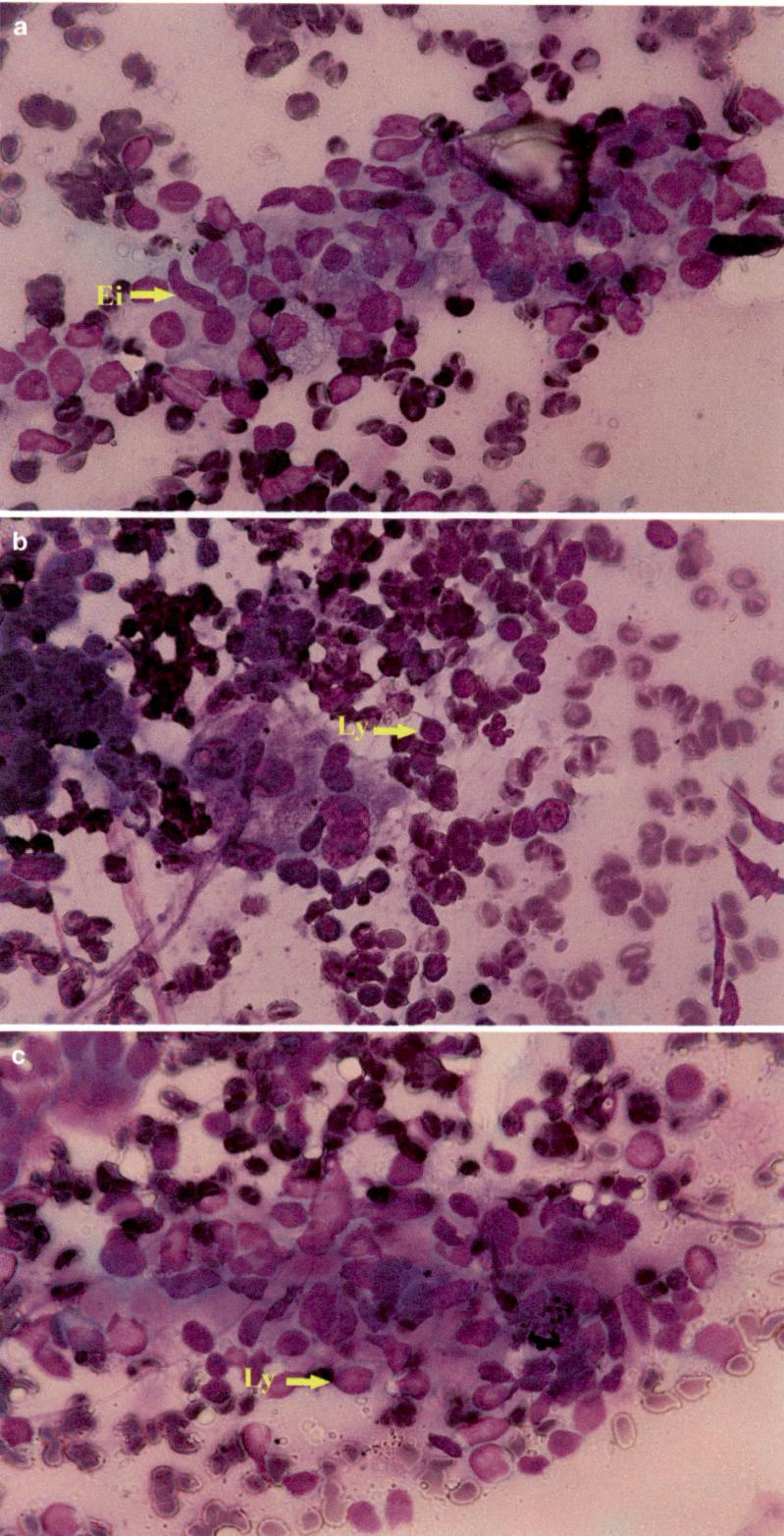

Fig. 4.14 (continued)

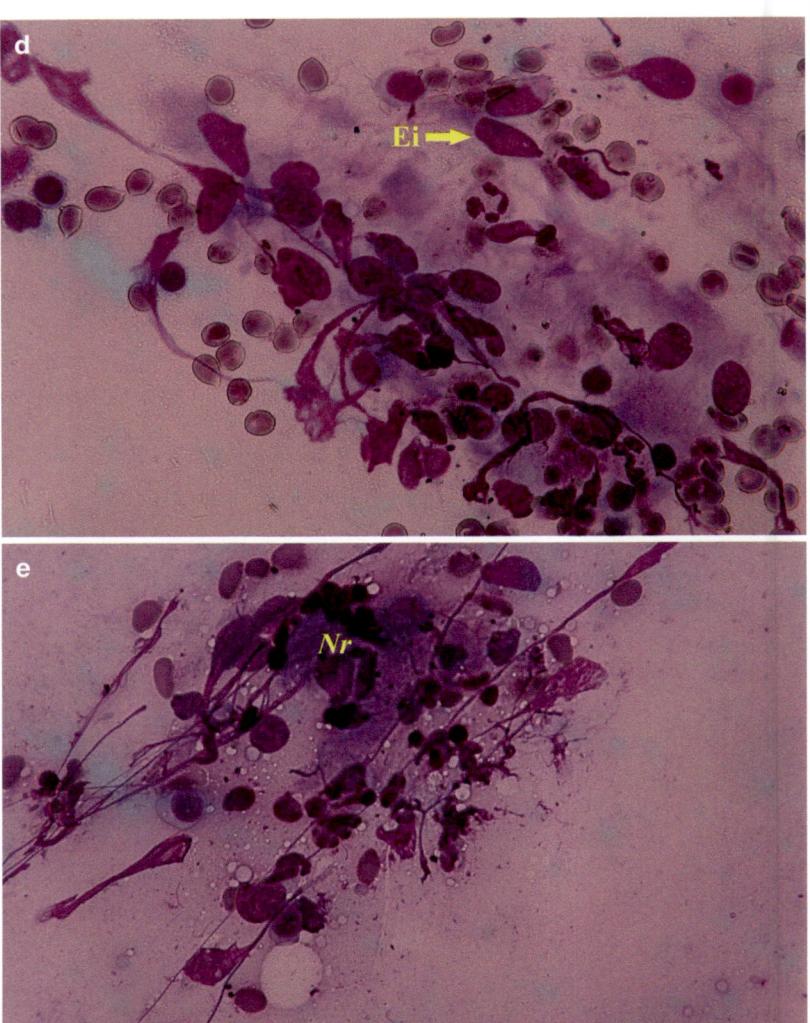

4.8 Sarcoidosis Case 8

Brief history: Female, 66 years old, persistent coughing with mild shortness of breath, clinically diagnosed as sarcoidosis.

Technology to obtain the target lesions: Transbronchial lung biopsy (TBLB).

The preparation of cytological slides for ROSE: Imprinting (rolling).

Clustering (categorizing) analysis in ROSE interpretation:

- "Inflammatory changes".
- Granulomatous inflammation.
- Lymphocyte-based immune inflammatory response.

Fig. 4.15 (a, b)
Enlargement of hilar and mediastinal lymph nodes and associated reticulonodular abnormalities involving both lungs, resulting from thickening of interlobular septa and intralobular irregular lines, distributed along the bronchovascular bundles

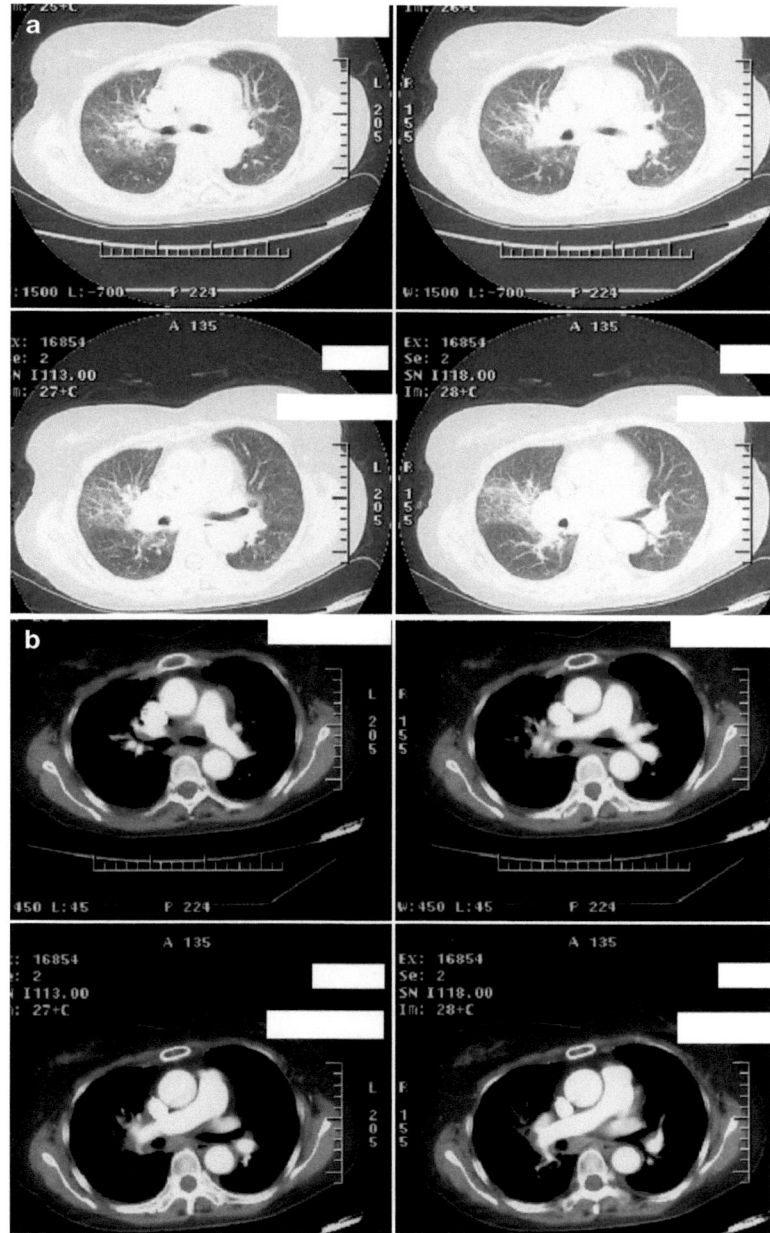

Fig. 4.16 (a–e)
Annotated at the figure
(yellow arrow)

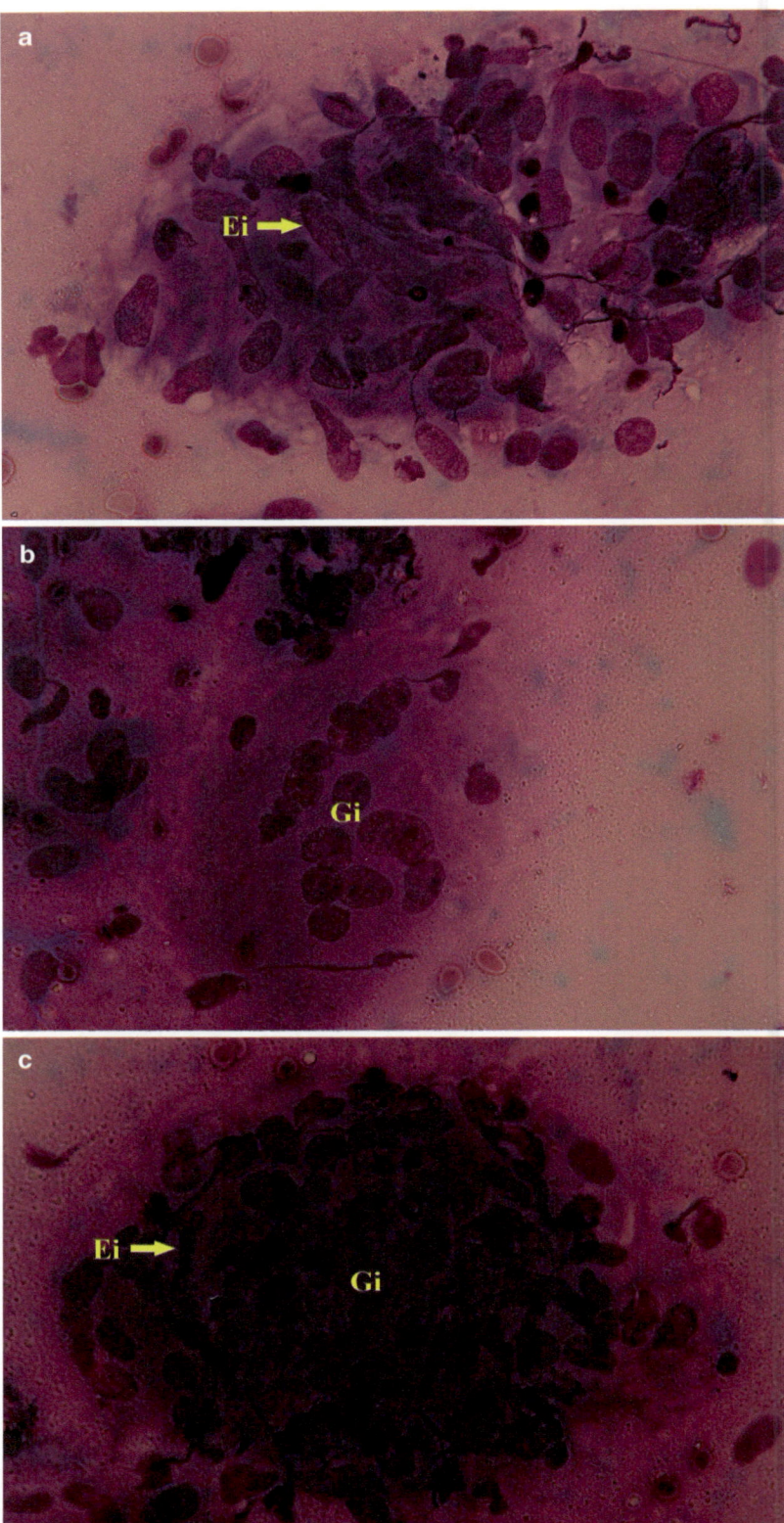

Fig. 4.16 (continued)

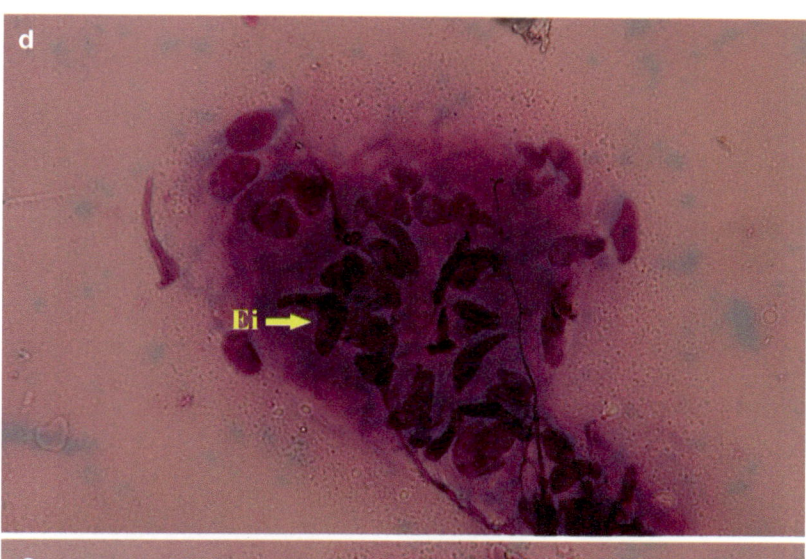

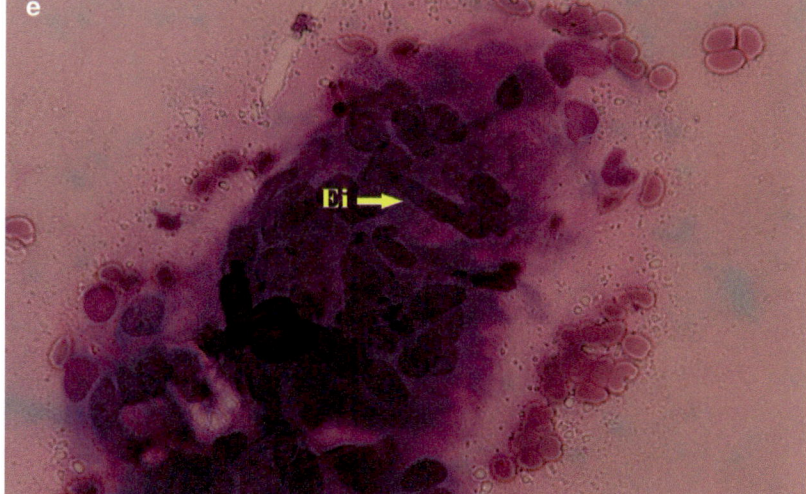

4.9   Sarcoidosis Case 9

Brief history: Male, 38 years old, persistent coughing with mild shortness of breath, clinically diagnosed as sarcoidosis.

Technology to obtain the target lesions: Transbronchial needle aspiration (TBNA).

The preparation of cytological slides for ROSE: Imprinting (rolling).

Clustering (categorizing) analysis in ROSE interpretation:

- "Inflammatory changes".
- Granulomatous inflammation.
- Lymphocyte-based immune inflammatory response.

Fig. 4.17 (a, b) Enlargement of hilar and mediastinal lymph nodes

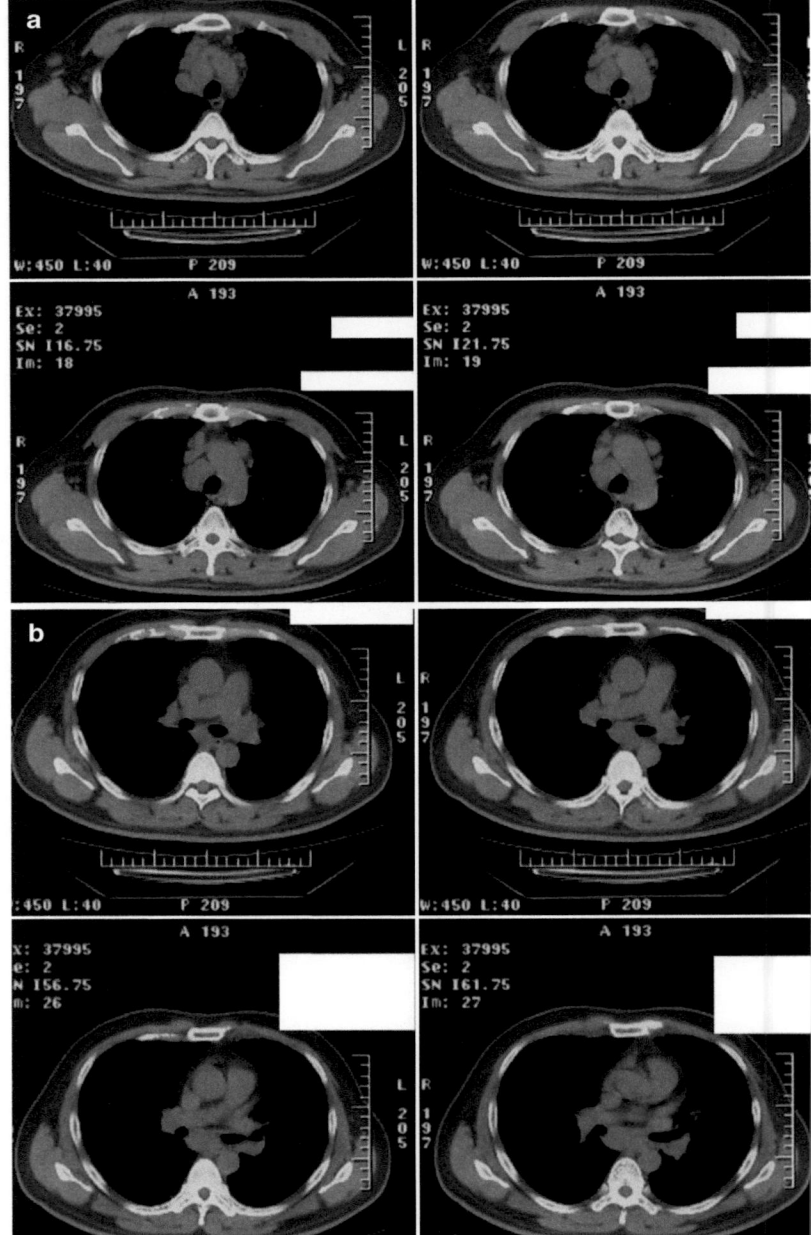

Fig. 4.18 (a–e)
Annotated at the figure
(yellow arrow)

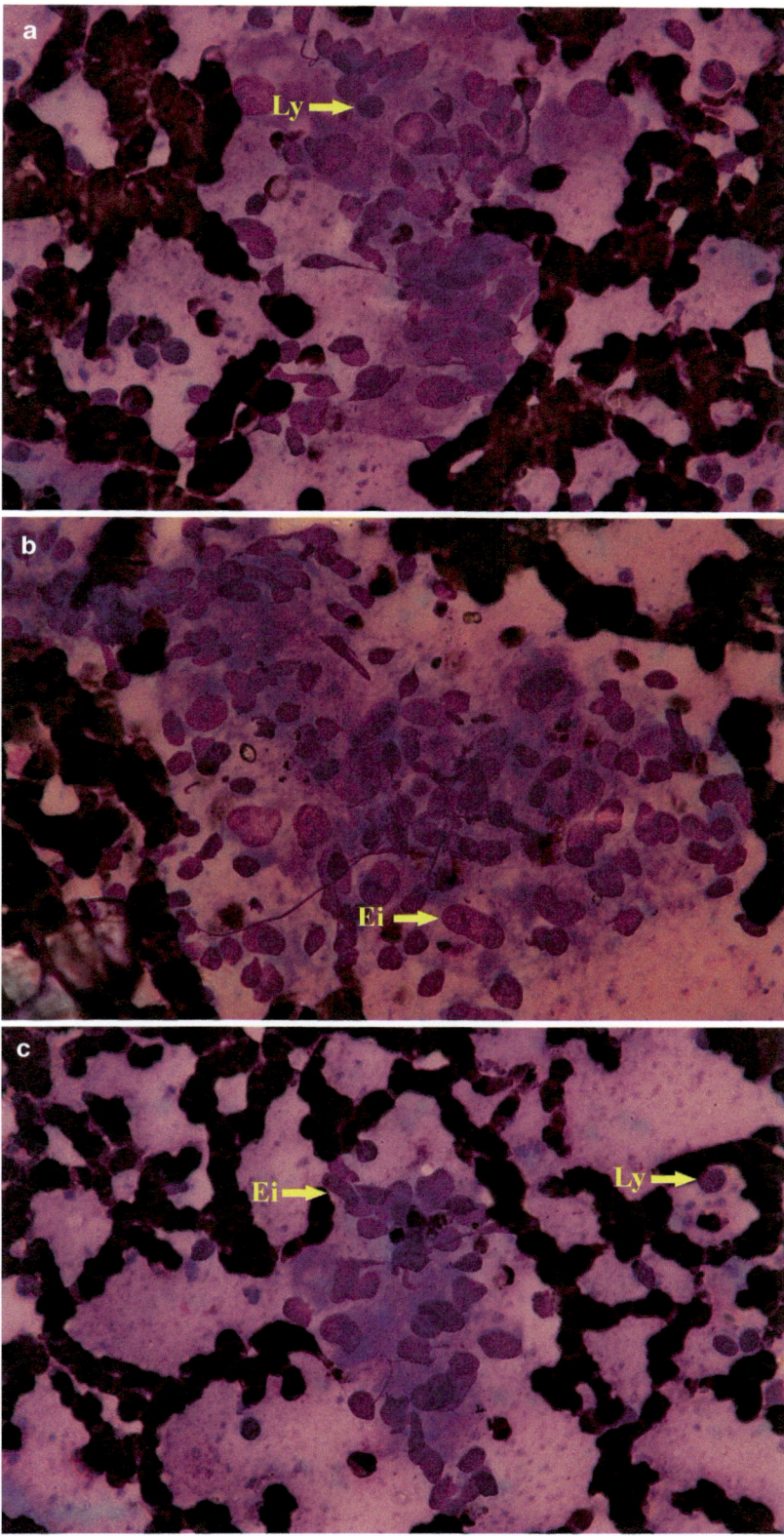

Fig. 4.18 (continued)

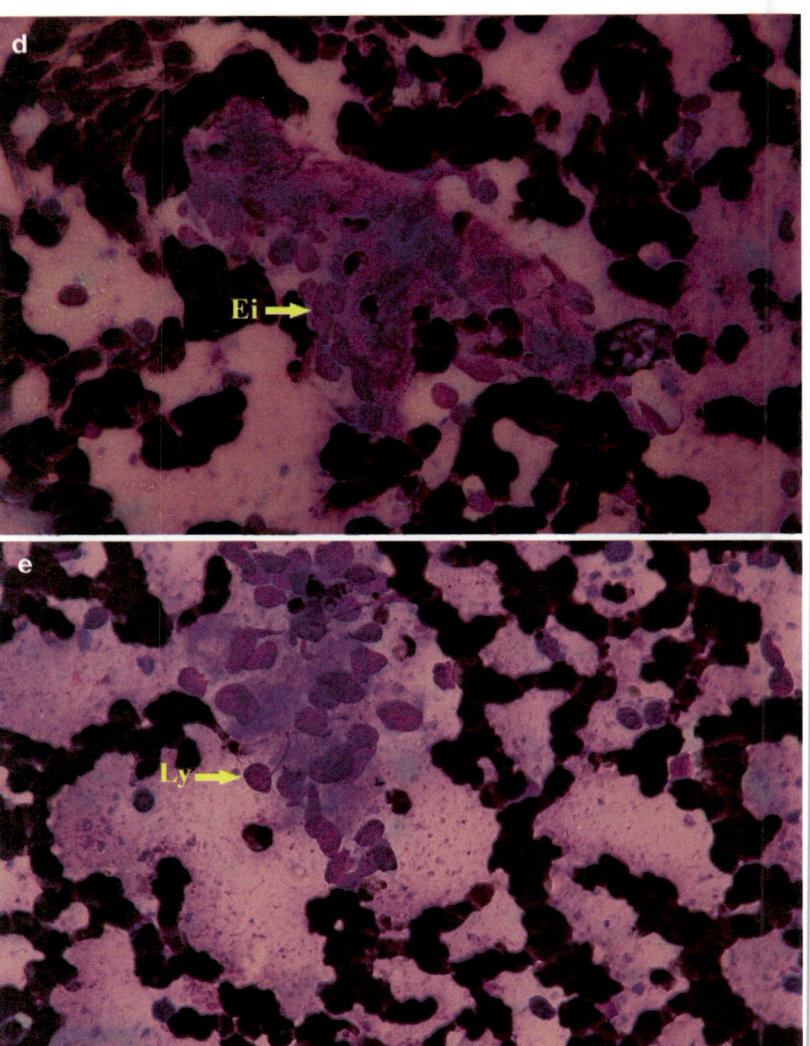

4.10   Sarcoidosis Case 10

Brief history: Female, 58 years old, persistent coughing with mild shortness of breath, clinically diagnosed as sarcoidosis.

Technology to obtain the target lesions: Transbronchial lung biopsy (TBLB).

The preparation of cytological slides for ROSE: Imprinting (rolling).

Clustering (categorizing) analysis in ROSE interpretation:

- "Inflammatory changes".
- Granulomatous inflammation.
- Lymphocyte-based immune inflammatory response.

Fig. 4.19 (**a, b**) Enlargement of hilar and mediastinal lymph nodes and associated reticulonodular abnormalities involving both lungs, resulting from thickening of interlobular septa and intralobular irregular lines, distributed along the bronchovascular bundles, ground-glass opacities in the right lung

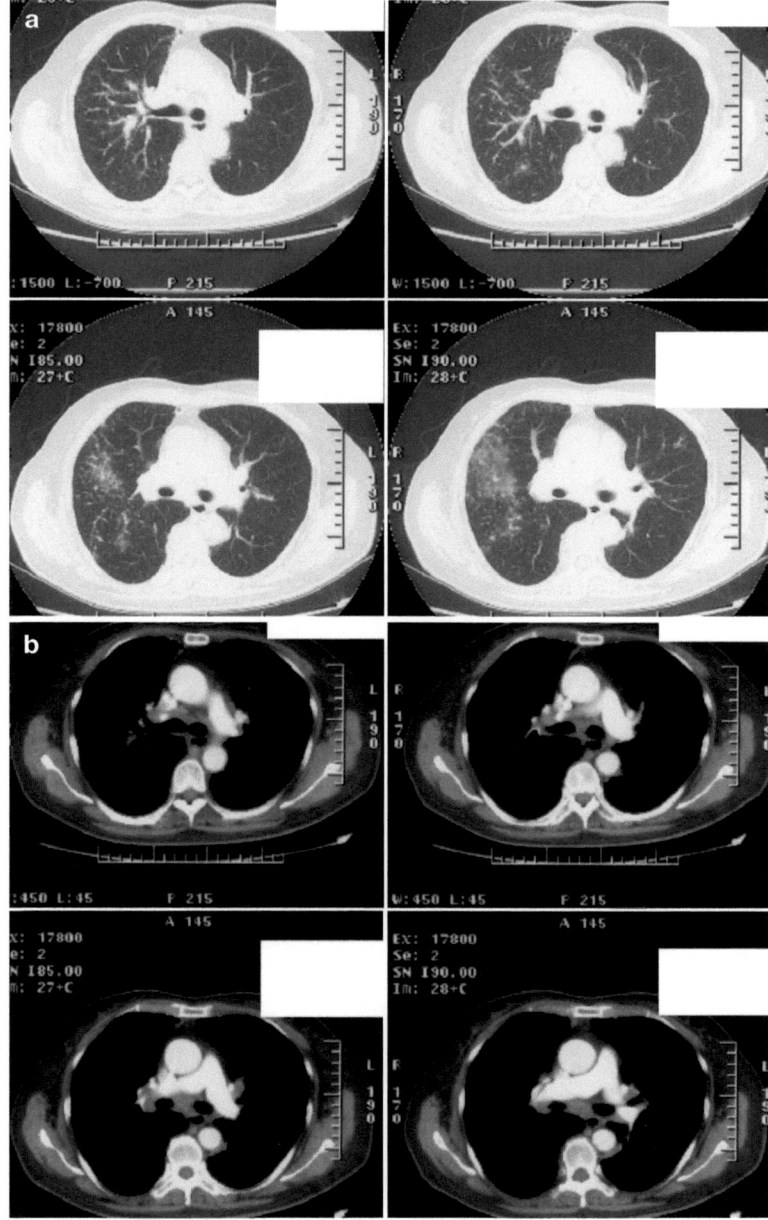

Fig. 4.20 (a–e)
Annotated at the figure
(yellow arrow)

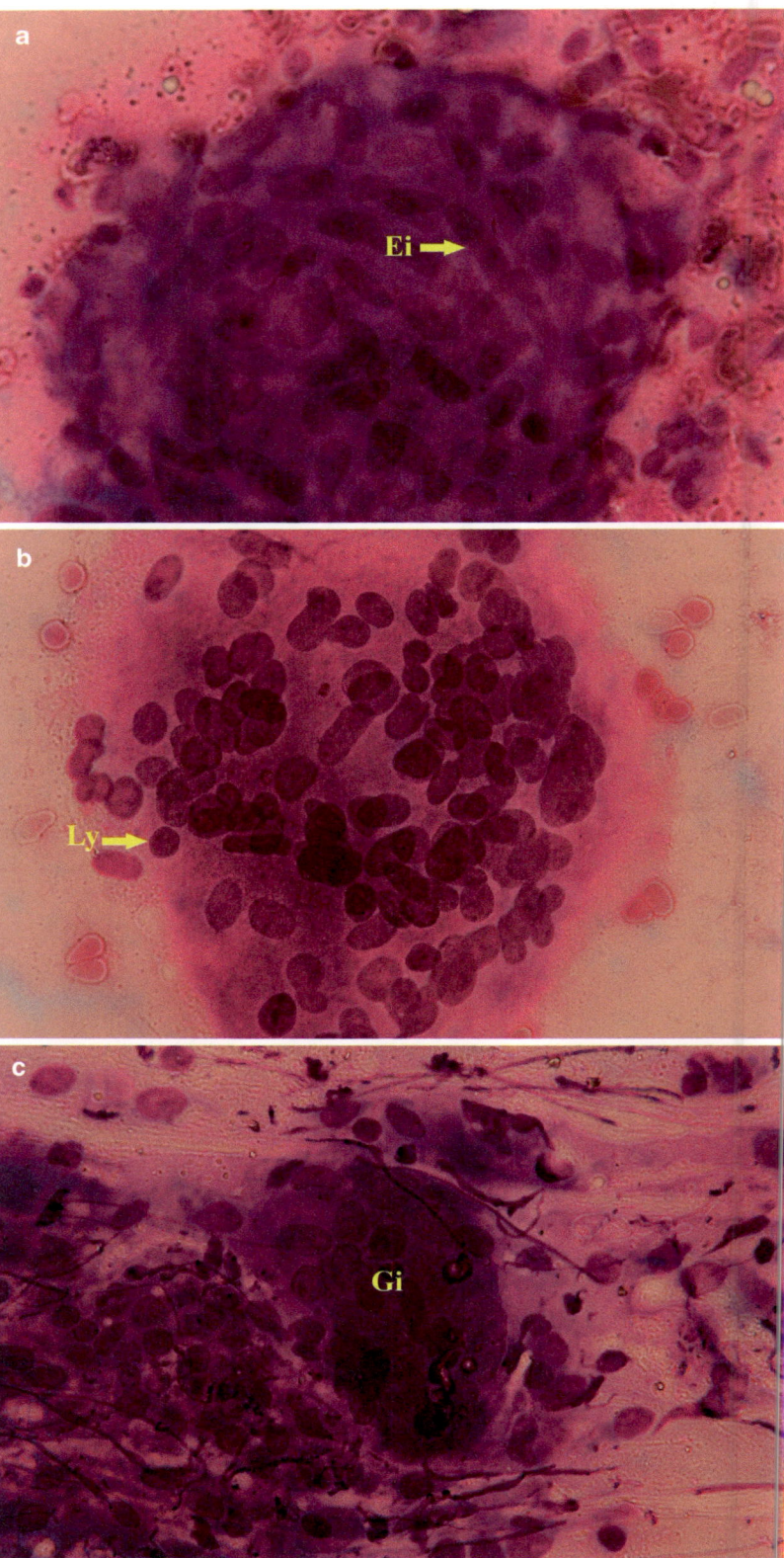

Fig. 4.20 (continued)

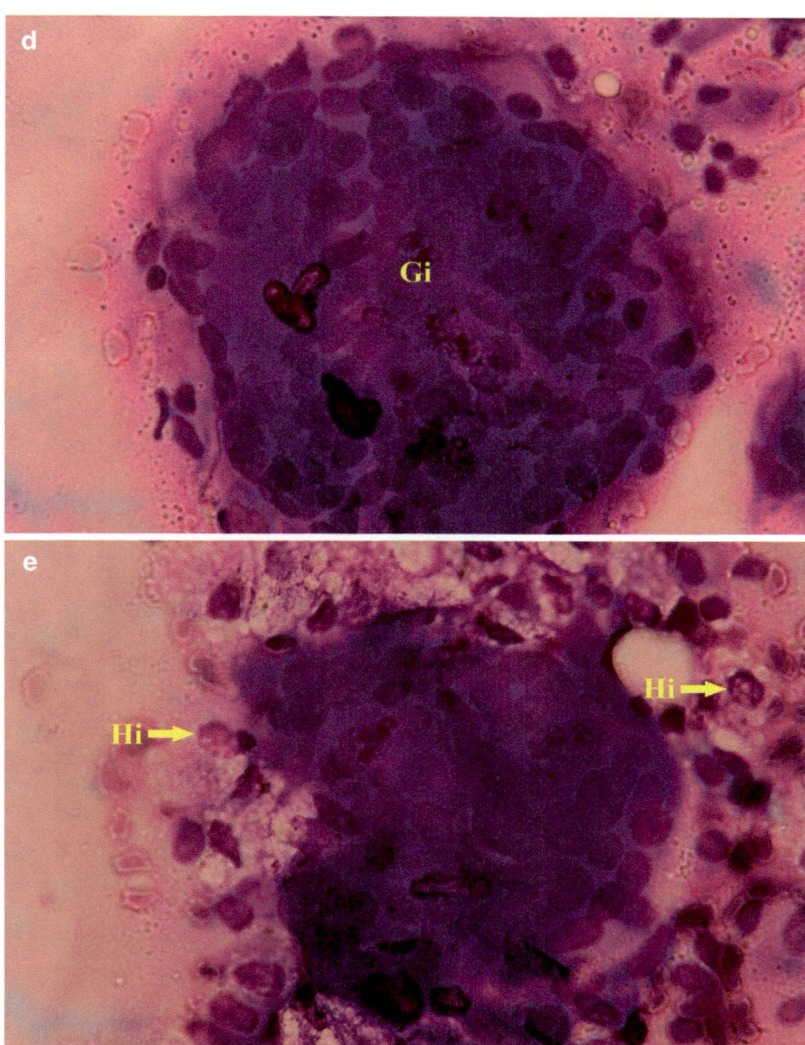

4.11 Sarcoidosis Case 11

Brief history: Female, 51 years old, persistent coughing with mild shortness of breath, clinically diagnosed as sarcoidosis.

Technology to obtain the target lesions: Transbronchial needle aspiration (TBNA).

The preparation of cytological slides for ROSE: Imprinting (rolling).

Clustering (categorizing) analysis in ROSE interpretation:

- "Inflammatory changes".
- Granulomatous inflammation.
- Lymphocyte-based immune inflammatory response.

Fig. 4.21 (a, b) Enlargement of hilar and mediastinal lymph nodes

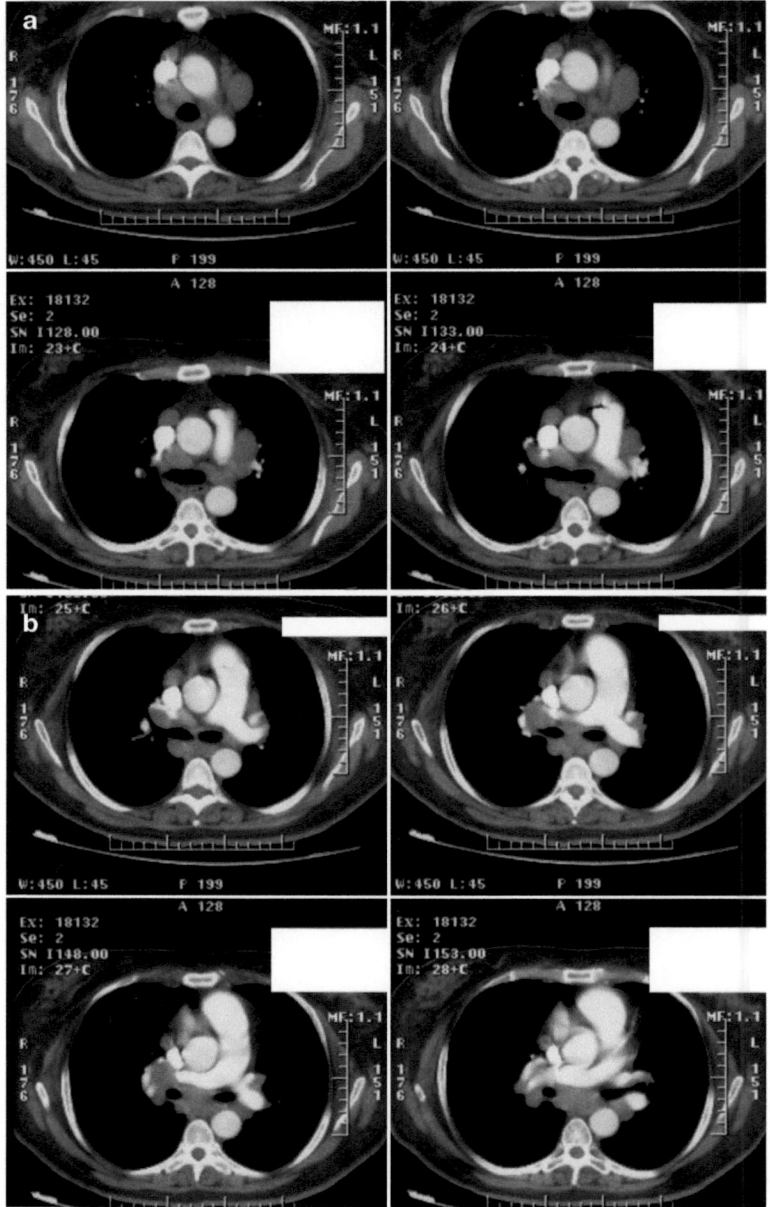

Fig. 4.22 (a–e)
Annotated at the figure
(yellow arrow)

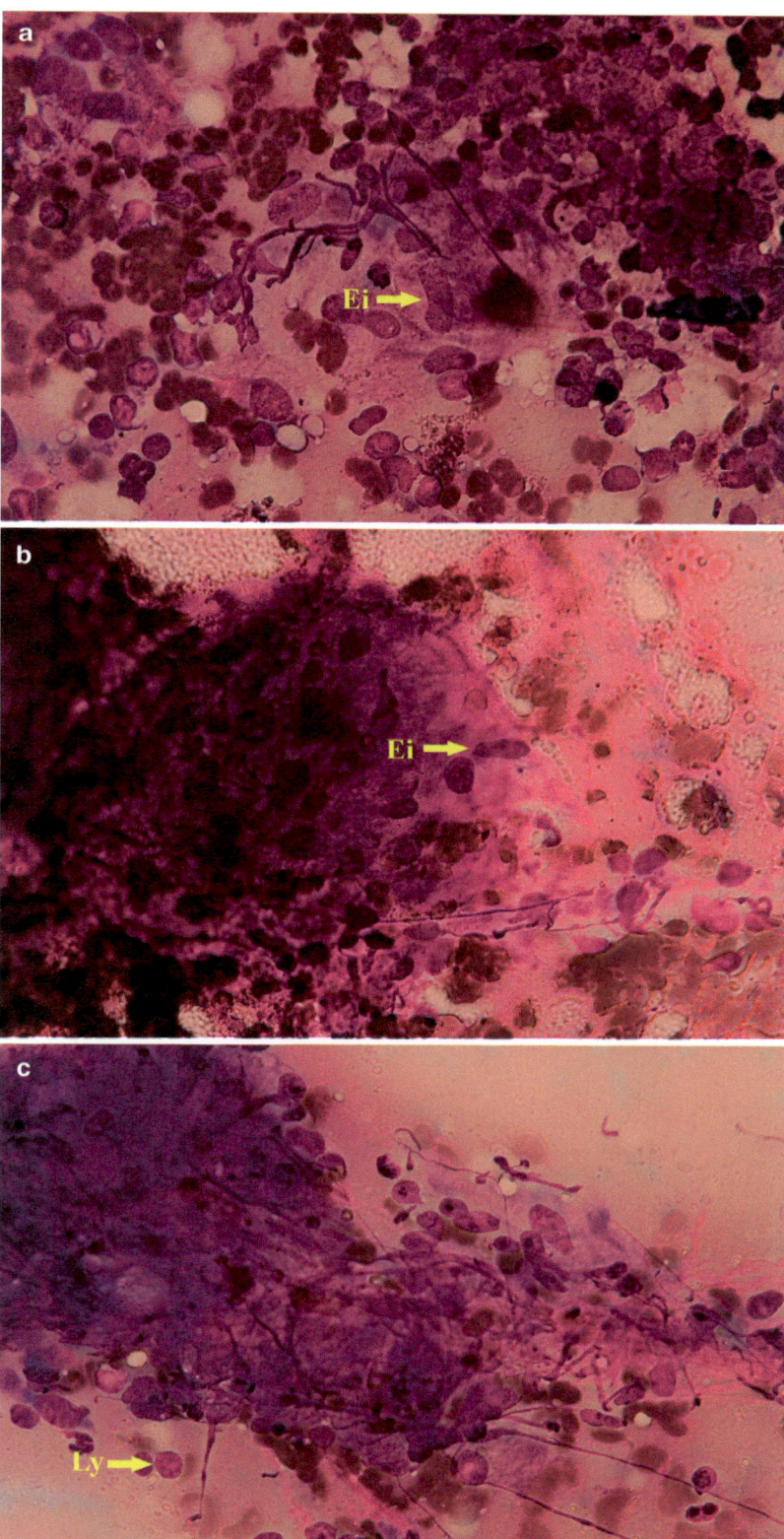

Fig. 4.22 (continued)

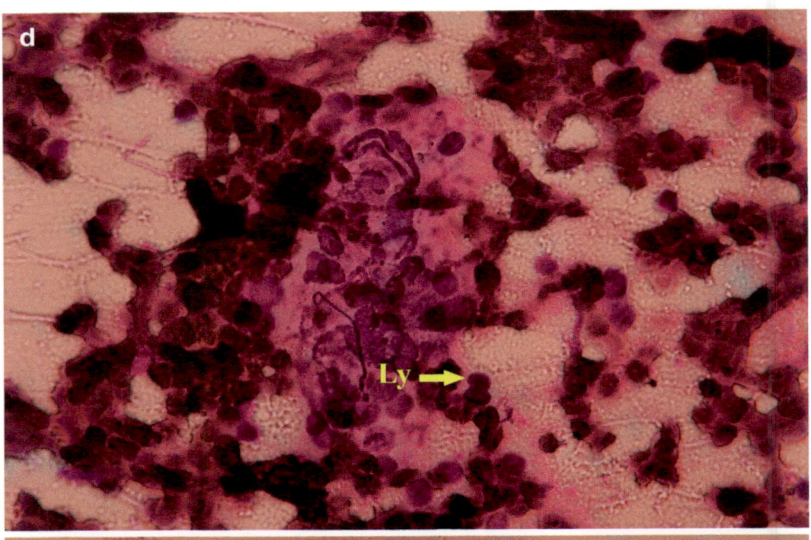

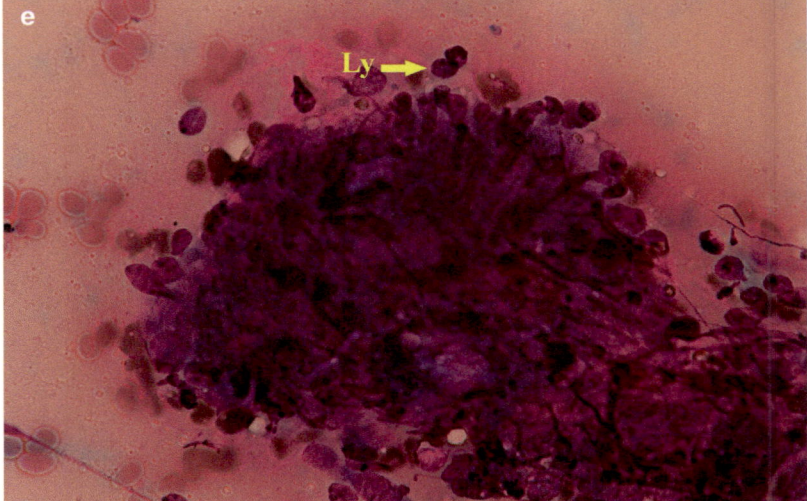

4.12   Final Diagnosis: Clinically Diagnosed as Sarcoidosis

Brief History.

Gender: Female.

Age: 51 years old.

Persistent coughing, shortness of breath.

Technology to obtain the target lesions: Transbronchial needle aspiration (TBNA).

Technology to obtain the target lesions: Transbronchial node forceps biopsy (TBNFB).

The preparation of cytological slides for ROSE: Imprinting (rolling).

Imaging Features.

Enlargement of hilar and mediastinal lymph nodes.

Technology to obtain the target lesions: Transbronchial node forceps biopsy (TBNFB).

Clustering (categorizing) analysis in ROSE interpretation:

- "Inflammatory changes".
- Granulomatous inflammation.
- Lymphocyte-based immune inflammatory response.

Fig. 4.23 (a, b) CT/x-ray/PET-CT

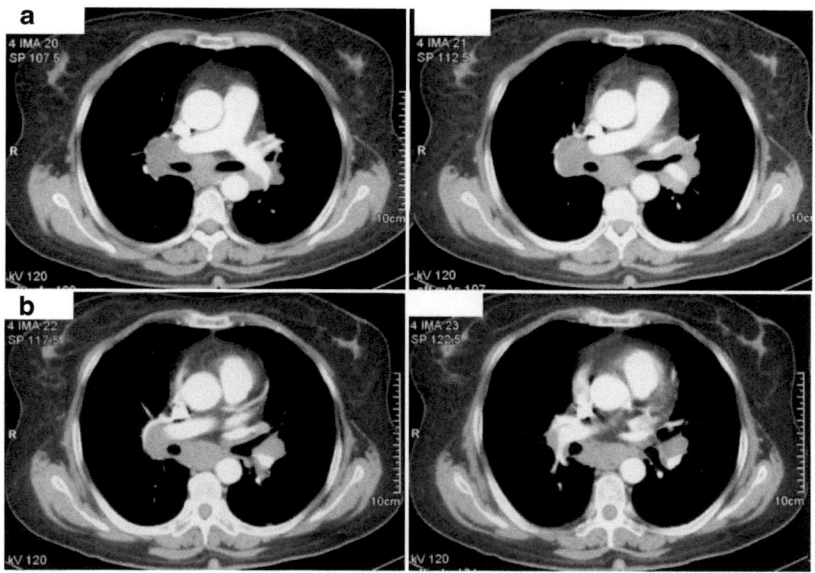

Fig. 4.24 (**a, b**) Under Direct Vision

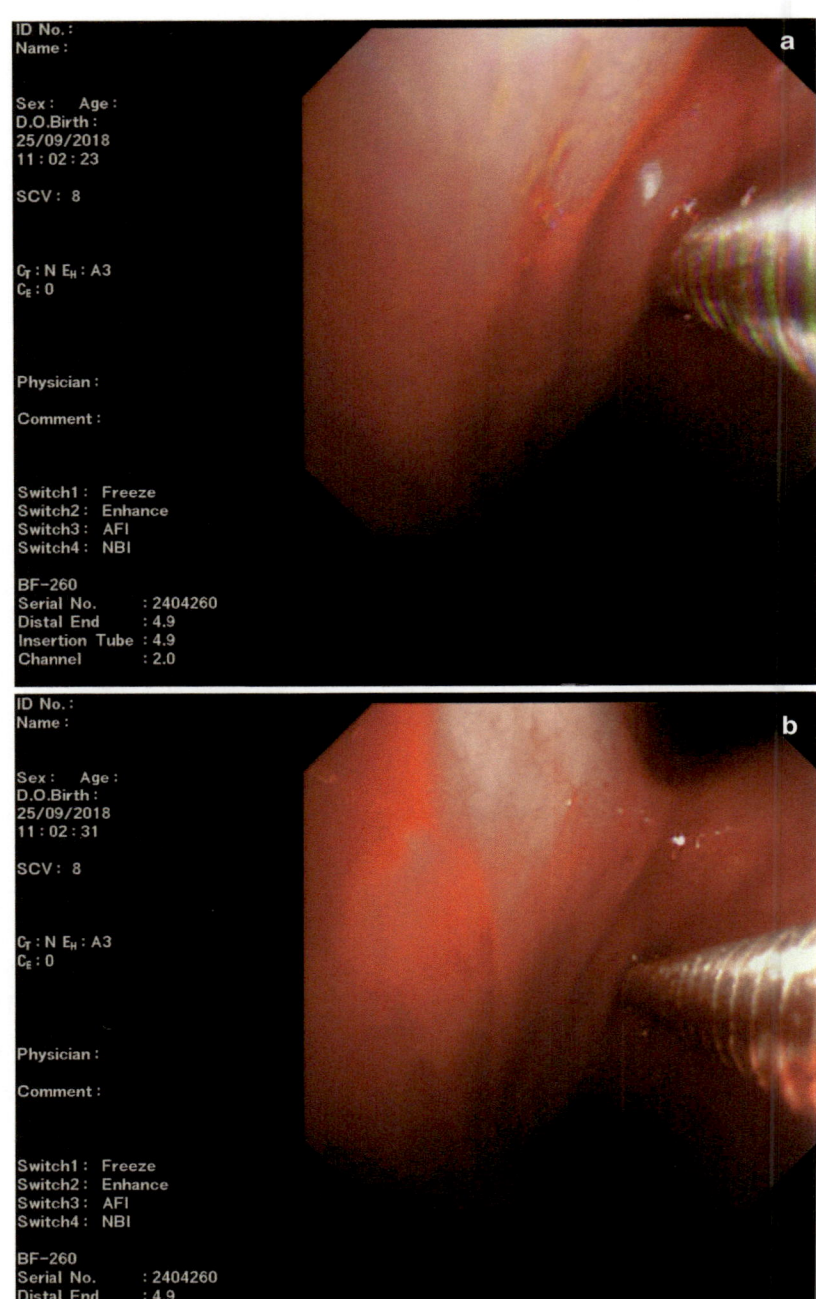

Fig. 4.25 (a–e)
Annotated at the figure
(yellow arrow)

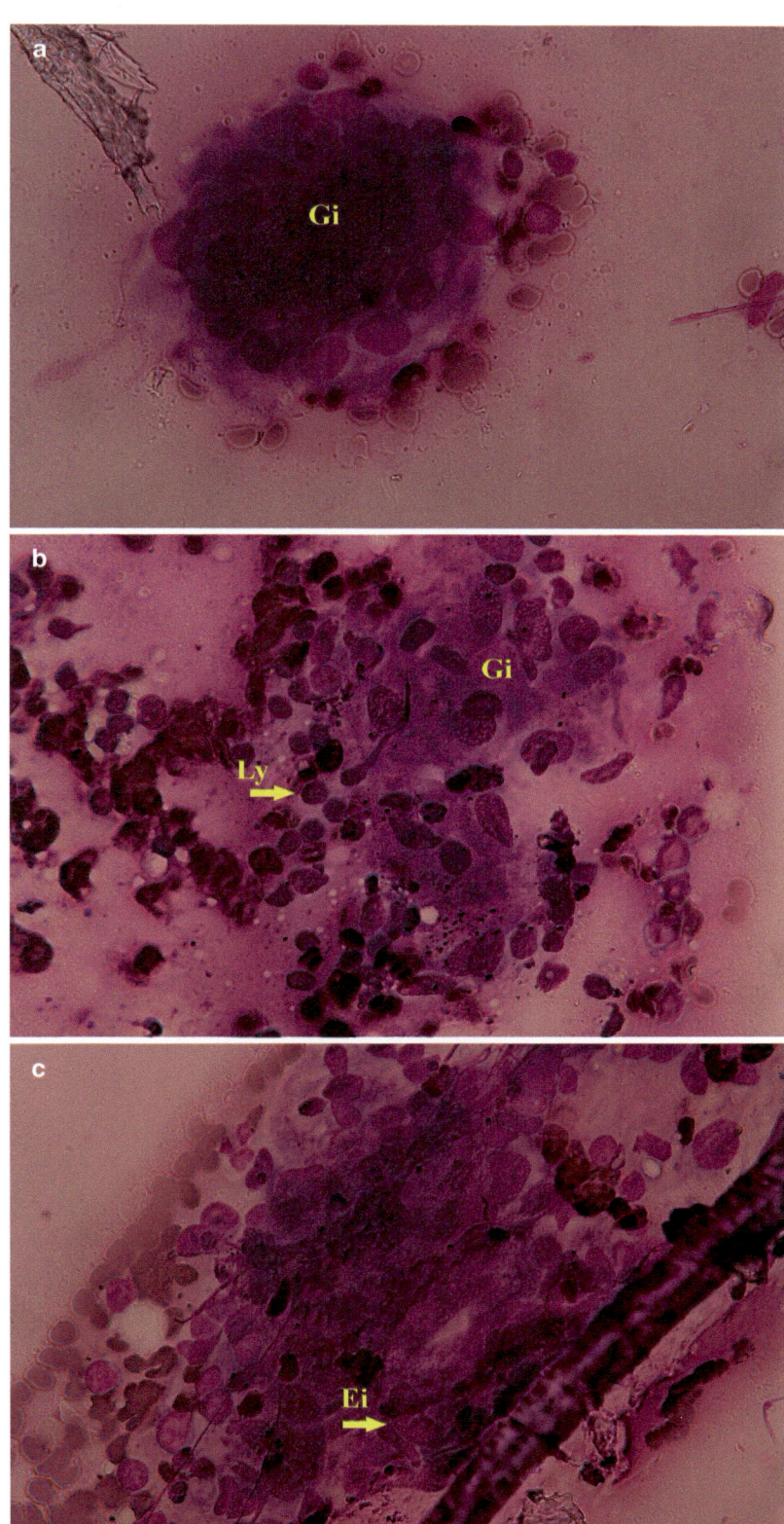

Fig. 4.25 (continued)

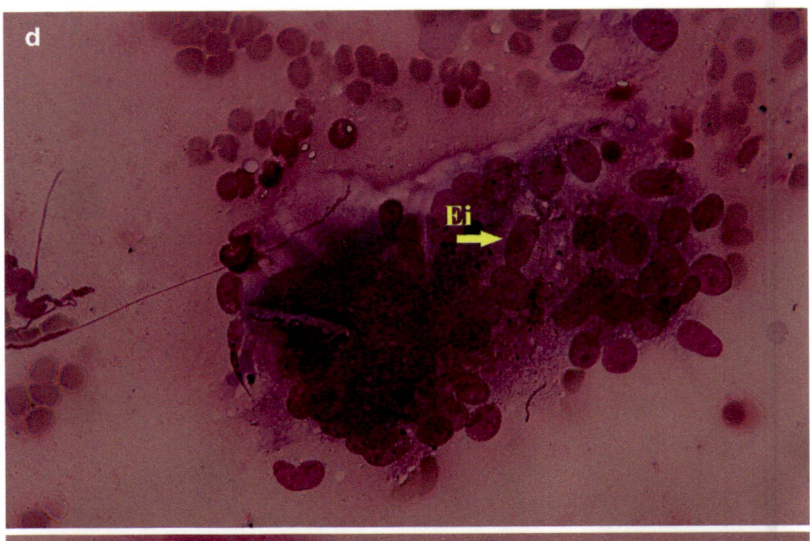

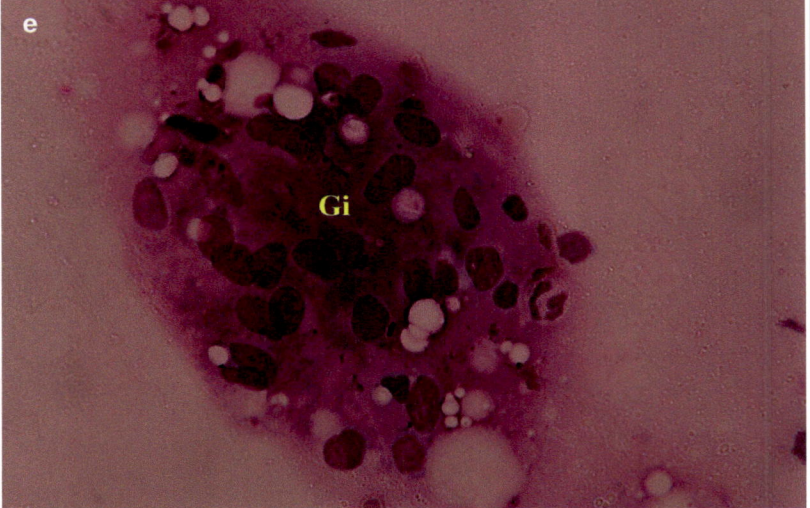

ROSE Cytopathology Cases of Pulmonary Involvement from Vasculitis

5

Jing Feng, Bo Wu, and Wen Ning

5.1 Pulmonary Involvement from ANCA-Associated Vasculitis Case 1

Brief history: Coughing with mild shortness of breath for more than 2 weeks, clinically diagnosed as ANCA-associated vasculitis.

Technology to obtain the target lesions: Transbronchial lung biopsy (TBLB).

The preparation of cytological slides for ROSE: Imprinting (rolling).

Clustering (categorizing) analysis in ROSE interpretation:

- "Inflammatory changes".
- May conform to organization.
- May conform to fibrosis (fibroblast dominant or fibrocyte dominant).
- Lymphocyte-based immune inflammatory response.

J. Feng
Pulmonary and Critical Care Medicine, Tianjin Medical University General Hospital, Tianjin, China
e-mail: zyyhxkfj@126.com

B. Wu
Lung Transplantation Group, Nanjing Medical University, Wuxi, China
e-mail: fyz333@126.com

W. Ning (✉)
College of Life Sciences, Nankai University, Tianjin, China
e-mail: ningwen108@nankai.edu.cn

© Springer Nature Singapore Pte Ltd. 2020
J. Feng et al. (eds.), *Rapid On-Site Evaluation (ROSE) in Diagnostic Interventional Pulmonology*,
https://doi.org/10.1007/978-981-15-0939-1_5

Fig. 5.1 (**a–c**) Initial CT, multiple patches, consolidation, and tree-in-bud sign in both lungs

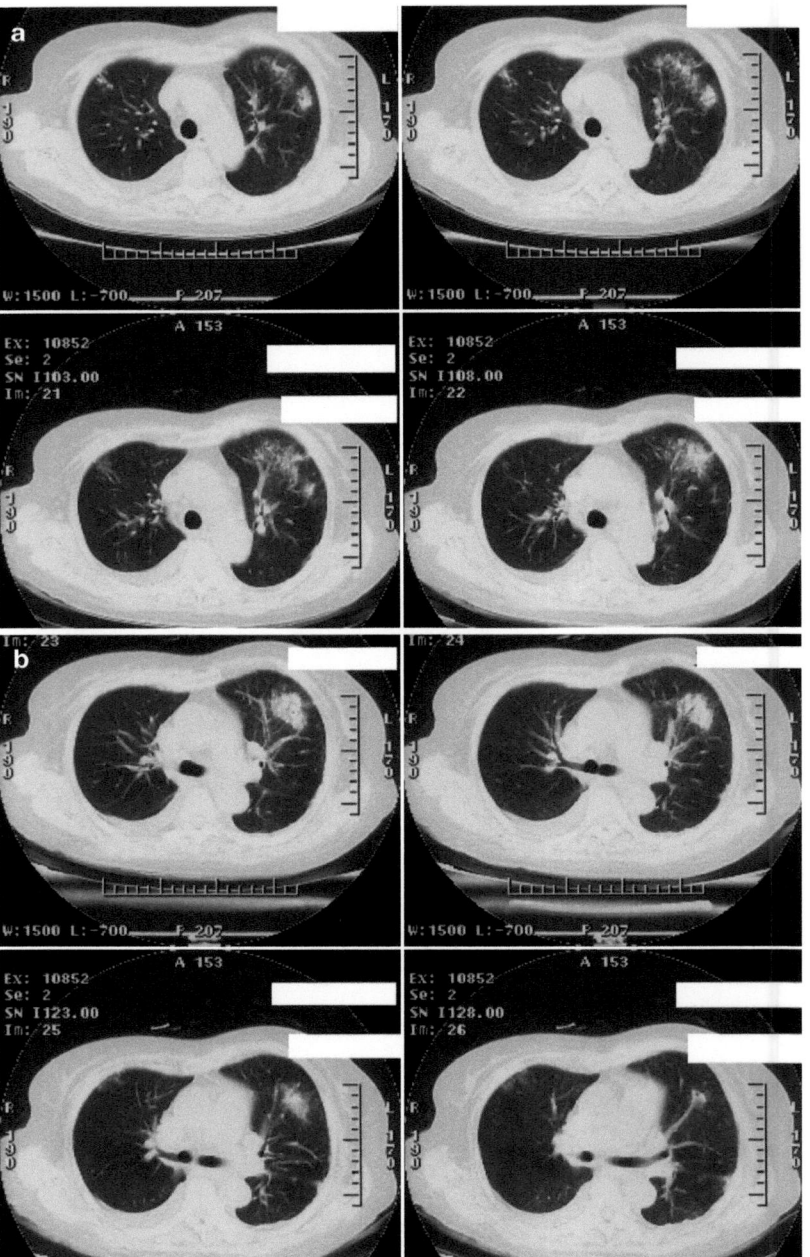

Fig. 5.1 (continued)

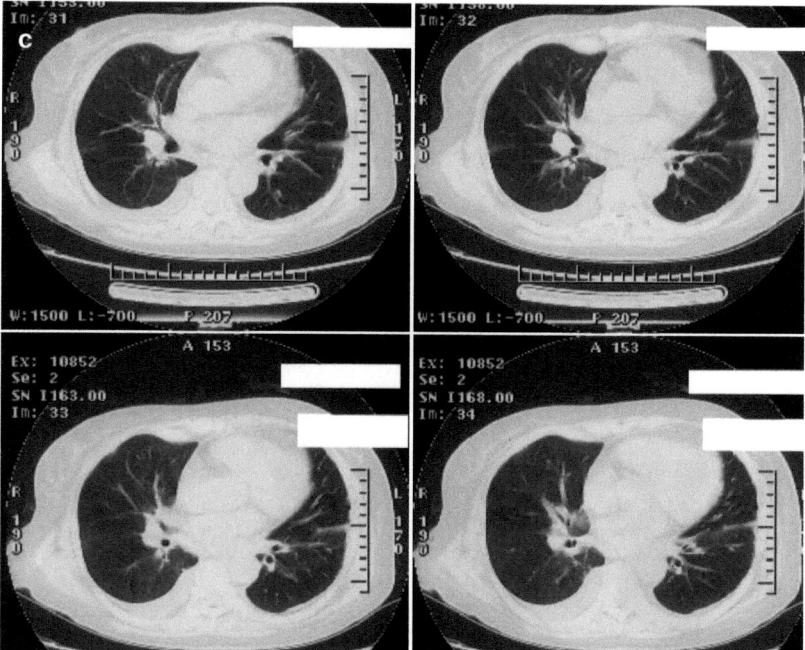

Fig. 5.2 (**a**–**c**) CT taken 40 days later, extensive ground-glass opacities and interstitial thickening, distributed along the bronchial vascular bundles

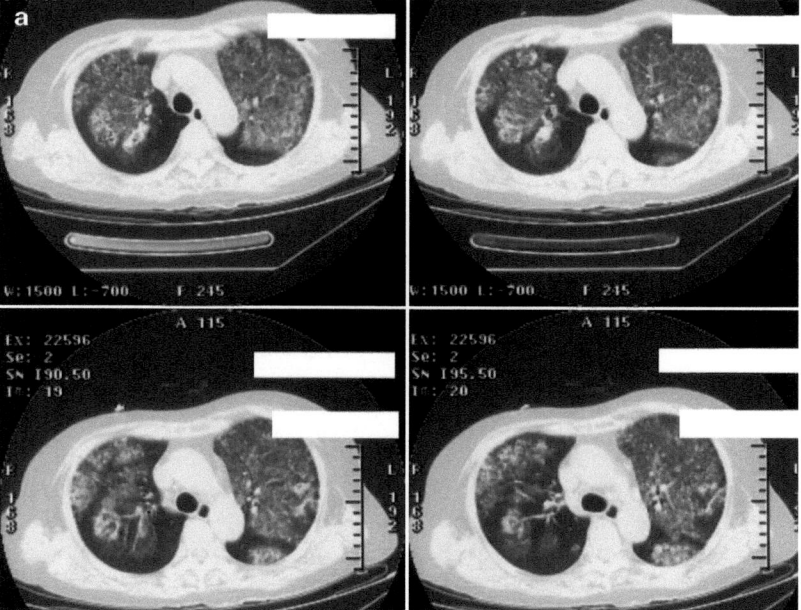

Fig. 5.2 (continued)

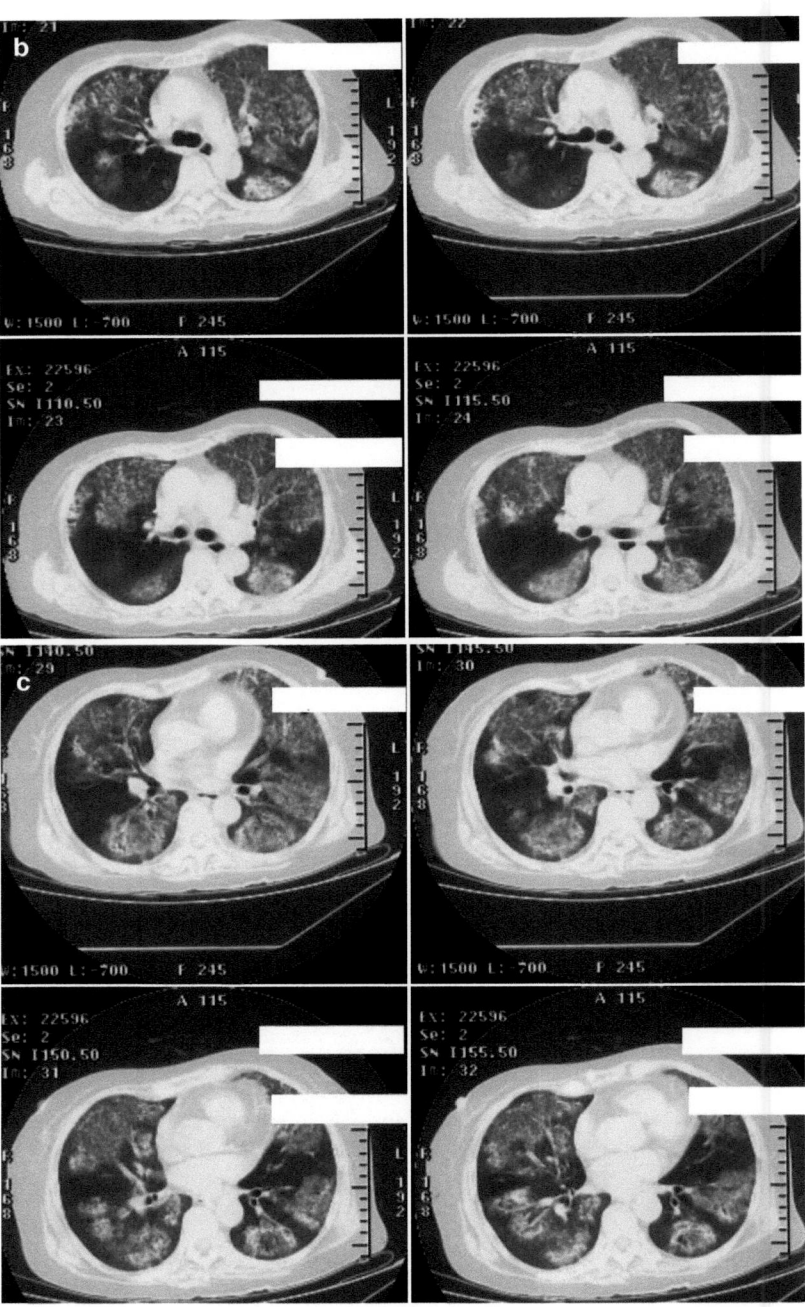

Fig. 5.3 (a–e)
Annotated at the figure
(yellow arrow)

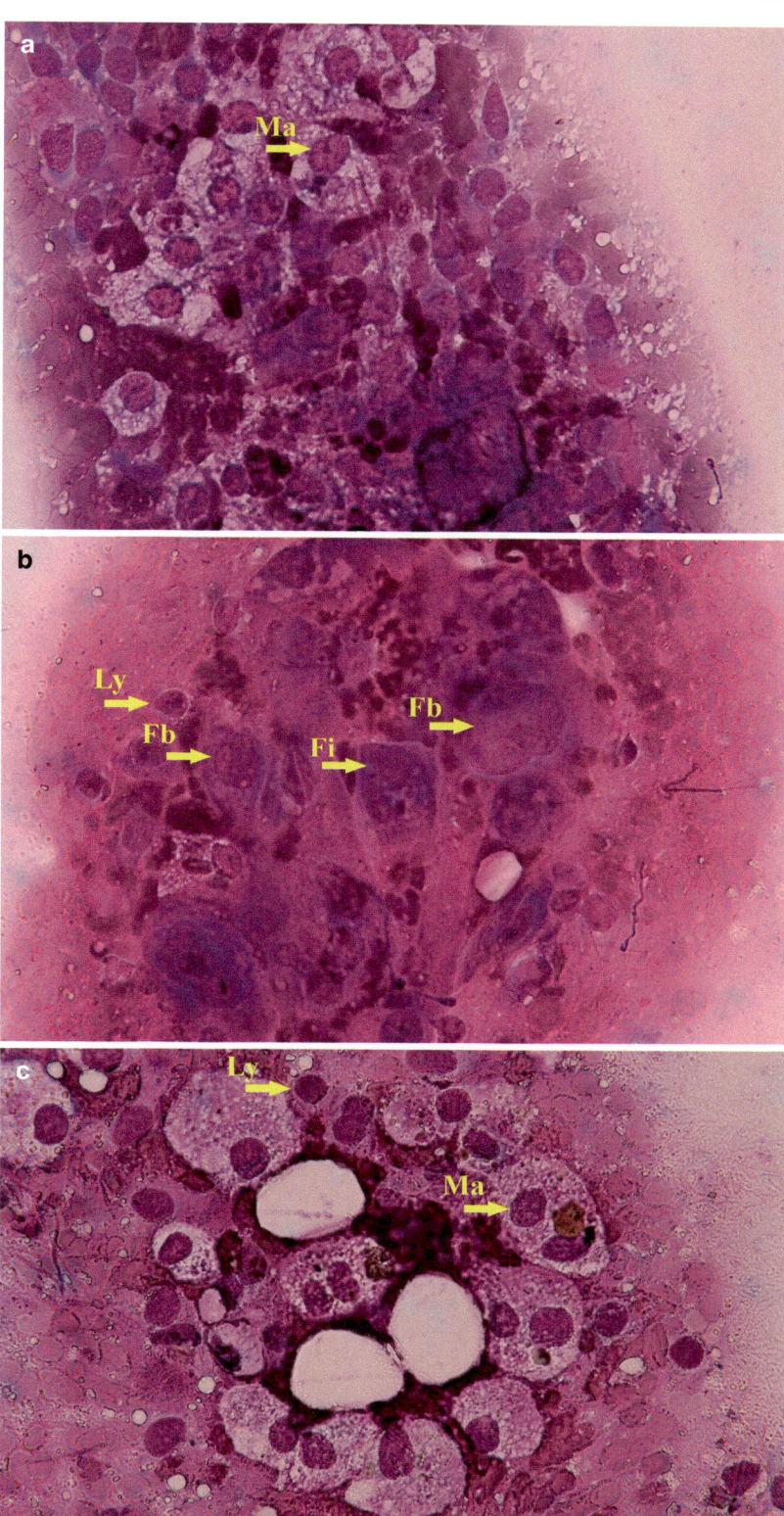

Fig. 5.3 (continued)

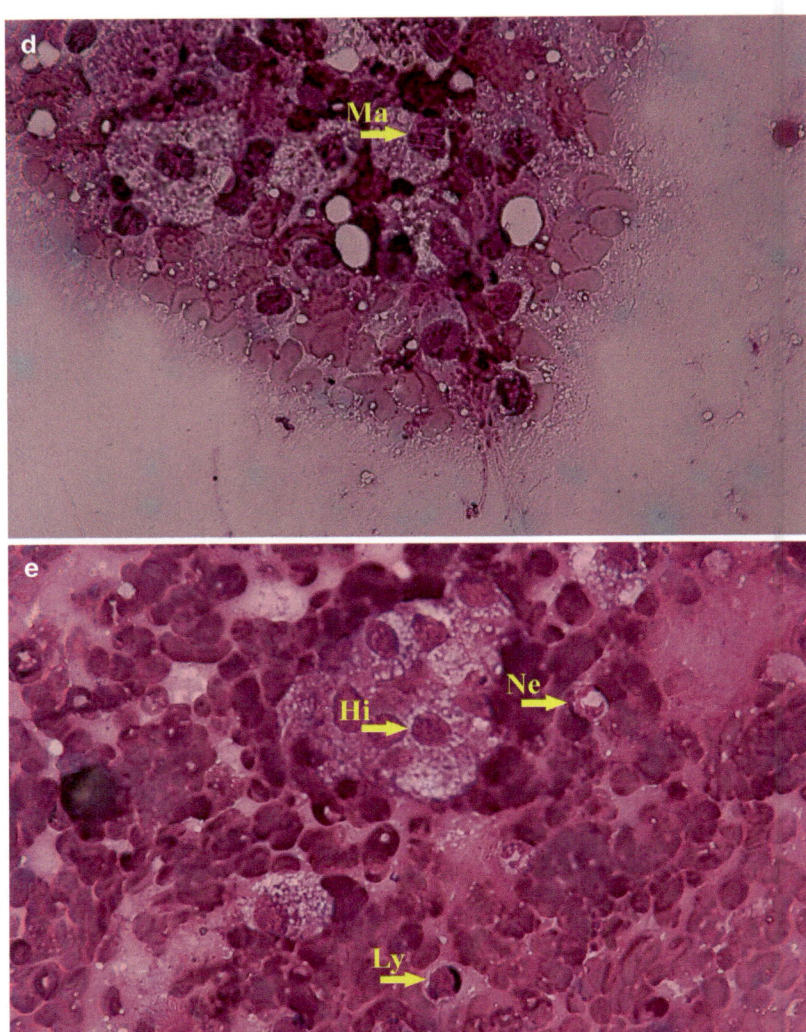

5.2 Pulmonary Involvement from ANCA-Associated Vasculitis Case 2

Brief history: Coughing with mild shortness of breath for more than 1 month, clinically diagnosed as ANCA-associated vasculitis.

Technology to obtain the target lesions: Transbronchial lung biopsy (TBLB).

The preparation of cytological slides for ROSE: Imprinting (rolling).

Clustering (categorizing) analysis in ROSE interpretation:

- "Inflammatory changes".
- Granulomatous inflammation.
- May conform to fibrosis (fibroblast dominant or fibrocyte dominant).
- Lymphocyte-based immune inflammatory response.

Fig. 5.4 (**a–c**) Multiple patches in both lungs, extensive ground-glass opacities, and interstitial thickening, distributed along the bronchial vascular bundles

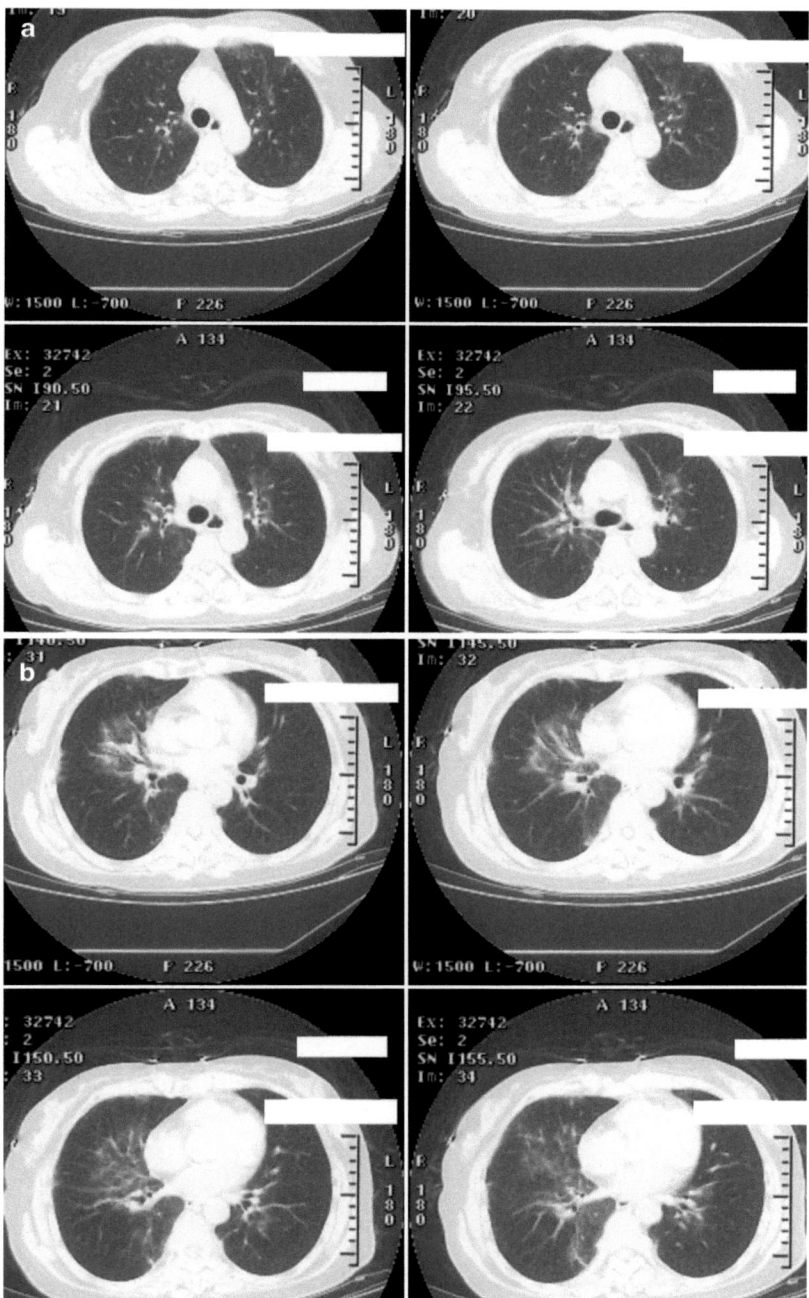

Fig. 5.4 (continued)

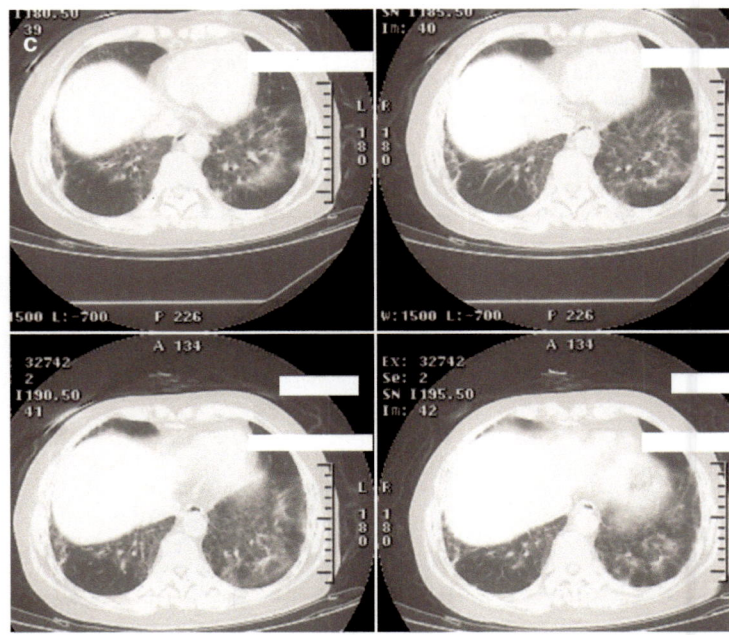

Fig. 5.5 (a–e) Annotated at the figure (yellow arrow)

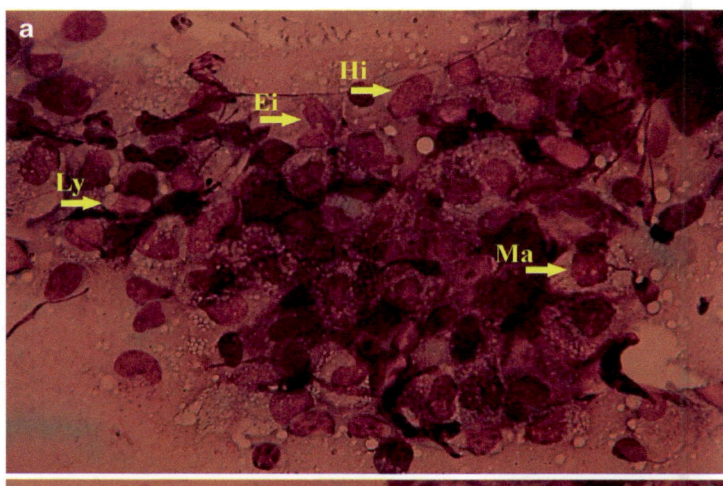

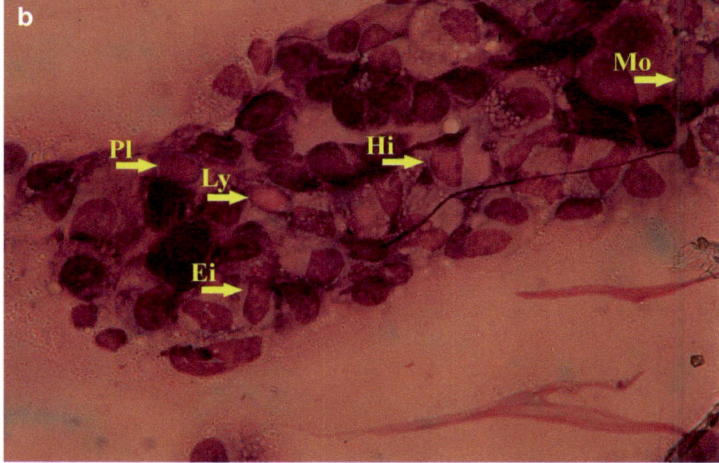

Fig. 5.5 (continued)

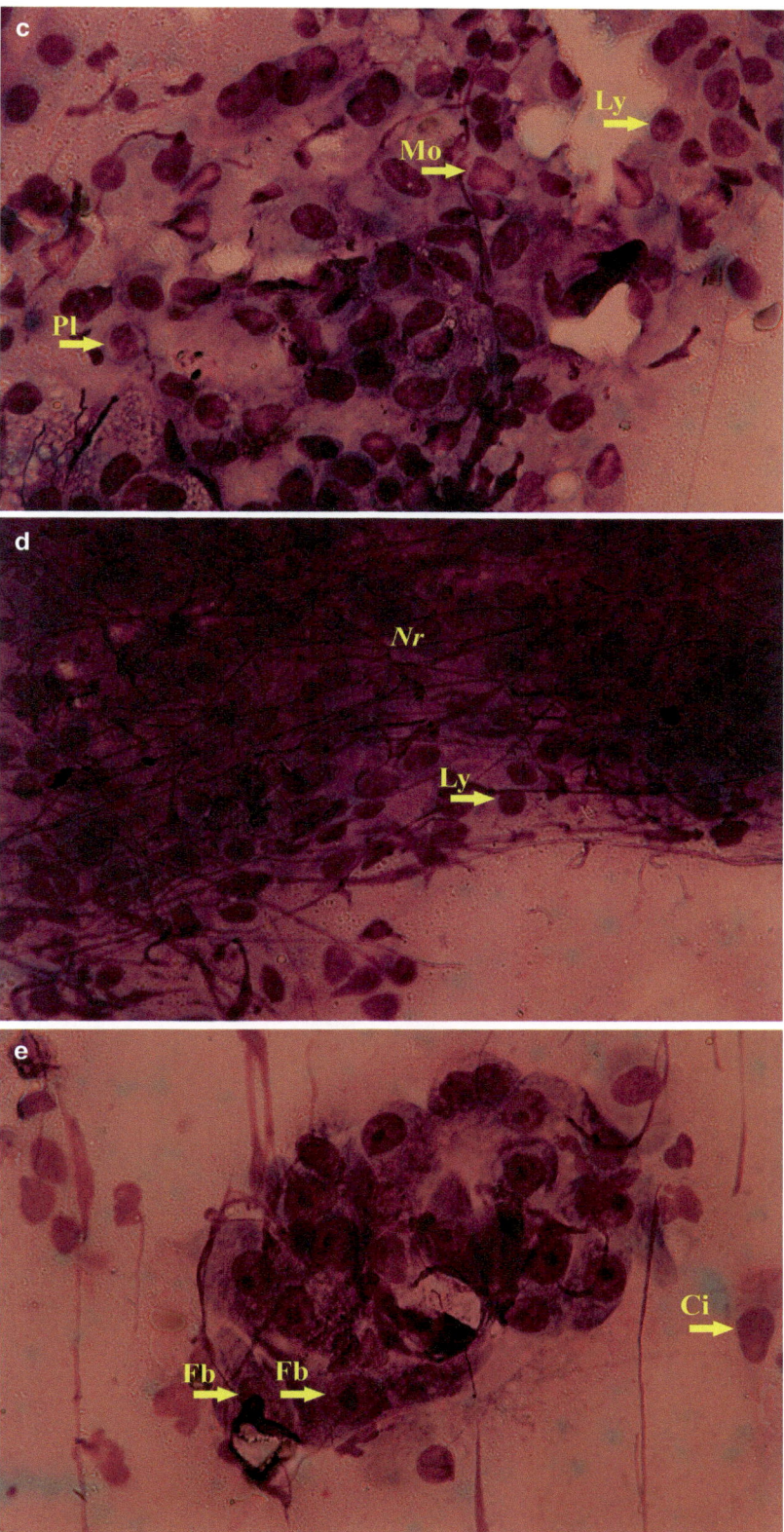

5.3 Pulmonary Involvement from ANCA-Associated Vasculitis Case 3

Brief history: Male, 64 years old, persistent coughing with mild shortness of breath for more than 3 months, clinically diagnosed as ANCA-associated vasculitis.

Technology to obtain the target lesions: Transbronchial lung biopsy (TBLB).

The preparation of cytological slides for ROSE: Imprinting (rolling).

Clustering (categorizing) analysis in ROSE interpretation:

- "Inflammatory changes".
- May conform to fibrosis (fibroblast dominant or fibrocyte dominant).
- Lymphocyte-based immune inflammatory response.

Fig. 5.6 (**a, b**) Extensive ground-glass opacities and slight interstitial thickening in both lungs, especially in subpleural areas

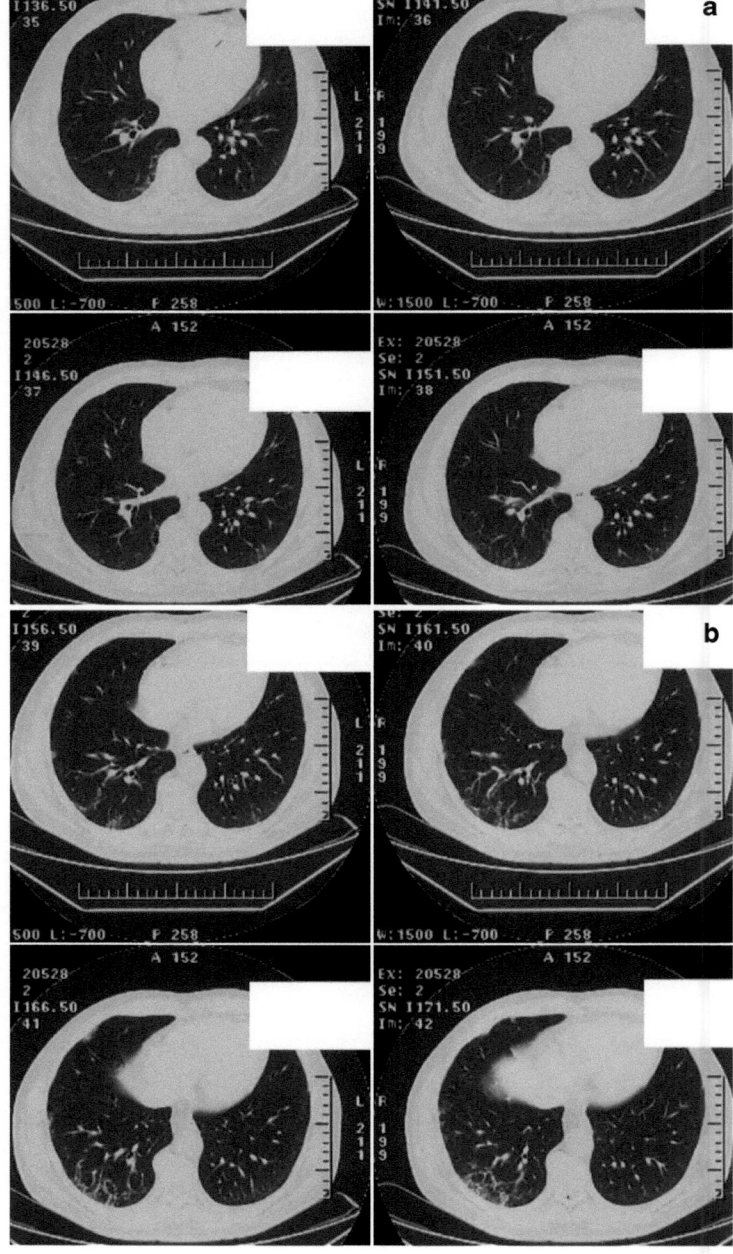

Fig. 5.7 (a–e)
Annotated at the figure
(yellow arrow)

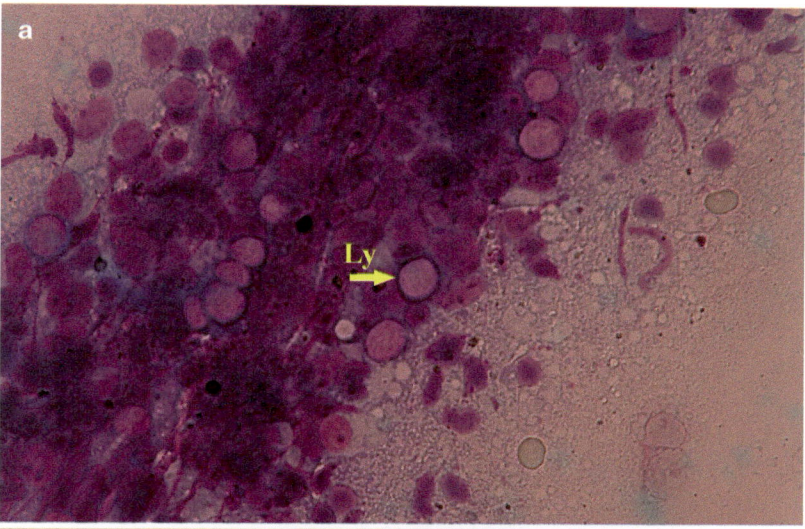

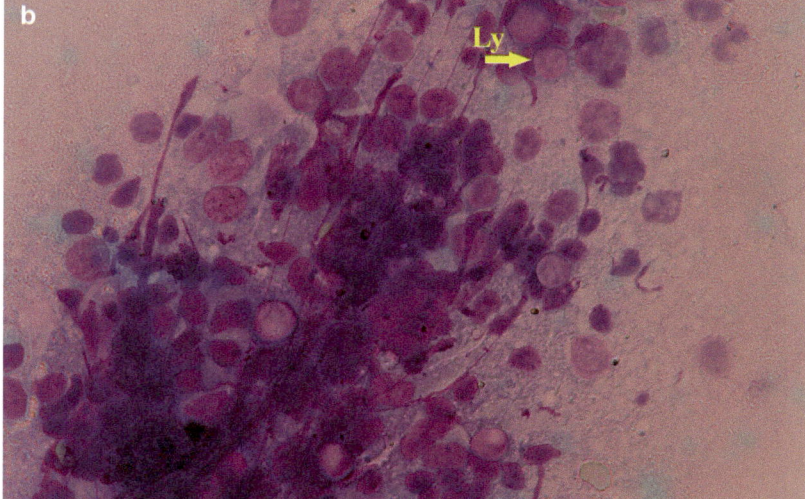

Fig. 5.7 (continued)

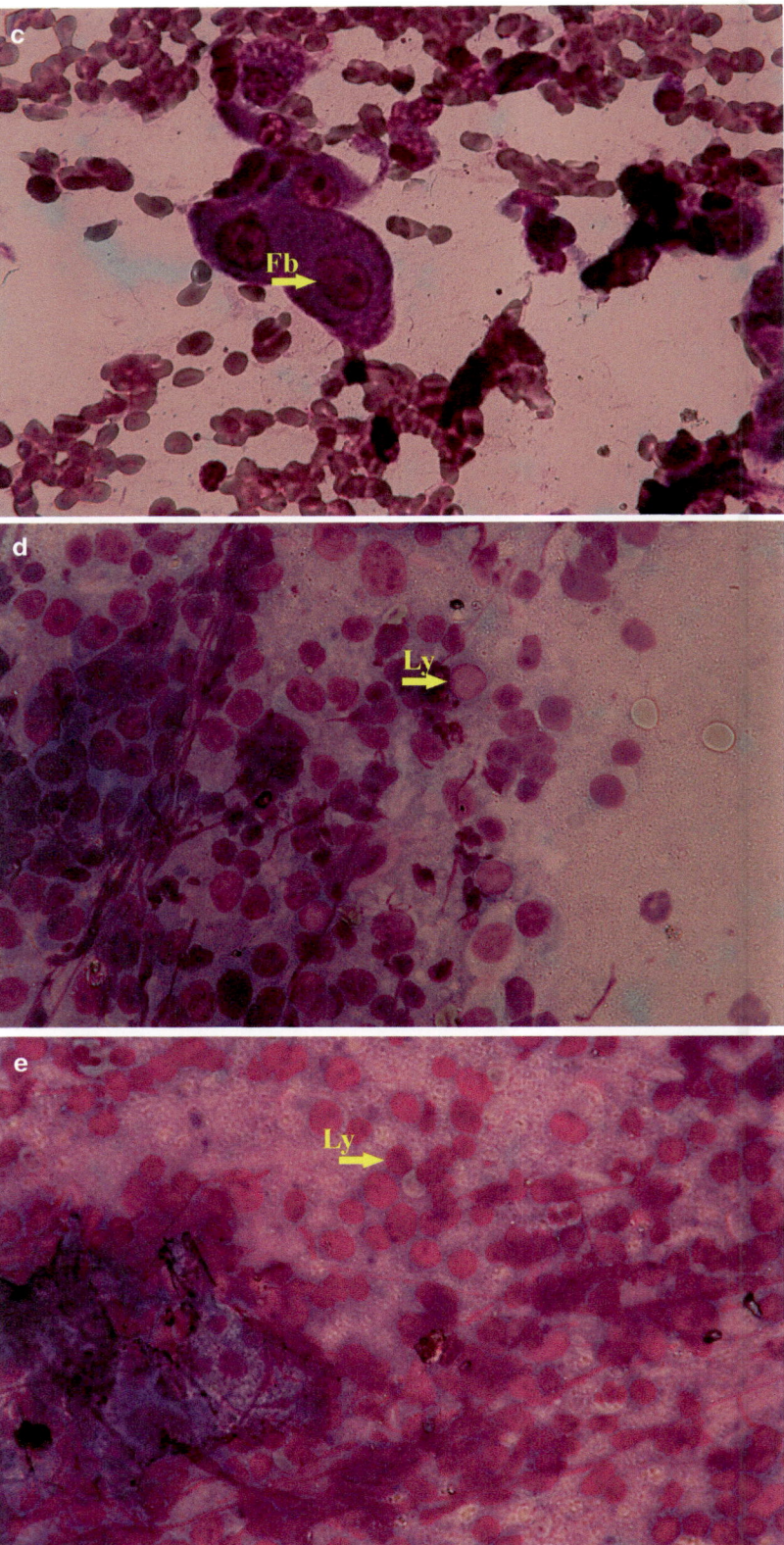

5.4   Pulmonary Involvement of ANCA-Associated Vasculitis

Brief history: Diagnosed as ANCA-associated vasculitis clinically, irritable dry cough with dyspnea.

Technology to obtain the target lesions: Transbronchial lung biopsy (TBLB).

The preparation of cytological slides for ROSE: Imprinting (rolling).

Clustering (categorizing) analysis in ROSE interpretation:

• "Inflammatory changes".
• Granulomatous inflammation.
• Lymphocyte-based immune inflammatory response.

Fig. 5.8 (**a**, **b**) Diffuse interstitial changes in both lungs, interlobular septal thickening, diffuse ground-glass opacities, and scattered patchy exudation

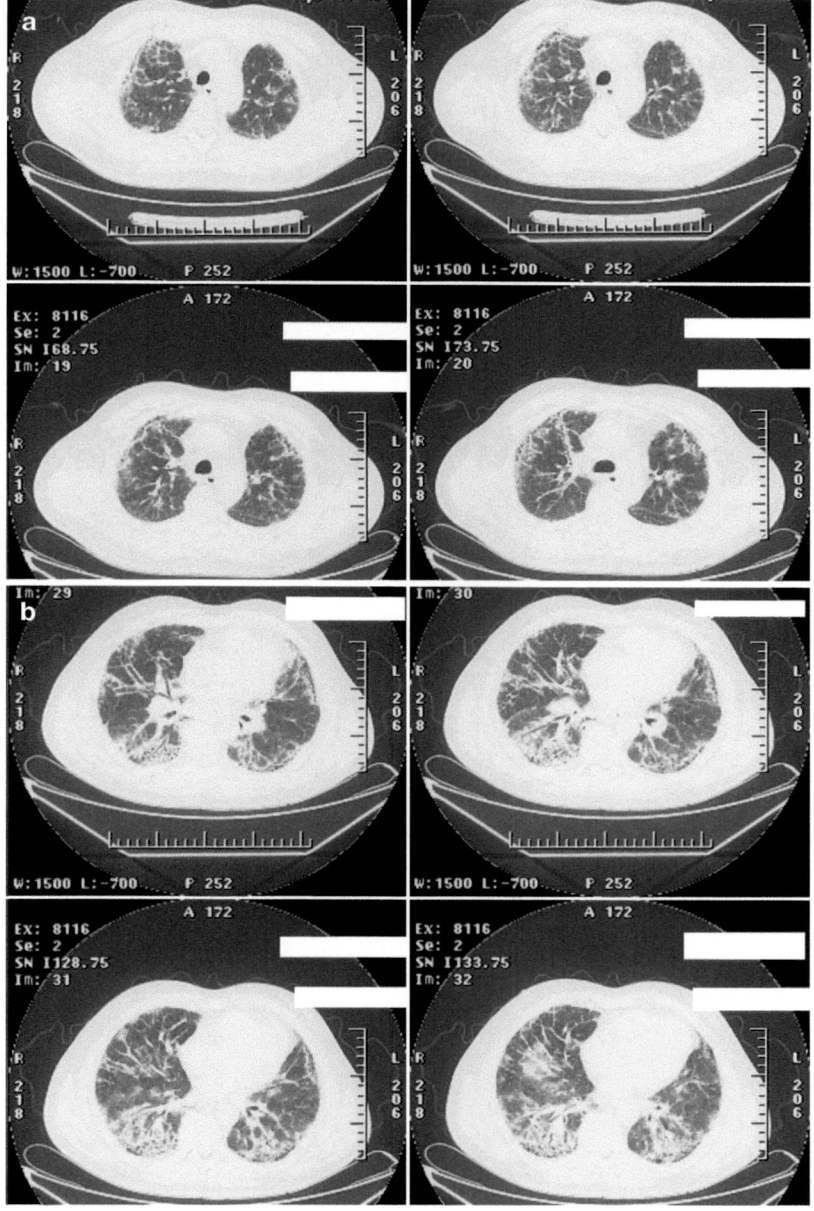

Fig. 5.9 Foamy macrophages (yellow arrow), hyperplastic type II alveolar epithelial cell (red arrow), reactive lymphocytes (green arrow), epithelioid cells (blue arrow), short columnar distal airway ciliated columnar epithelial cells (pink arrow), and degeneration, denaturation, and necrosis from some epithelial cells (brown arrow)

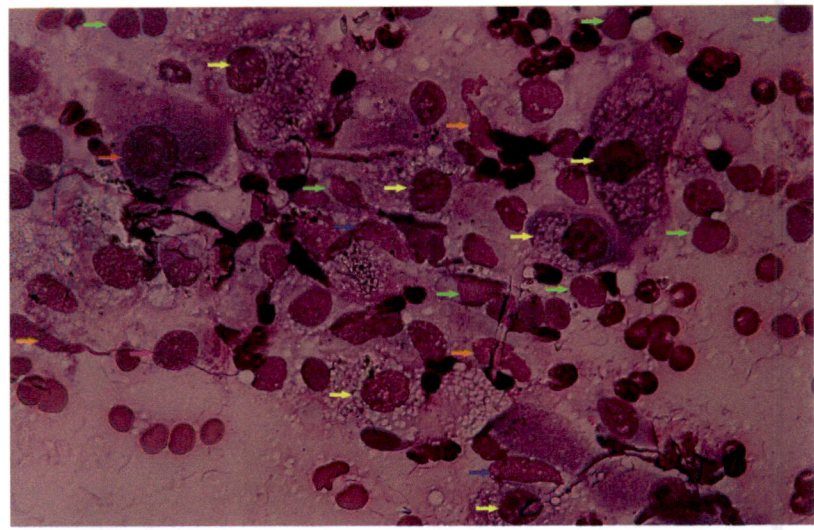

Fig. 5.10 Foamy macrophages (yellow arrow), hyperplastic type II alveolar epithelial cell (red arrow), reactive lymphocytes (green arrow), ciliated columnar epithelial cells (blue arrow), and degeneration, denaturation, and necrosis from some epithelial cells (pink arrow)

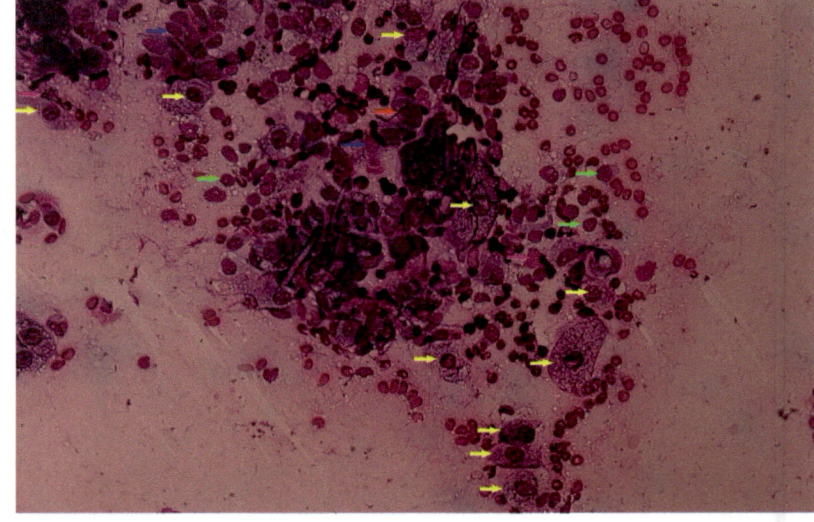

Fig. 5.11 Foamy macrophages (yellow arrow), hyperplastic type II alveolar epithelial cells (red arrow), reactive lymphocytes (green arrow), epithelioid cells (blue arrow), and ciliated columnar epithelial cells (pink arrow)

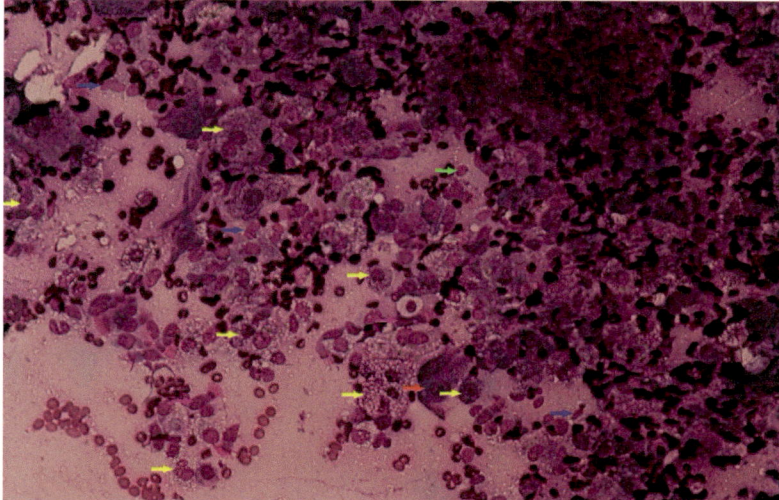

Fig. 5.12 Reactive lymphocytes (yellow arrow)

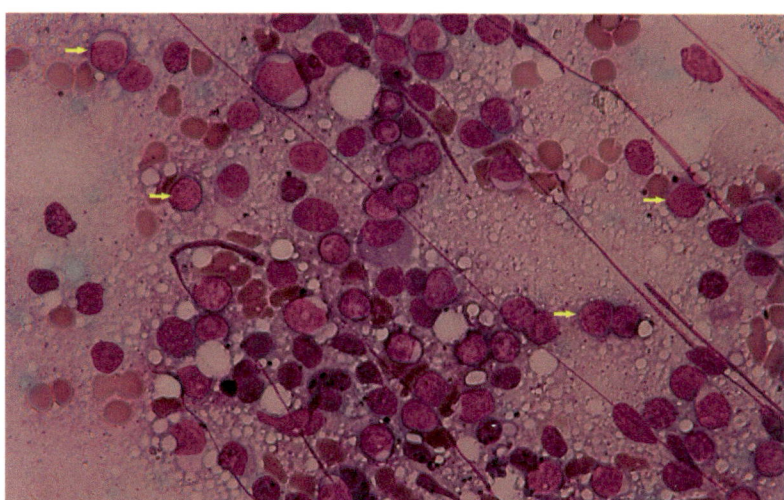

Fig. 5.13 Reactive lymphocytes (yellow arrow), plasmocytes (red arrow), and degeneration, denaturation, and necrosis from some lymphocytes (green arrow)

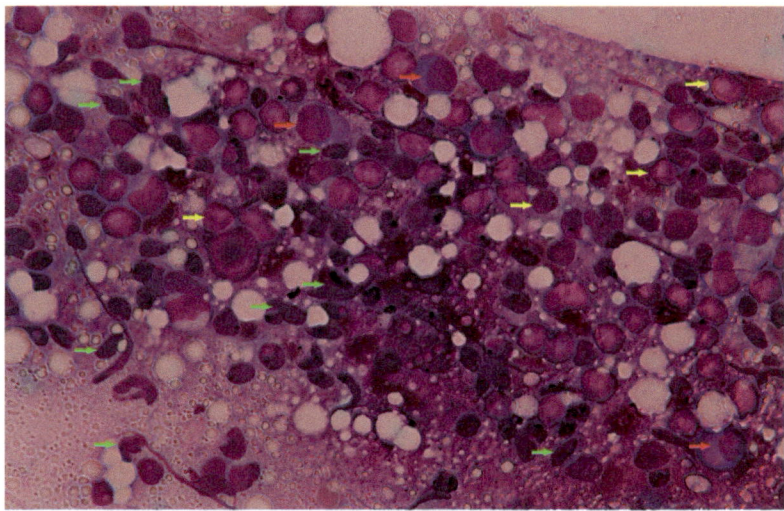

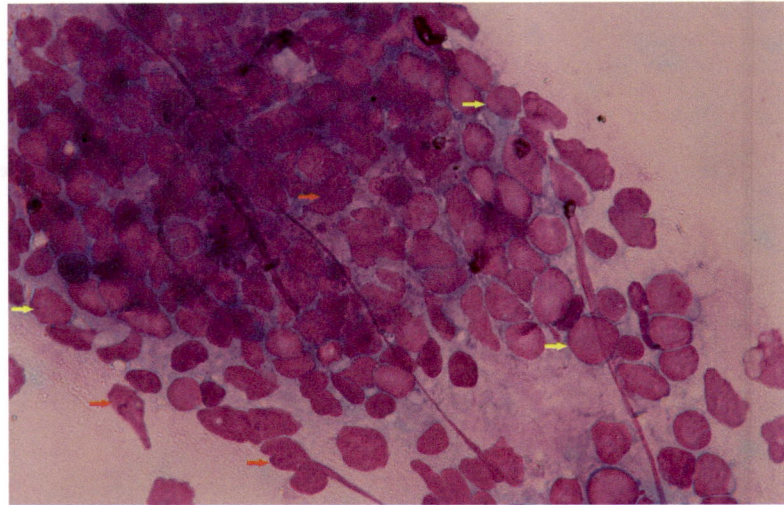

Fig. 5.14 Reactive lymphocytes (yellow arrow) and degeneration, denaturation, and necrosis from some lymphocytes (red arrow)

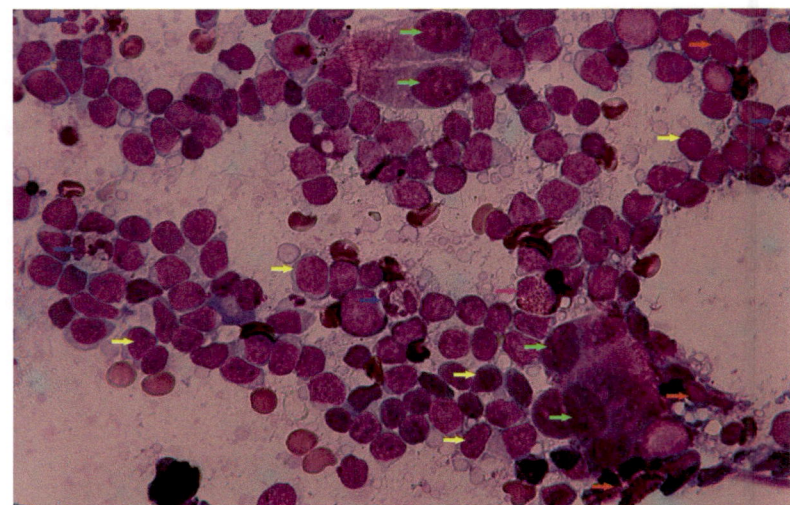

Fig. 5.15 Reactive lymphocytes (yellow arrow); degeneration, denaturation, and necrosis from some lymphocytes (red arrow); ciliated columnar epithelial cells (green arrow); scattered neutrophils (blue arrow); and scattered eosinophils (pink arrow)

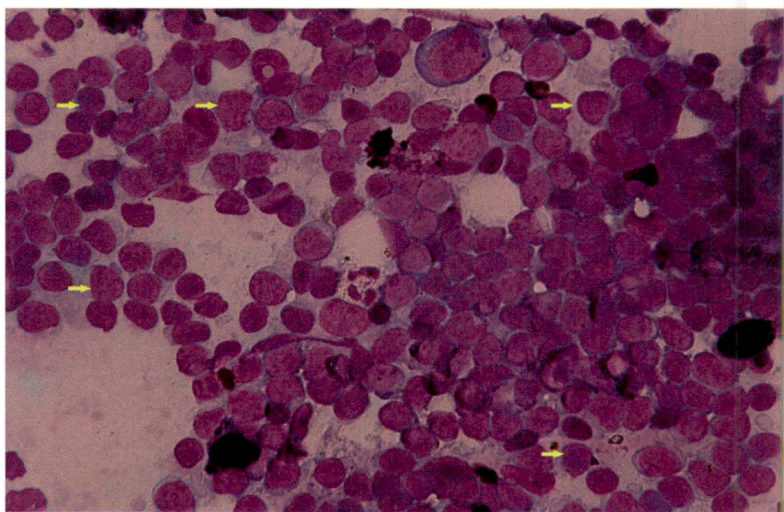

Fig. 5.16 Reactive lymphocytes (yellow arrow)

Fig. 5.17   Reactive lymphocytes (yellow arrow) and active hyperplasia and lymphocyte mitotic figure (red arrow)

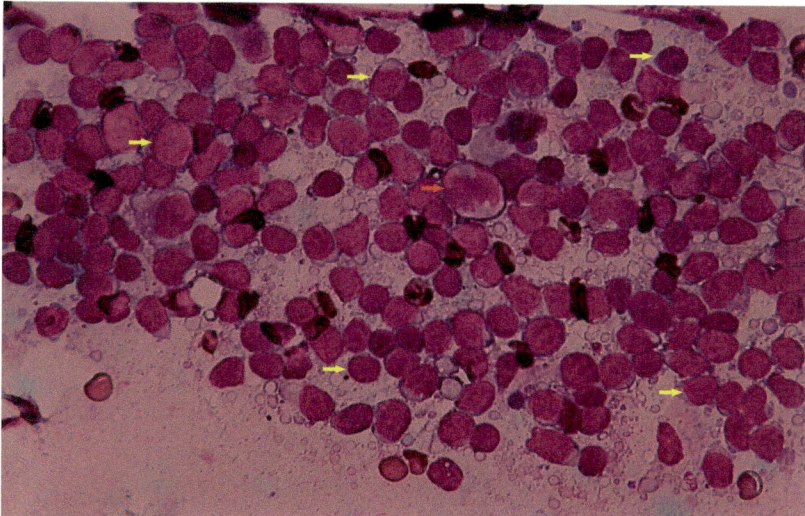

Fig. 5.18   (**a–c**) Reactive lymphocytes (yellow arrow) and degeneration, denaturation, and necrosis from some lymphocytes (red arrow)

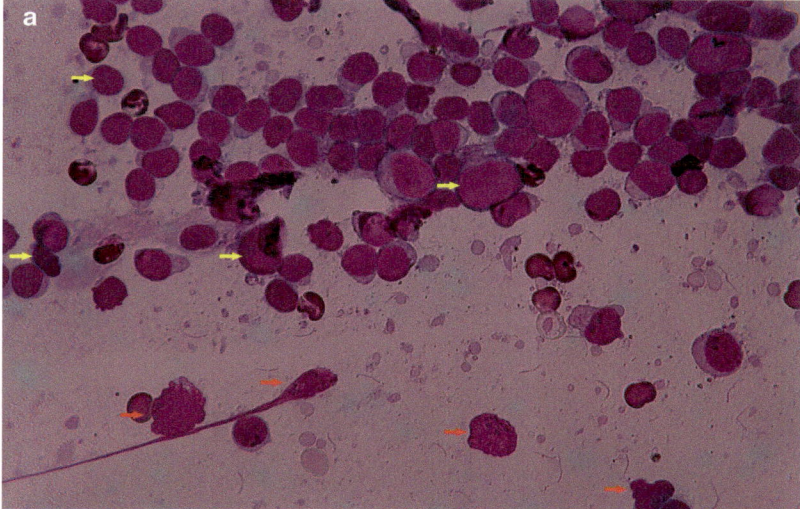

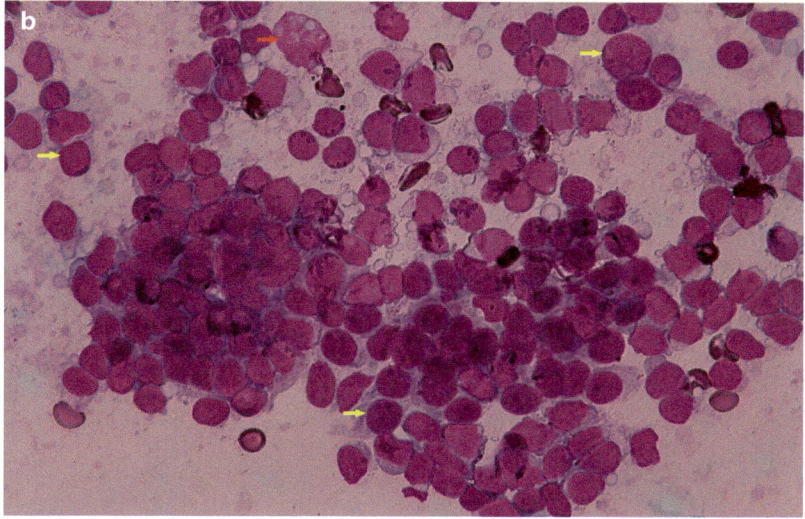

Fig. 5.18 (continued)

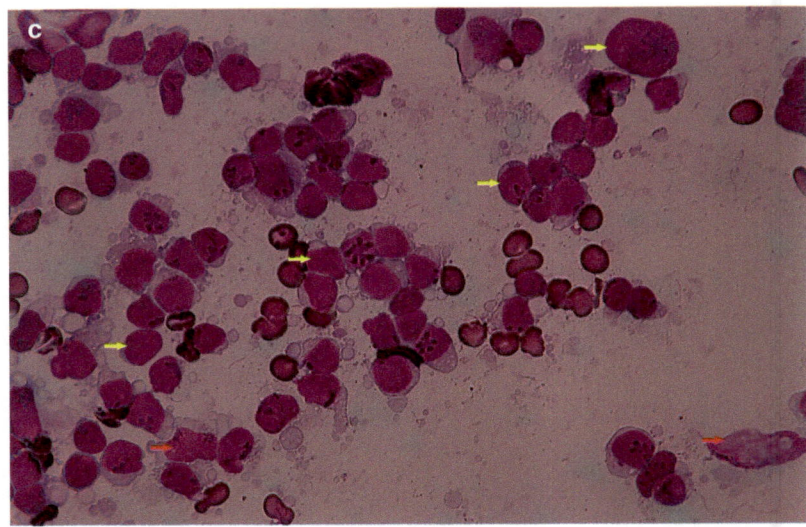

Fig. 5.19 (a, b)
Reactive lymphocytes
(yellow arrow);
degeneration,
denaturation, and
necrosis from some
lymphocytes (red
arrow); and ciliated
columnar epithelial cells
(green arrow)

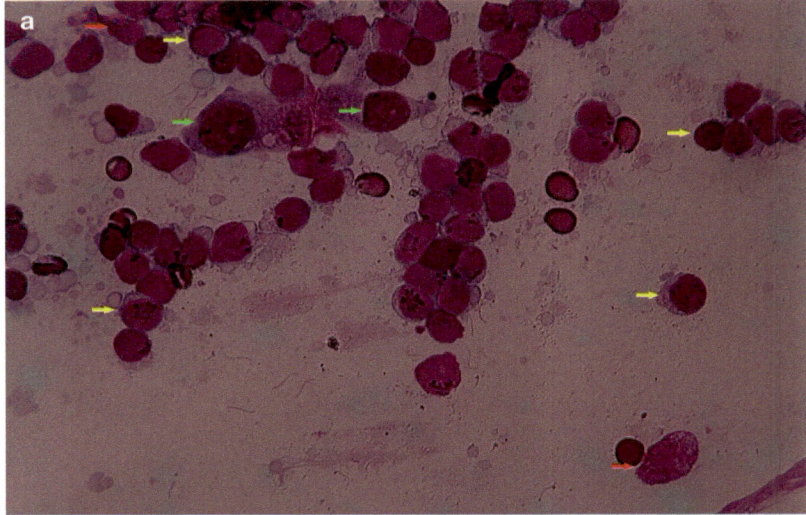

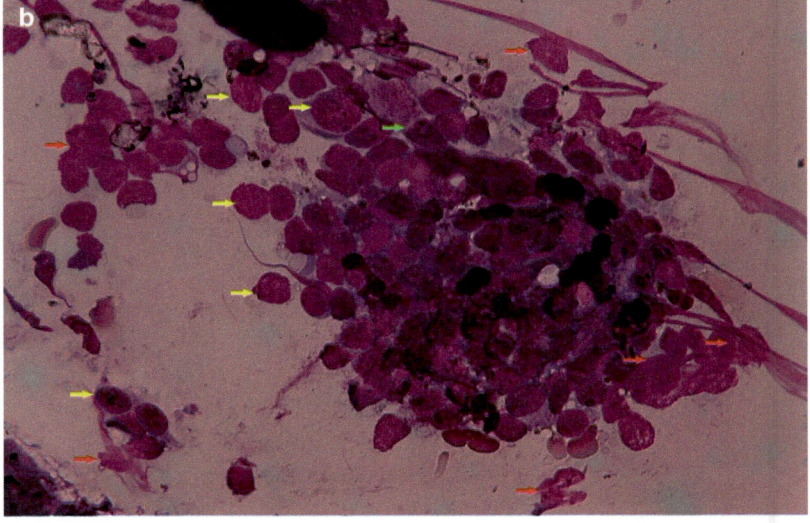

Fig. 5.20 Reactive lymphocytes (yellow arrow); degeneration, denaturation, and necrosis from some lymphocytes (red arrow); and scattered neutrophils (green arrow)

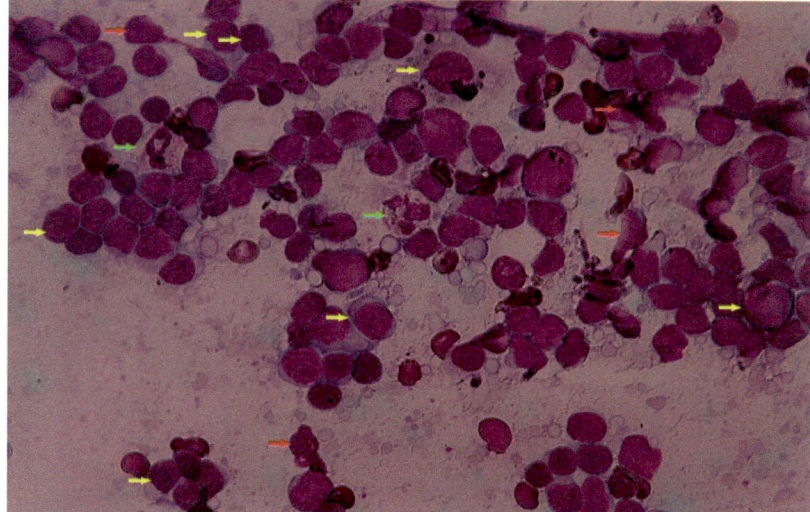

Fig. 5.21 (**a–c**) Ciliated columnar epithelial cells (yellow arrow) and goblet cells (red arrows) suggesting mucus hypersecretion

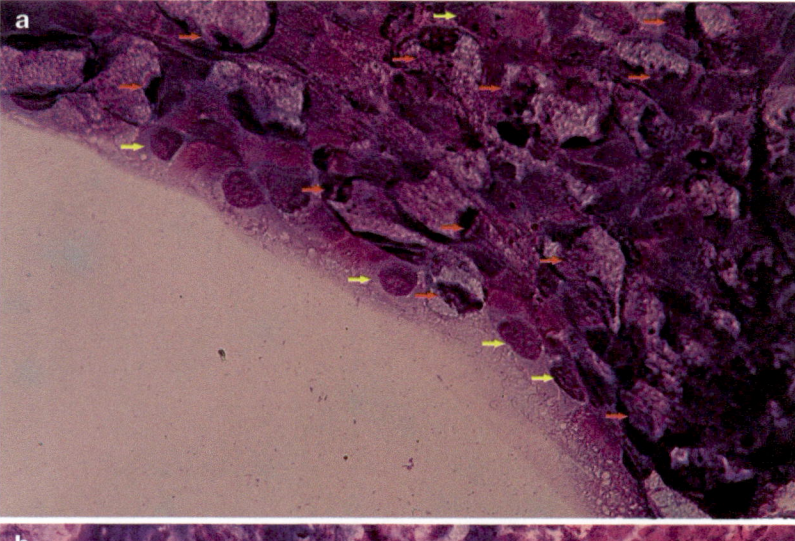

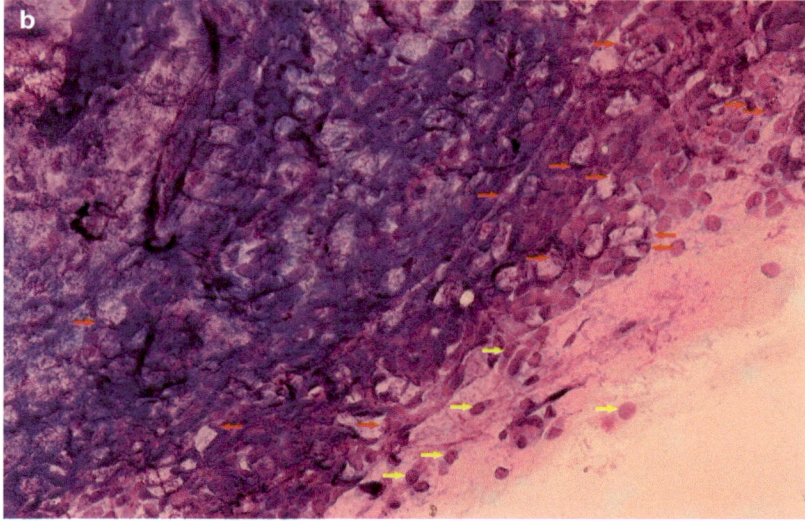

Fig. 5.21 (continued)

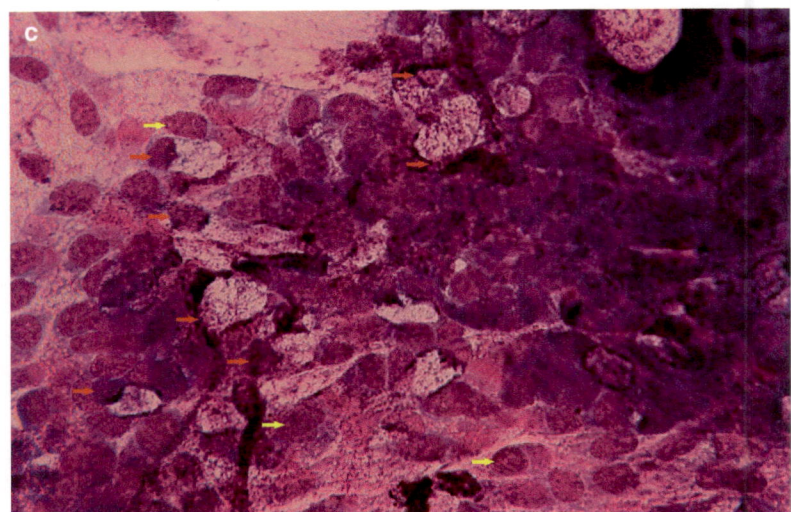

Fig. 5.22 Distal airway
epithelial cell
hyperplasia (yellow
arrow) and necrosis
from epithelial cells (red
arrow)

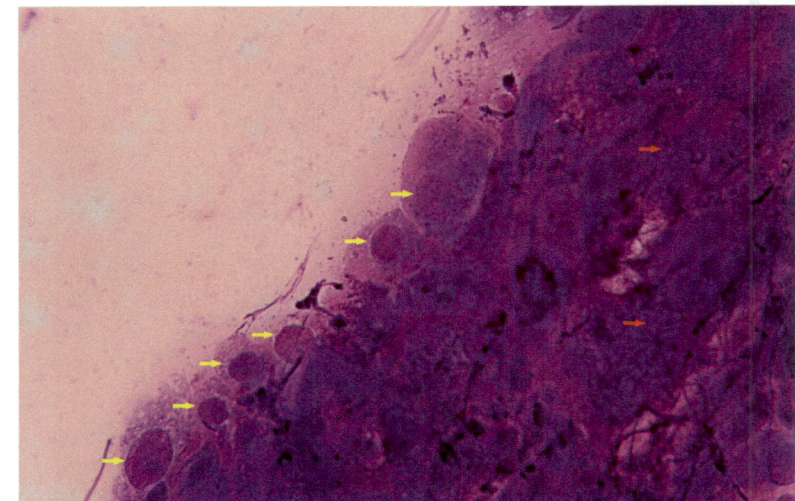

Fig. 5.23 Ciliated
columnar epithelial cells
(yellow arrow), goblet
cells (red arrow), and
hyperplasia and
degeneration of the
distal airway epithelial
cells (green arrow)

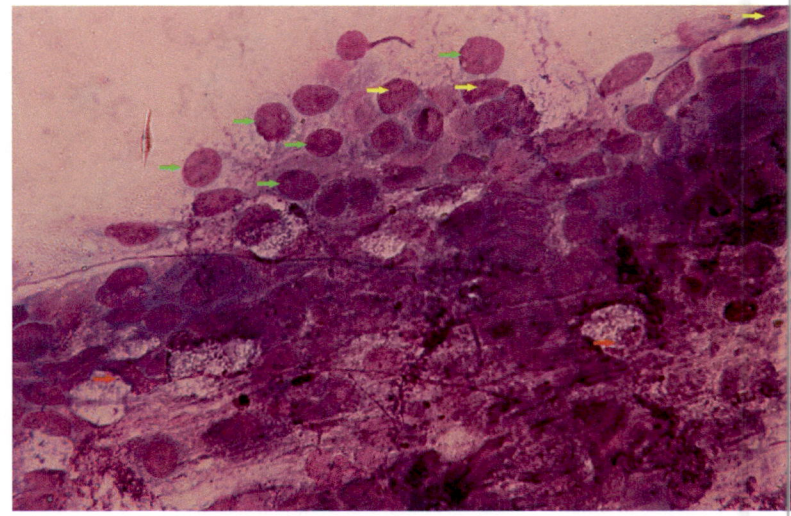

Fig. 5.24 Ciliated columnar epithelial cells (yellow arrow), goblet cells (red arrow), and denaturation and degeneration of the distal airway epithelial cells (green arrow)

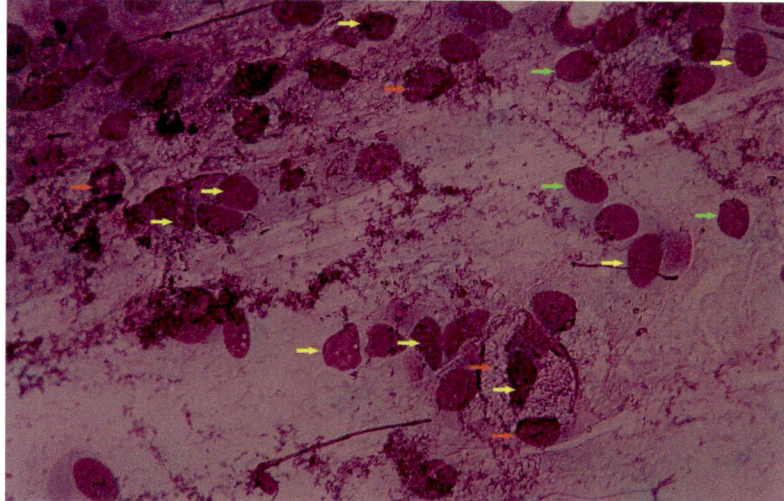

Fig. 5.25 Ciliated columnar epithelial cells (yellow arrow), goblet cells (red arrow), and hyperplasia, degeneration, denaturation, and necrosis of distal airway epithelial cells (green arrow)

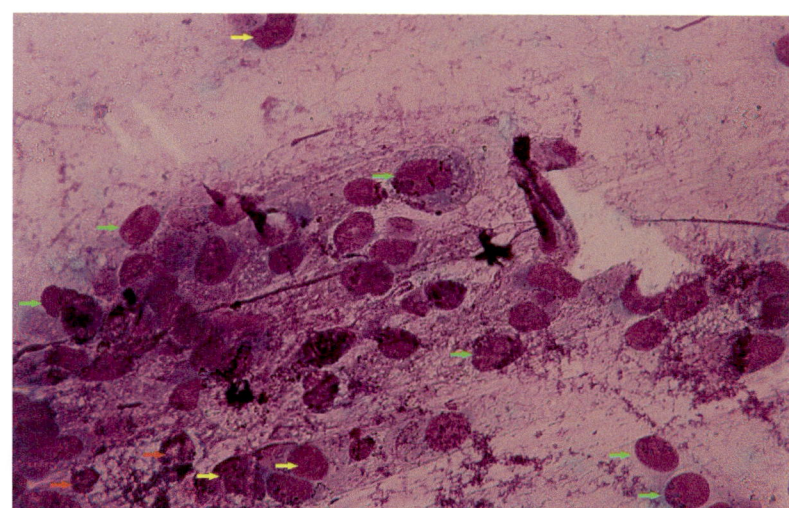

Fig. 5.26 Ciliated columnar epithelial cells (yellow arrow) and hyperplasia, degeneration, denaturation, and necrosis of distal airway epithelial cells (red arrow)

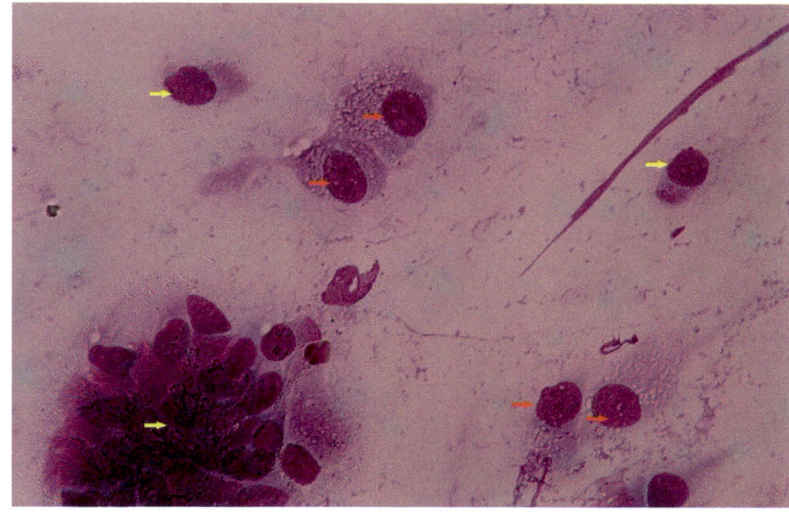

Fig. 5.27 Ciliated columnar epithelial cells (yellow arrow), distal airway epithelial cells (red arrow), fusion of macrophages (green arrow), and hyperplasia of type II alveolar epithelial cells (blue arrow)

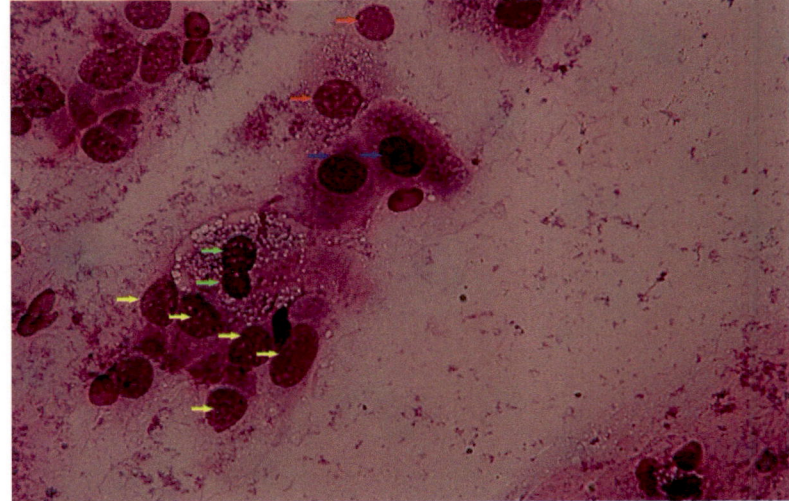

Fig. 5.28 Reactive lymphocytes (yellow arrow), plasmocytes (red arrow), and scattered neutrophils (green arrow)

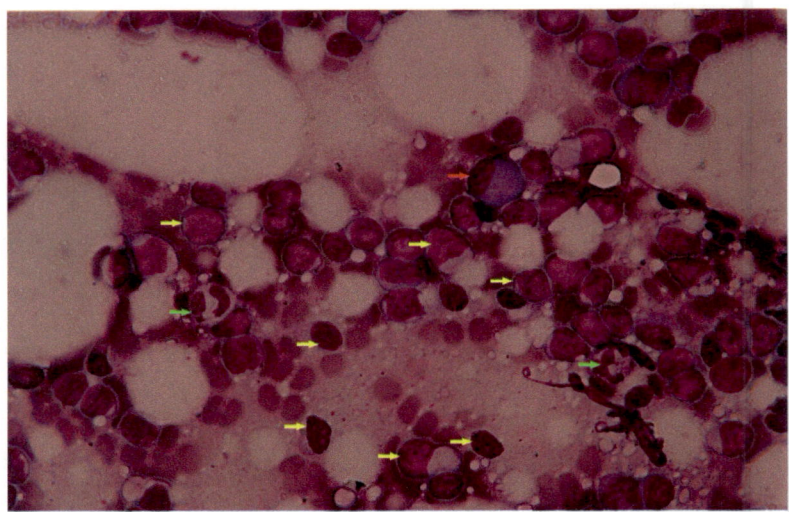

Fig. 5.29 Fibroblasts (yellow arrow) and hyperplasia, degeneration, denaturation, and necrosis of distal airway epithelial cells (red arrow)

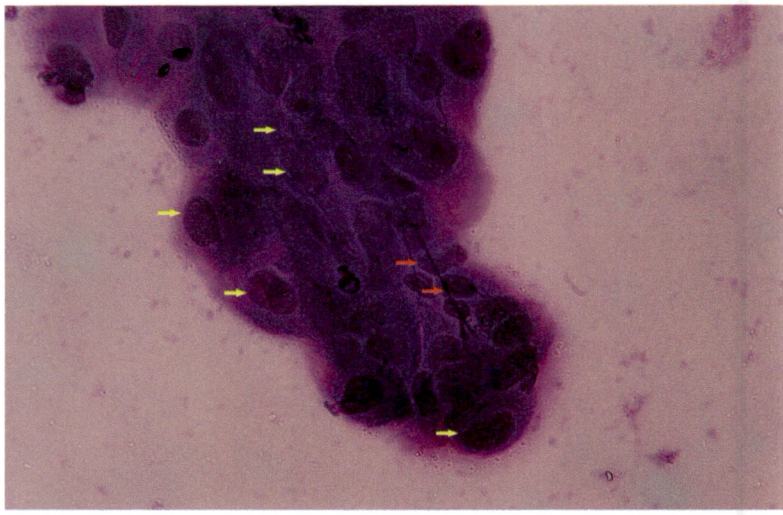

Fig. 5.30 Ciliated columnar epithelial cells (yellow arrow), brush cells (red arrow), and hyperplasia, degeneration, denaturation, and necrosis of distal airway epithelial cells

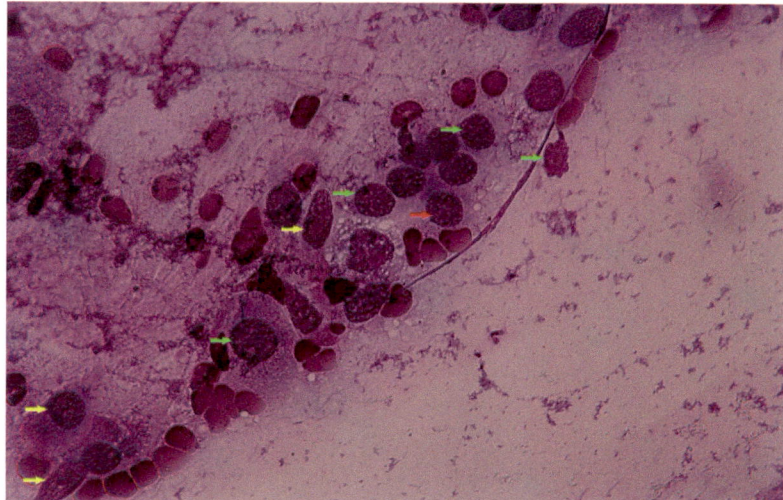

Fig. 5.31 Fusion of macrophages (yellow arrow), macrophages (red arrow), hyperplastic type II alveolar epithelial cells (green arrow), and hyperplasia, degeneration, denaturation, and necrosis of distal airway epithelial cells (blue arrow)

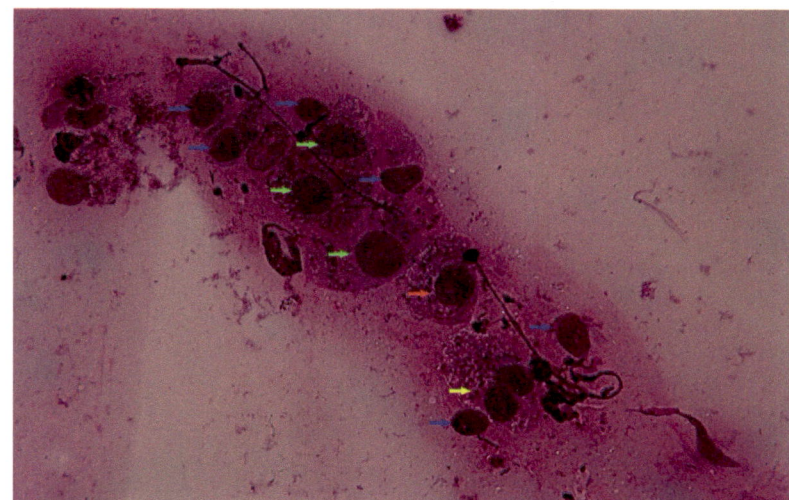

Fig. 5.32 Hyperplasia, degeneration, denaturation, and necrosis of distal airway epithelial cells (yellow arrow) and brush cells (red arrow)

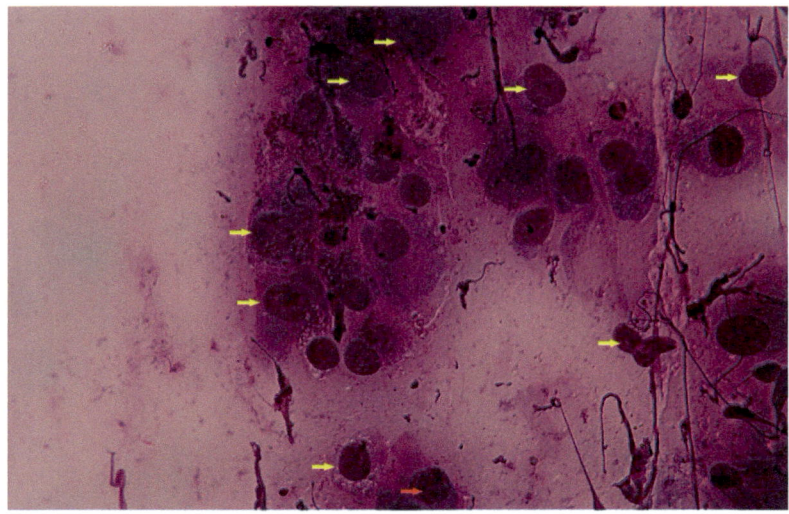

Fig. 5.33 Histiocytes (yellow arrow) and epithelioid cells (red arrow), a tendency to form atypical granulomas

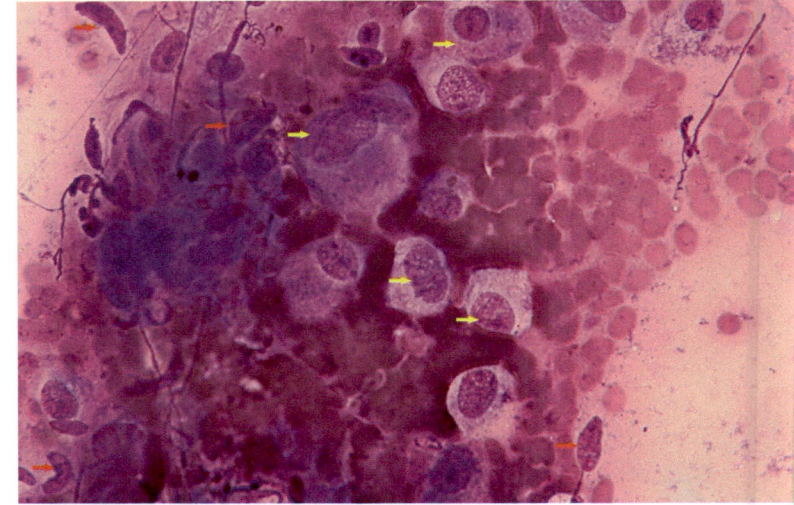

Fig. 5.34 Macrophages, some transforming into histiocytes (yellow arrow), cytoplasmic fusion from macrophages (red arrow), type II alveolar epithelial cell hyperplasia (green arrow), fusiform fibroblasts (blue arrow), distal airway epithelial cells (pink arrow), and degeneration and necrosis from epithelial cells

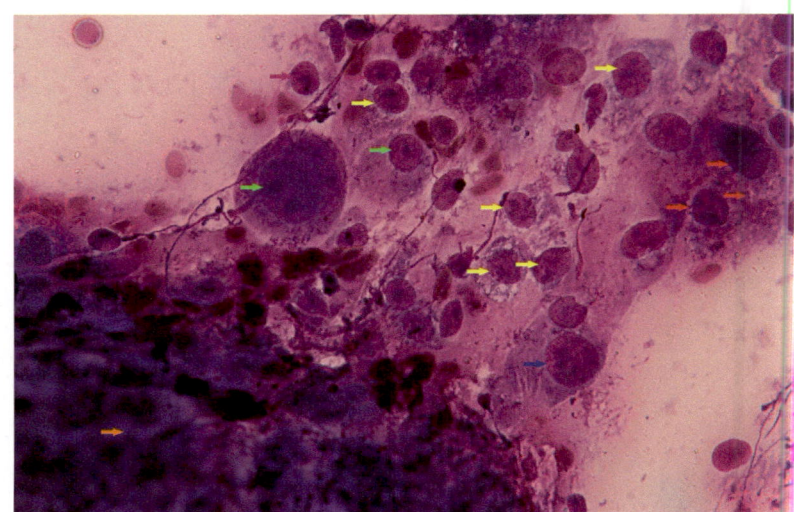

Fig. 5.35 Ciliated columnar epithelial cells (yellow arrow), macrophages (red arrow), and degeneration and necrosis from some epithelial cells (green arrow)

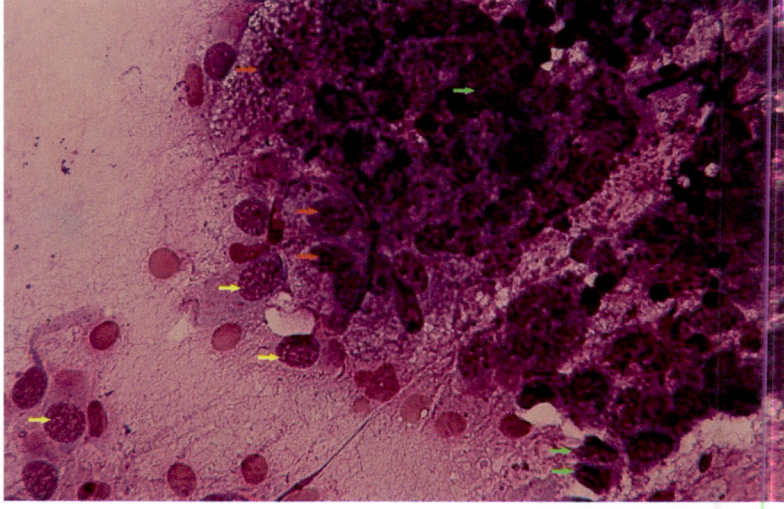

Fig. 5.36 Aggregation of foamy macrophages (yellow arrow) surrounded by amorphous necrosis (red arrow)

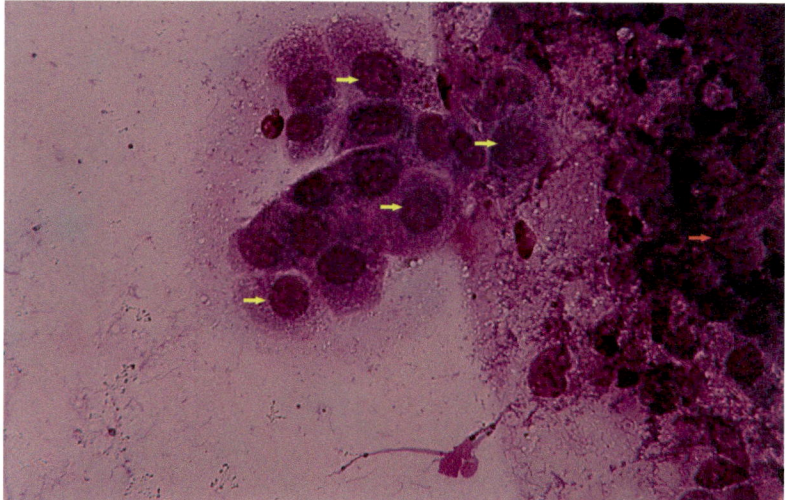

Fig. 5.37 Aggregation of foamy macrophages (yellow arrow), brush cells (red arrow), and distal airway epithelial cells (green arrow)

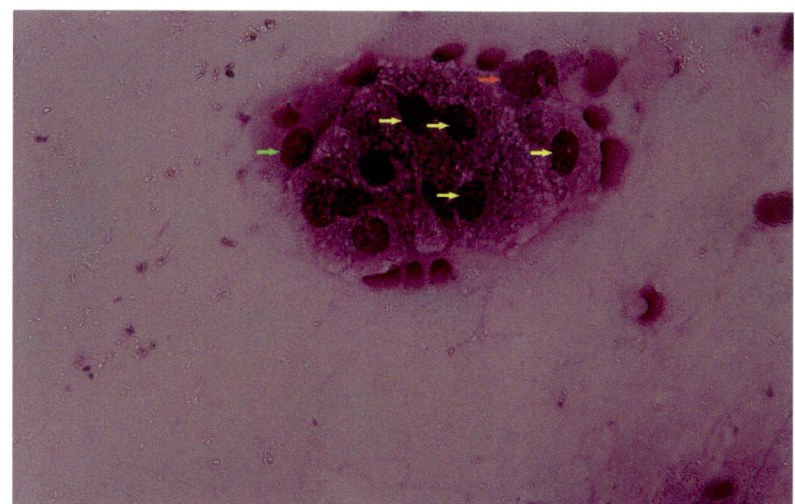

Fig. 5.38 Amorphous necrosis and exudation, neutrophils (yellow arrow), and distal airway epithelial cells (red arrow)

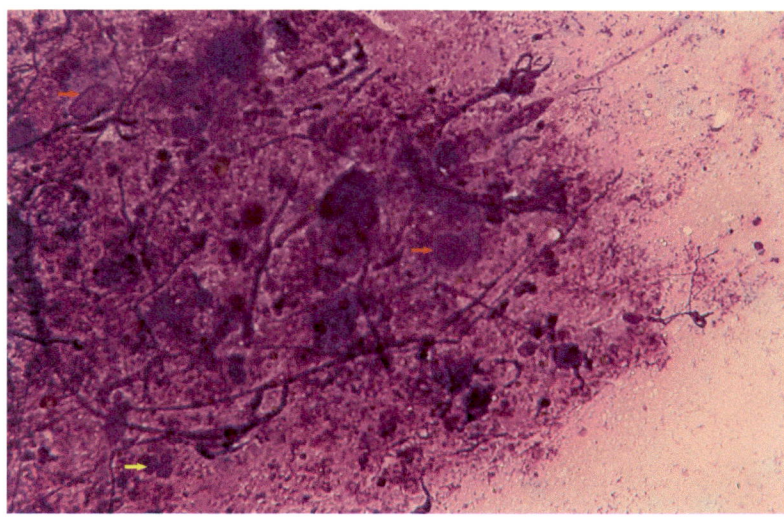

Fig. 5.39 Amorphous
necrosis; degeneration,
denaturation, and
necrosis of epithelial
cells (yellow arrow); and
degeneration of distal
airway epithelial cells
(red arrow)

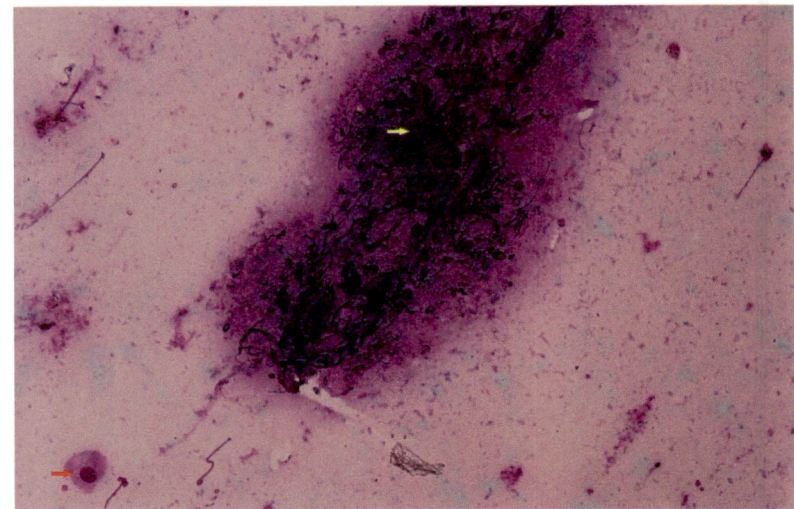

Fig. 5.40 Amorphous
necrosis and
degeneration,
denaturation, and
necrosis of epithelial
cells (yellow arrow)

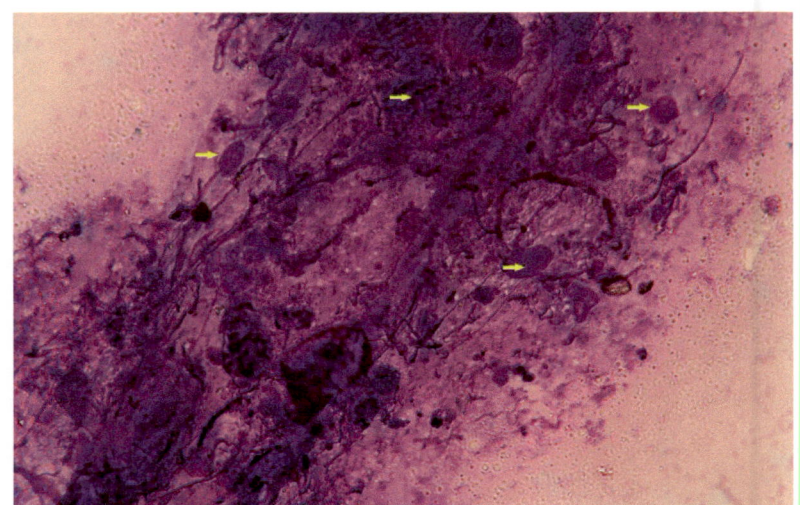

Fig. 5.41 Brush cells
(yellow arrow) and
hyperplasia,
degeneration,
denaturation, and
necrosis of distal airway
epithelial cells (red
arrow)

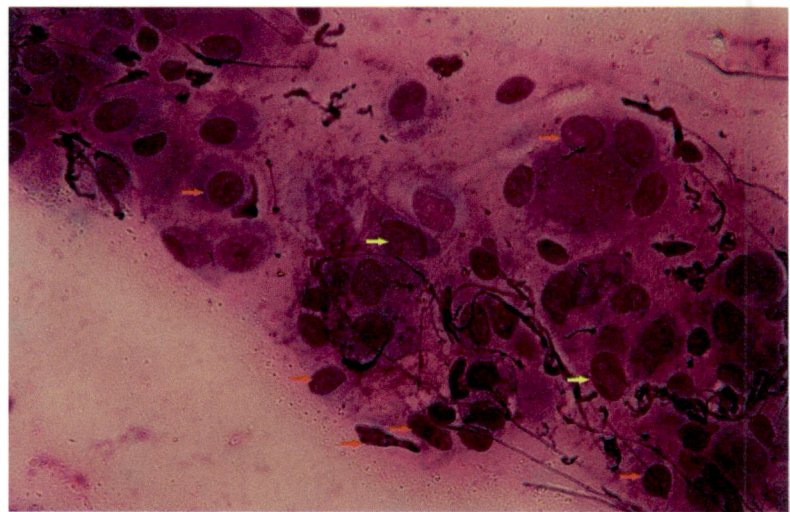

Fig. 5.42 Macrophages, some transforming into histiocytes (yellow arrow), and hyperplasia, degeneration, denaturation, and necrosis of distal airway epithelial cells (red arrow)

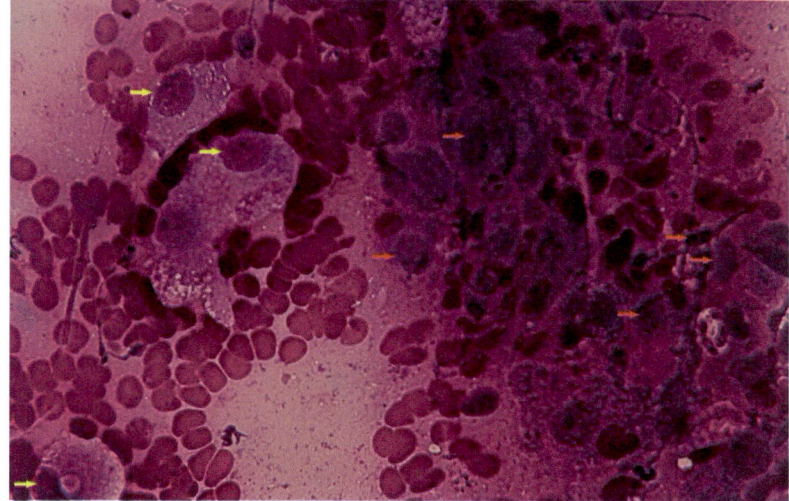

Fig. 5.43 Macrophages, some transforming into histiocytes (yellow arrow); hyperplasia, degeneration, denaturation, and necrosis of distal airway epithelial cells (red arrow), scattered neutrophils (green arrow)

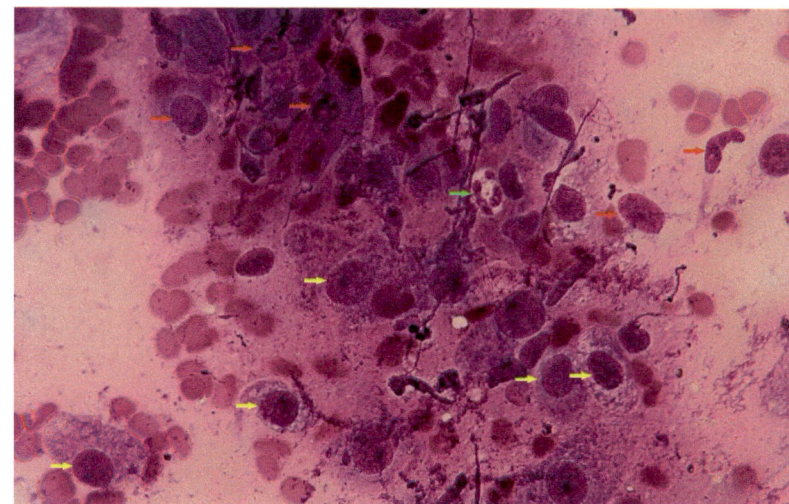

Fig. 5.44 Macrophages, some transforming into histiocytes (yellow arrow); hyperplasia, degeneration, denaturation, and necrosis of distal airway epithelial cells (red arrow); and type II alveolar epithelial cell hyperplasia (green arrow)

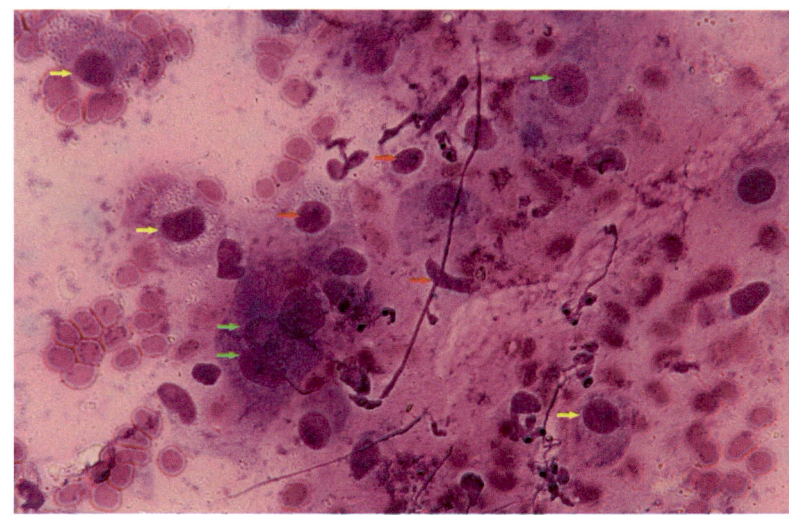

Fig. 5.45 Macrophages, some transforming into histiocytes (yellow arrow), some further evolving into epithelioid cells (red arrows), and scattered neutrophils (green arrow)

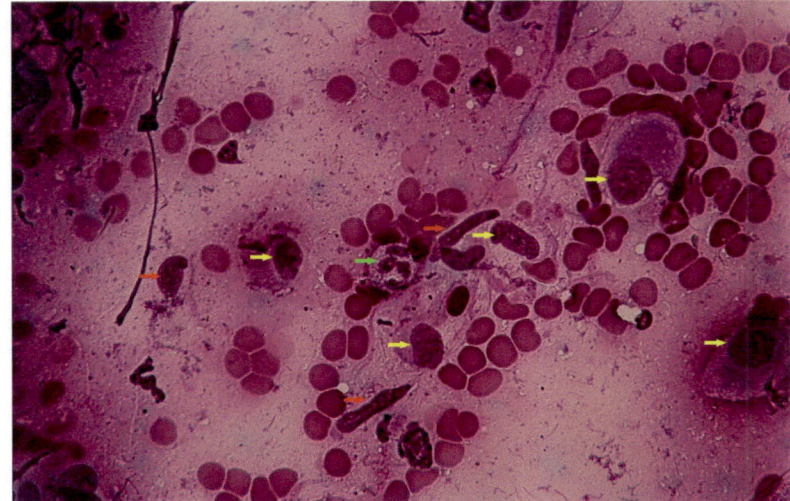

Fig. 5.46 Ciliated columnar epithelial cells (yellow arrow); hyperplasia, degeneration, denaturation, and necrosis of distal airway epithelial cells (red arrow); and fibroblasts (green arrow)

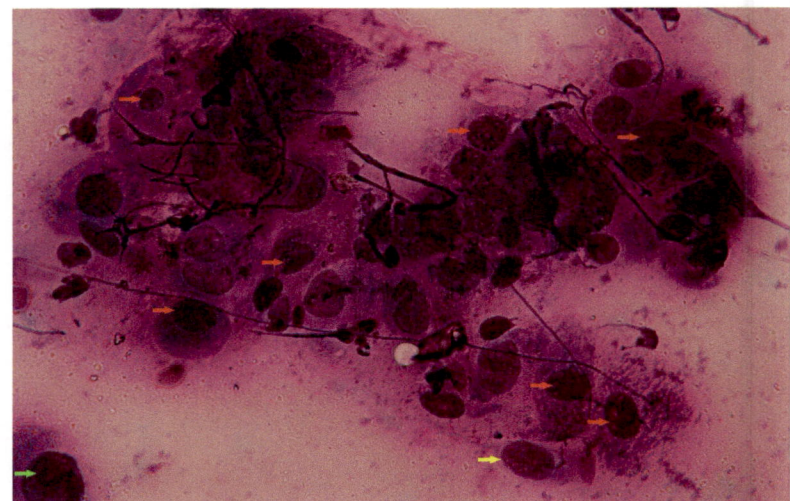

Fig. 5.47 Aggregation of foamy macrophages (yellow arrow), reactive lymphocytes (red arrow), fibroblasts (green arrow), and distal airway epithelial cells (blue arrow)

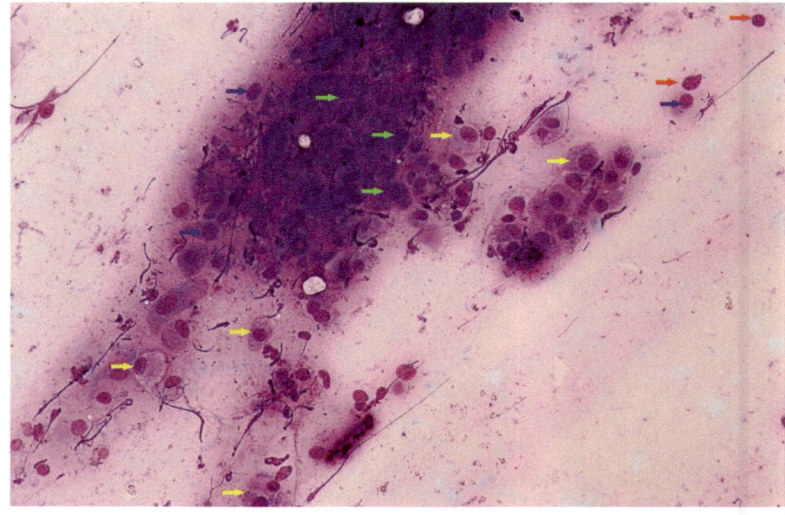

5.5   Pulmonary Involvement of ANCA-Associated Vasculitis

Brief history: Male, 66 years old, clinically diagnosed as ANCA-associated vasculitis, coughing, and dyspnea for 1 week.

Technology to obtain the target lesions: Transbronchial lung biopsy (TBLB).

The preparation of cytological slides for ROSE: Imprinting (rolling).

Fig. 5.48 (a, b) Subpleural interstitial thickening and extensive ground-glass opacities in both lungs

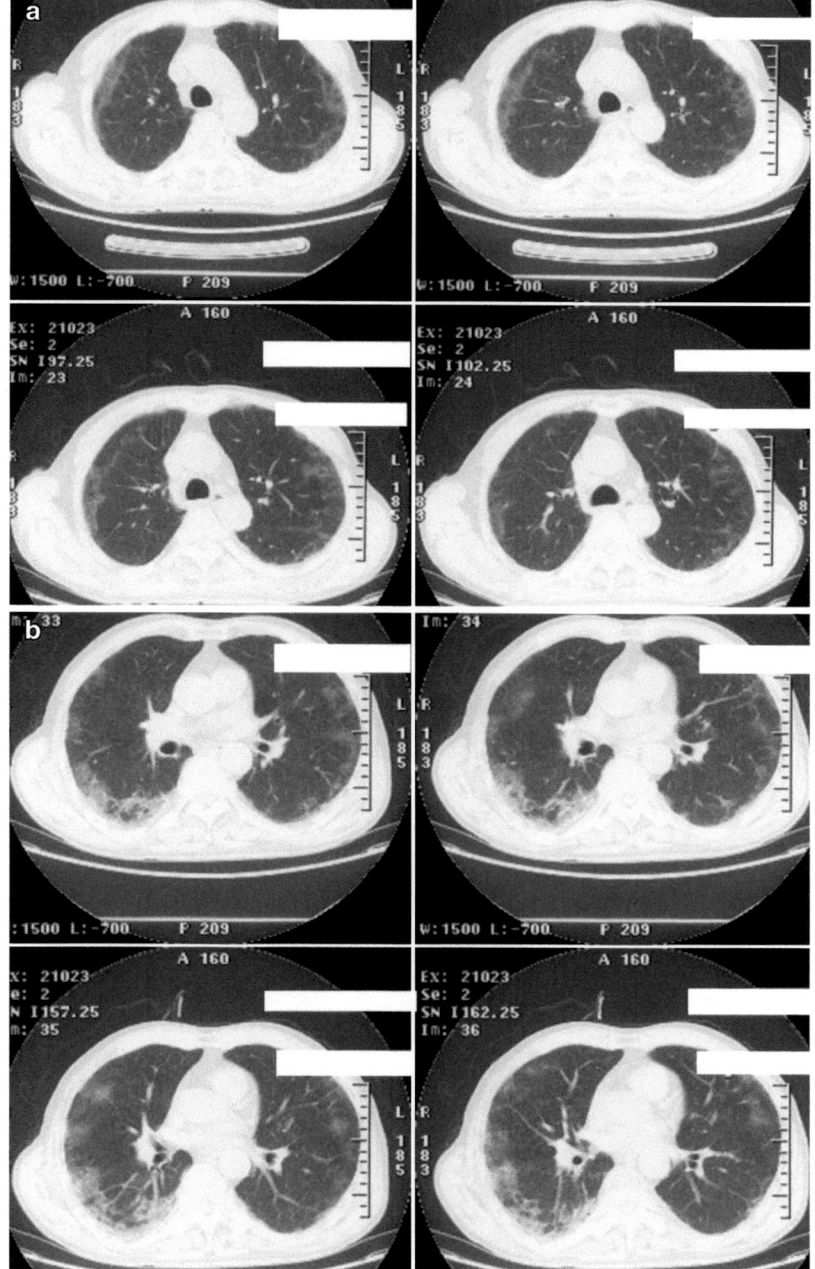

Fig. 5.49 (a–h)
Annotated at the figure
(yellow arrow)

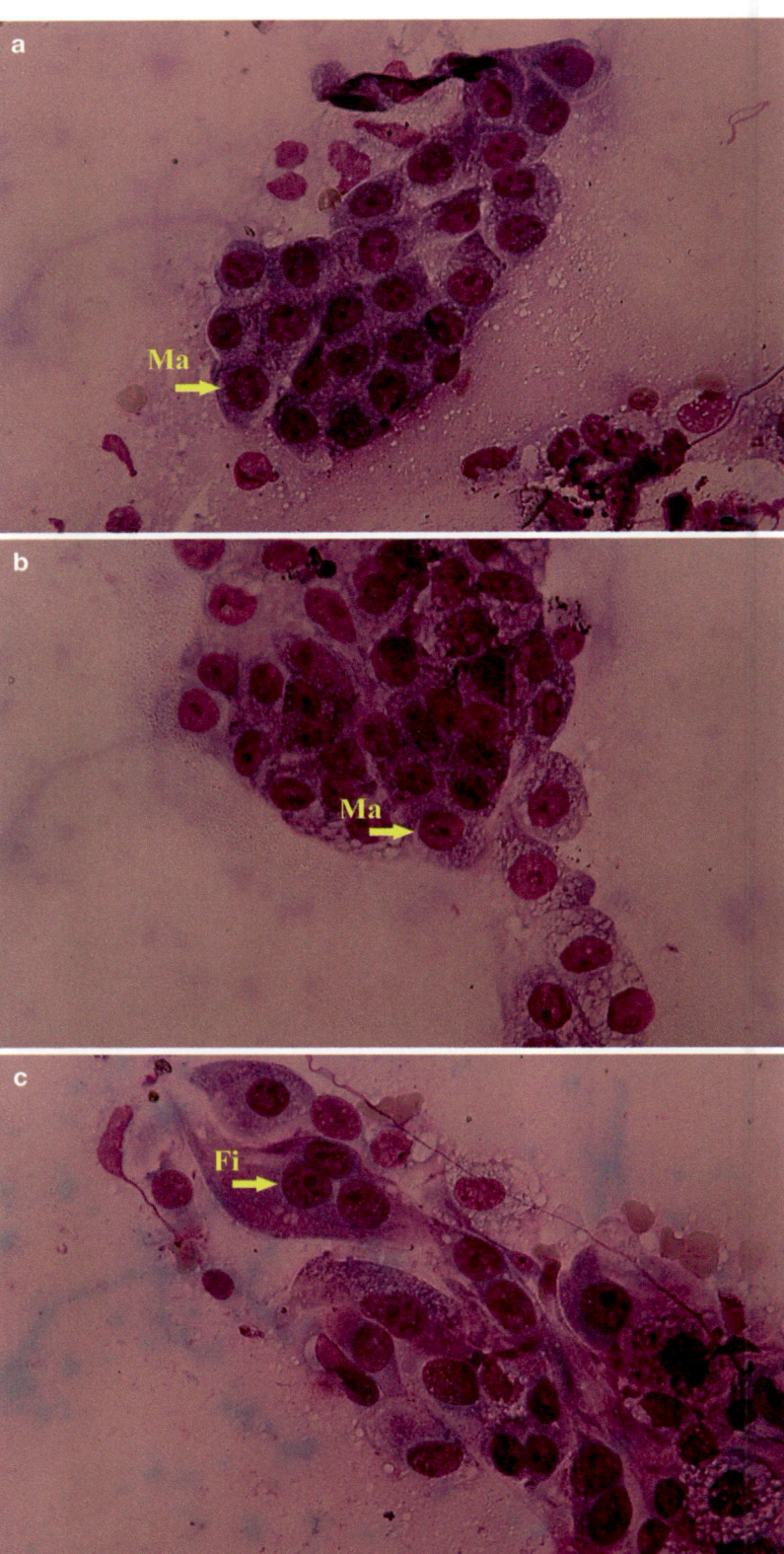

Fig. 5.49   (continued)

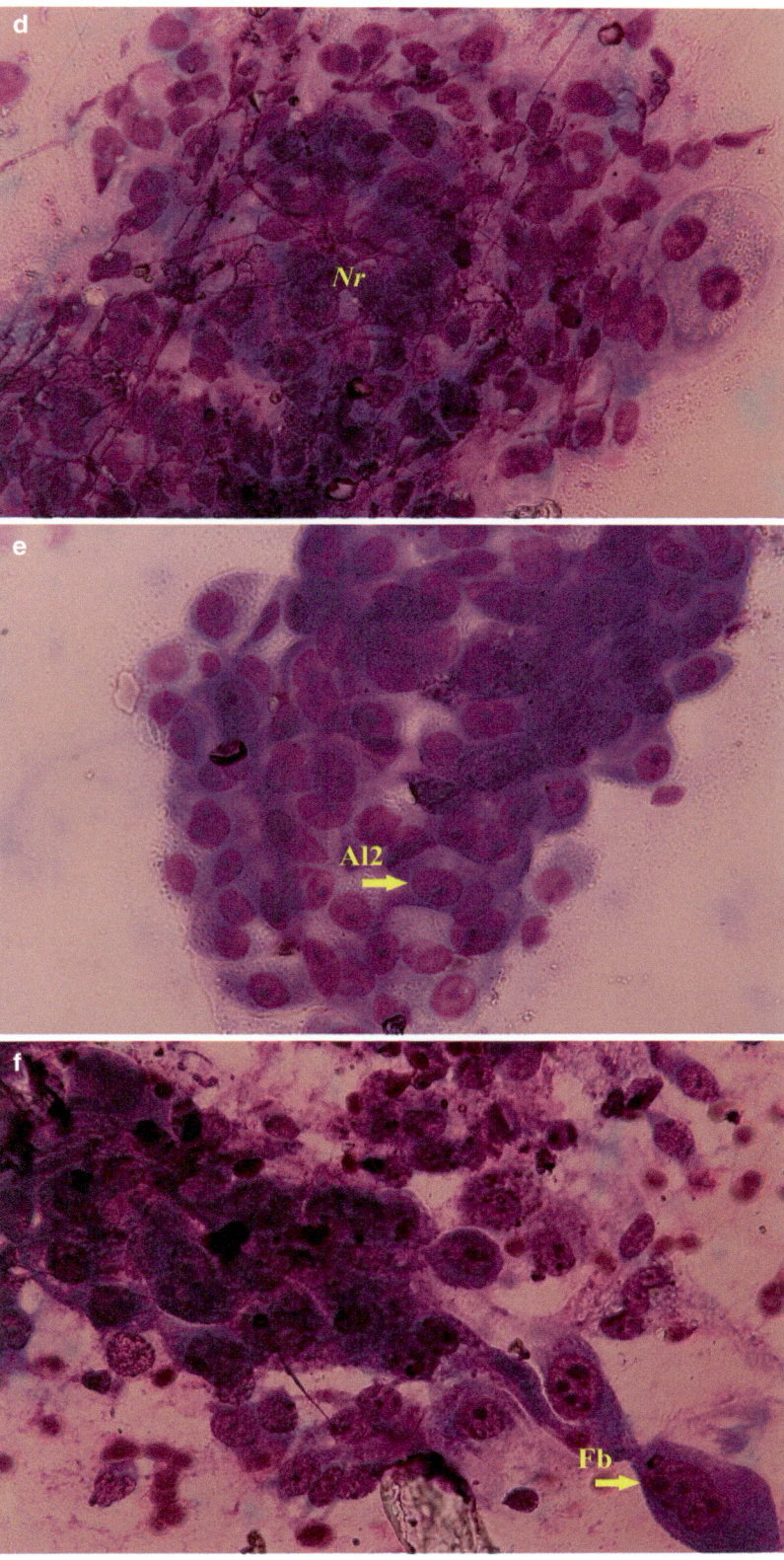

Fig. 5.49 (continued)

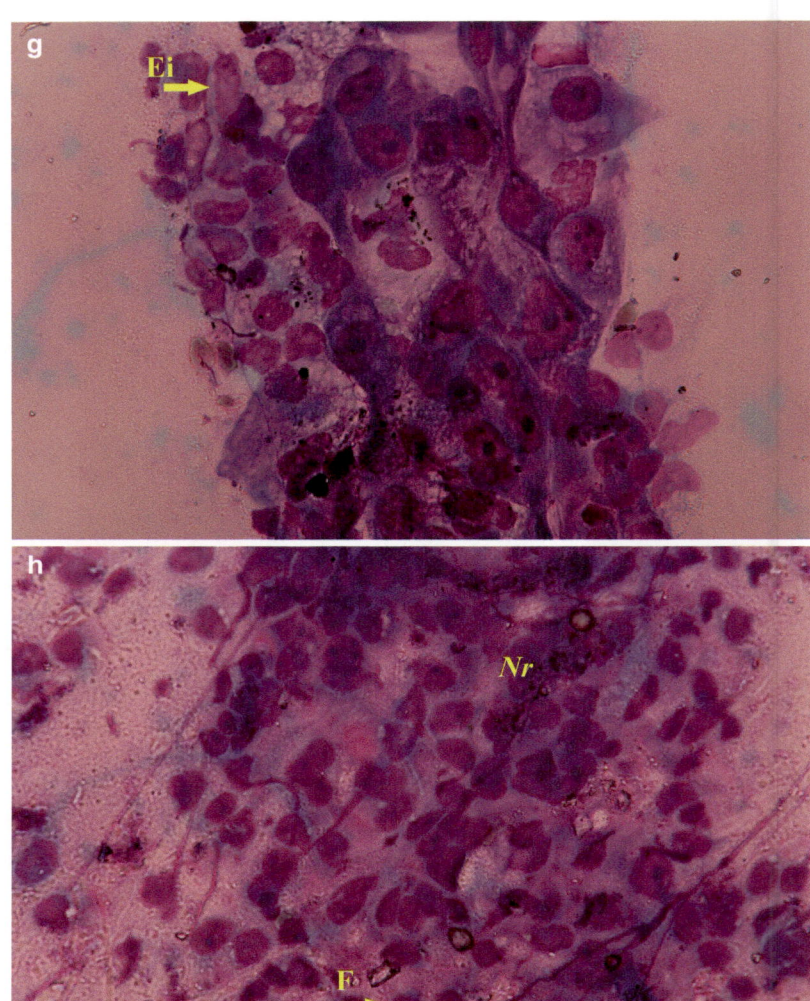

5.6   Pulmonary Involvement from Vasculitis

Brief history: Clinically diagnosed as vasculitis, irritable dry coughing for 1 month.

Technology to obtain the target lesions: Transbronchial lung biopsy (TBLB).

The preparation of cytological slides for ROSE: Imprinting (rolling).

Clustering (categorizing) analysis in ROSE interpretation:

- "Inflammatory changes"
- Granulomatous inflammation.
- May conform to organization.
- Lymphocyte-based immune inflammatory response.

Fig. 5.50 (**a, b**) Subpleural lobular interstitial thickening and interstitial thickening, the lower lobes more obvious than those in the upper lobes, especially in the right side

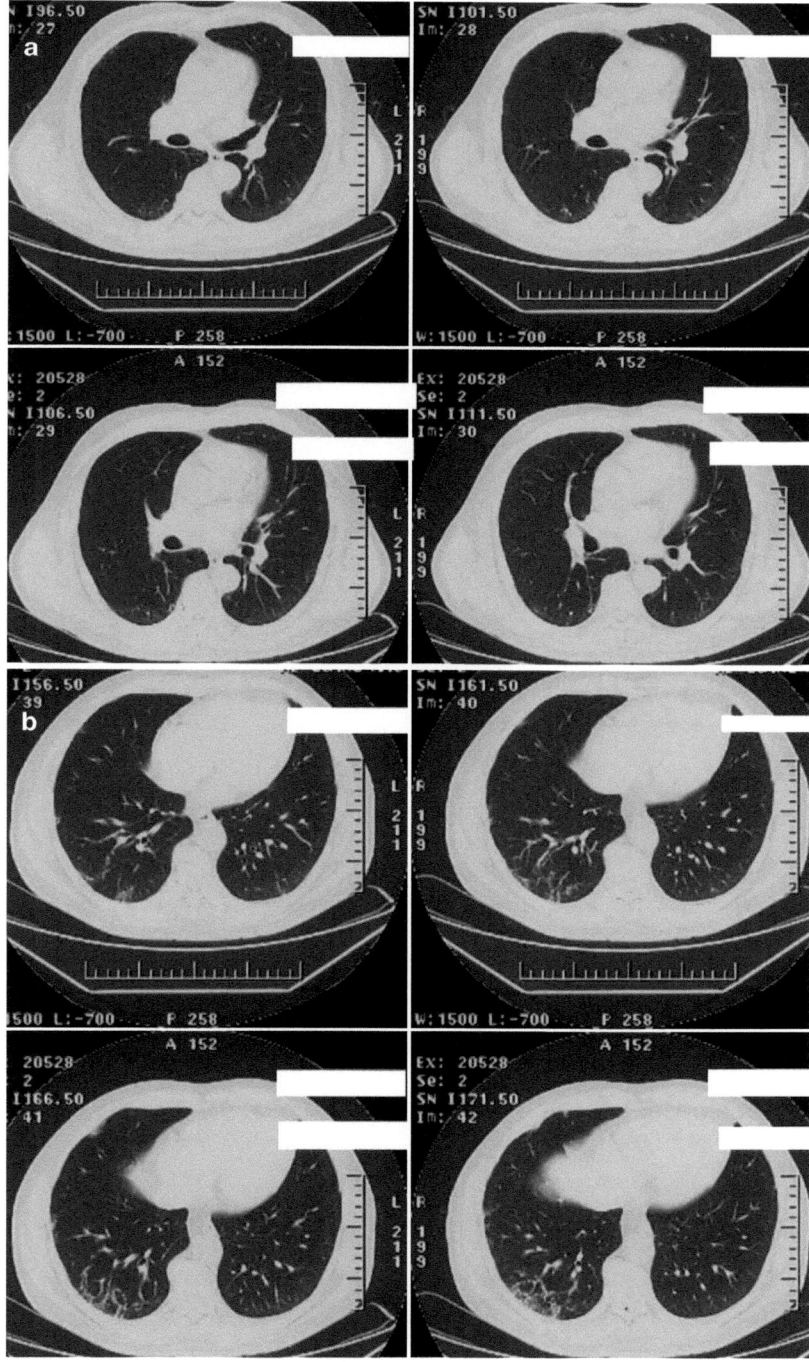

Fig. 5.51 Lots of reactive lymphocytes (yellow arrow) and nuclear filaments from necrotic cells (red arrow)

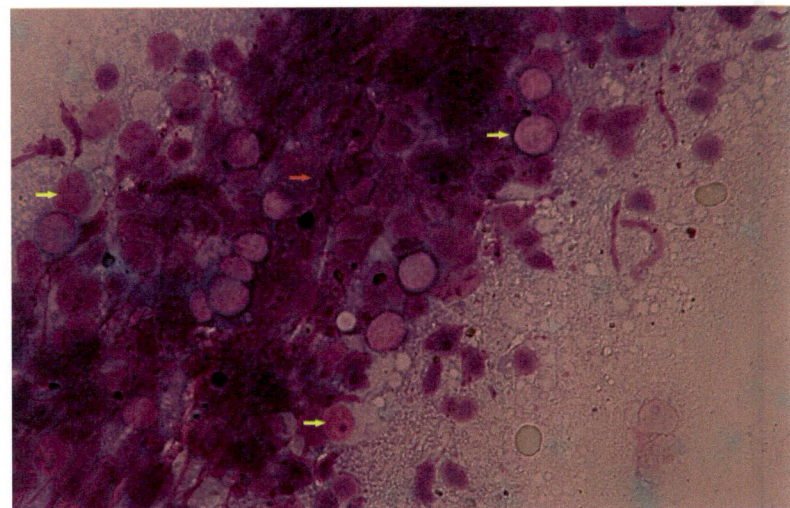

Fig. 5.52 Aggregation of macrophages, some evolving into histiocytes (yellow arrow) and lots of lymphocytes among them (red arrow)

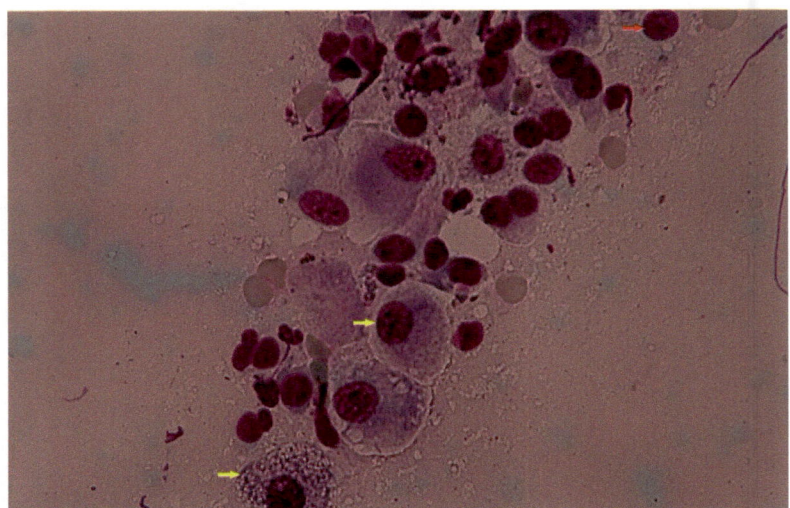

Fig. 5.53 Lots of reactive lymphocytes (yellow arrow), macrophages (red arrow), and type II alveolar epithelial cells (green arrow)

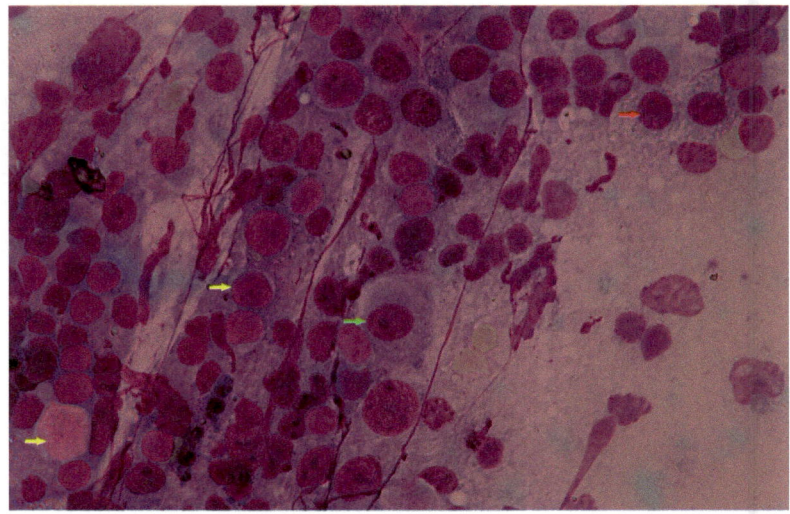

Fig. 5.54 Lots of reactive lymphocytes (yellow arrow) and distal airway epithelial cells (red arrow)

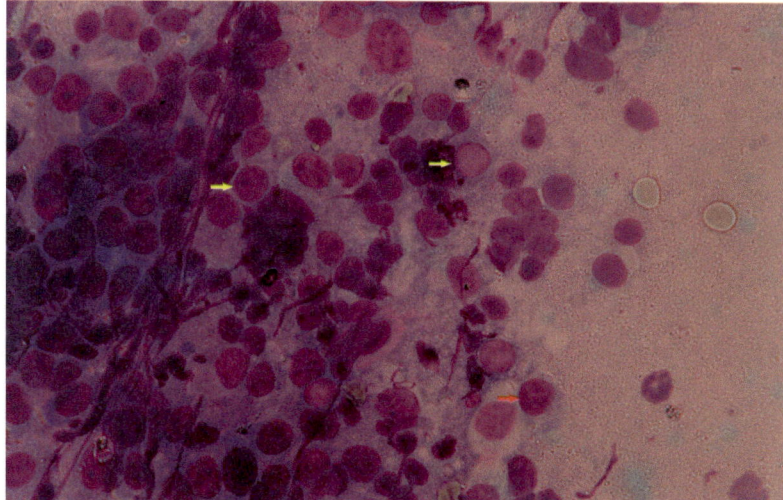

Fig. 5.55 Aggregation of macrophages, some evolving into histiocytes (yellow arrow), even epithelioid cells (red arrow), reactive lymphocytes (green arrow), and distal airway epithelial cells (blue arrow)

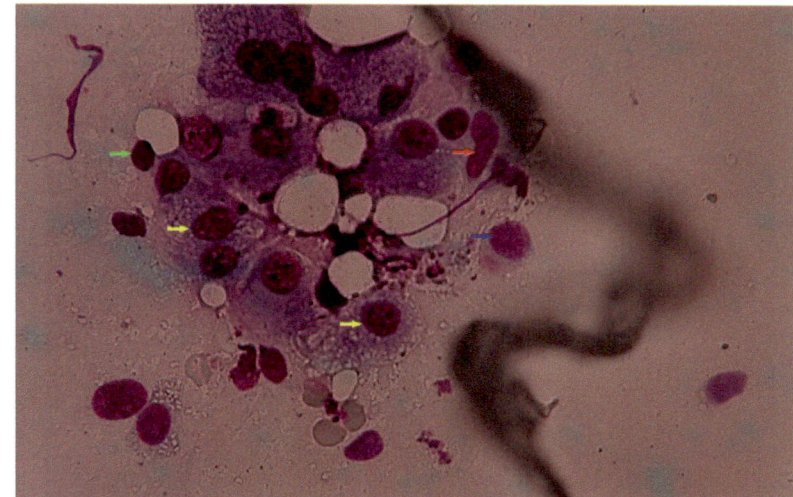

Fig. 5.56 Lots of reactive lymphocytes (yellow arrow) and aggregation of macrophages (red arrow)

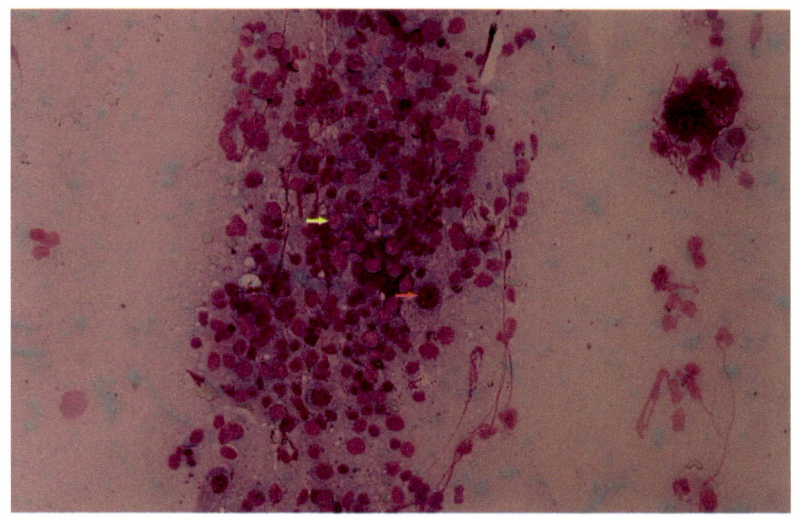

Fig. 5.57 Lots of reactive lymphocytes (yellow arrow) and nuclear filaments from necrotic cells (red arrow)

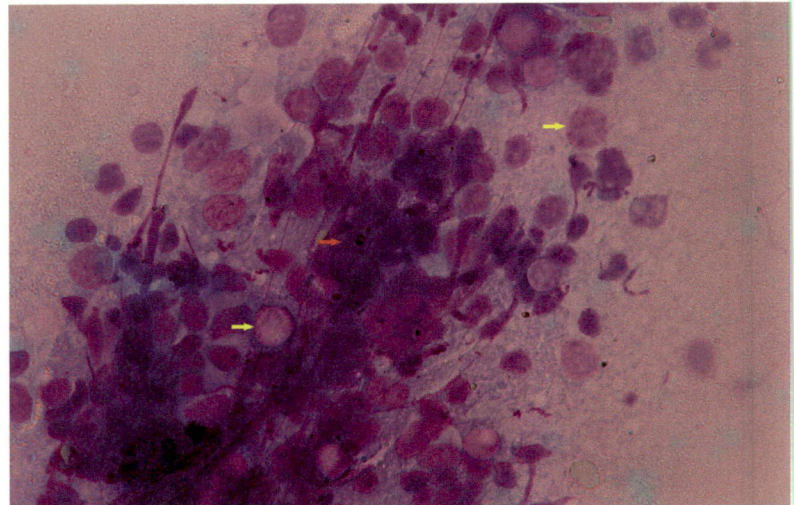

Fig. 5.58 Fibroblasts (yellow arrow) and foamy macrophages (red arrow)

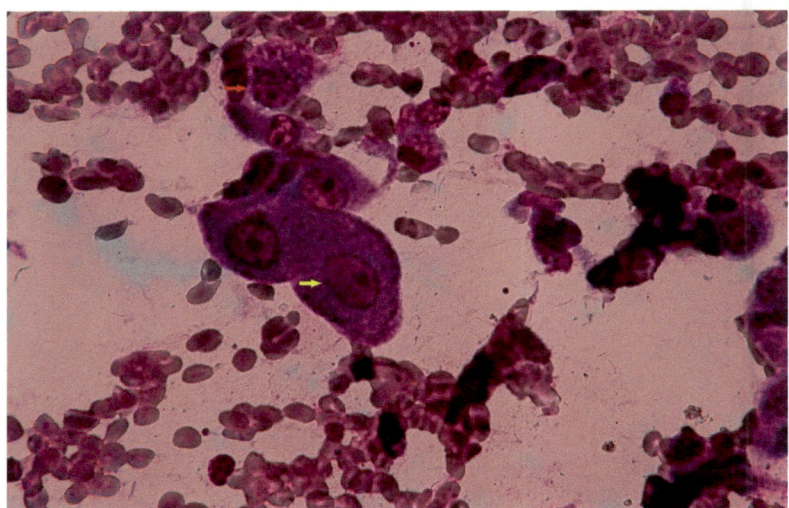

Fig. 5.59 (a, b) Aggregation of foamy macrophages (yellow arrow), some evolving into histiocytes (red arrow), and reactive lymphocytes (green arrow)

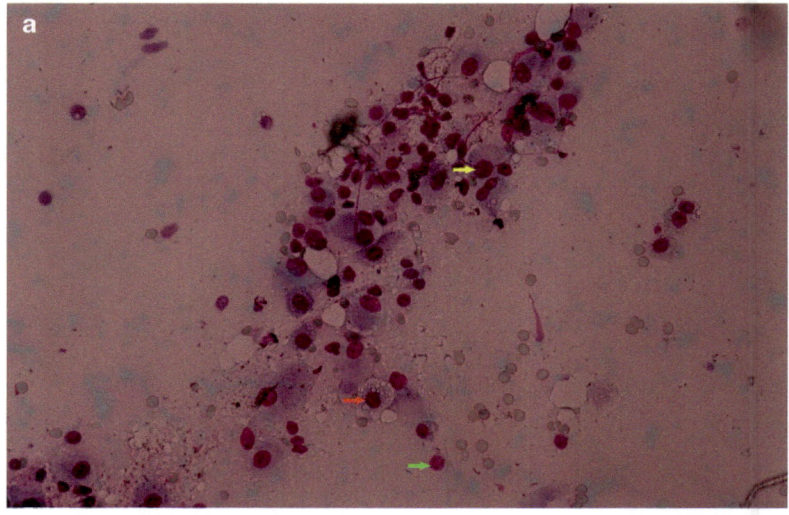

Fig. 5.59 (continued)

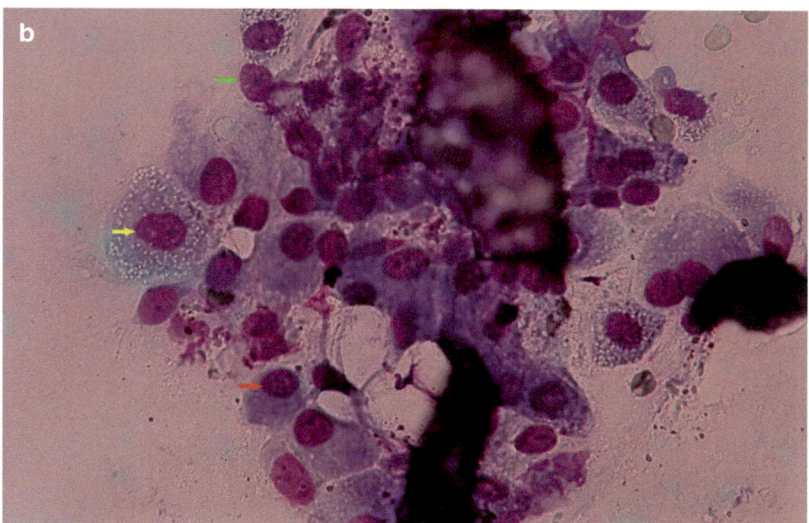

Fig. 5.60 Lots of reactive lymphocytes (yellow arrow), nuclear filaments from necrotic cells (red arrow), and aggregation of foamy macrophages (green arrow)

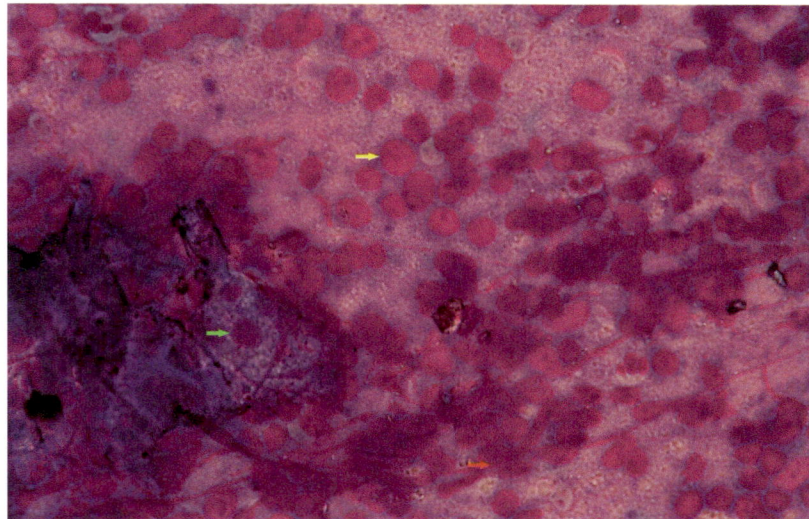

5.7   Pulmonary Involvement from Connective Tissue Disease (Vasculitis)

Brief history: Clinically diagnosed as connective tissue disease (vasculitis), coughing for more than 2 months, with obvious dyspnea.

Technology to obtain the target lesions: Transbronchial lung biopsy (TBLB).

The preparation of cytological slides for ROSE: Imprinting (rolling).

Clustering (categorizing) analysis in ROSE interpretation:

- Granulomatous inflammation.
- Lymphocyte-based immune inflammatory response.
- Necrotic "inflammatory changes".

Fig. 5.61 (a, b) Extensive ground-glass opacities in both lungs, lower lungs predominant, especially right lower lobe, showing a paving sign

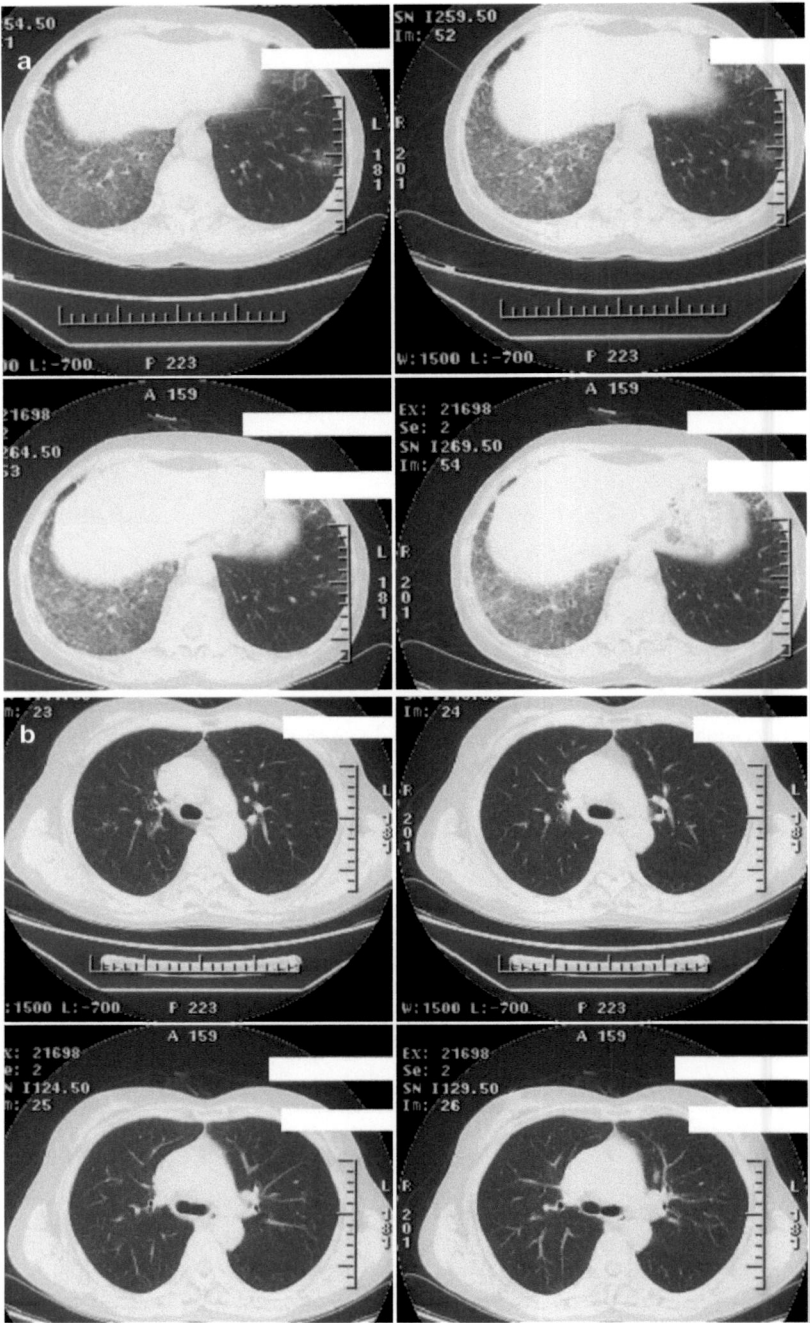

Fig. 5.62 (a–f)
Annotated at the figure
(yellow arrow)

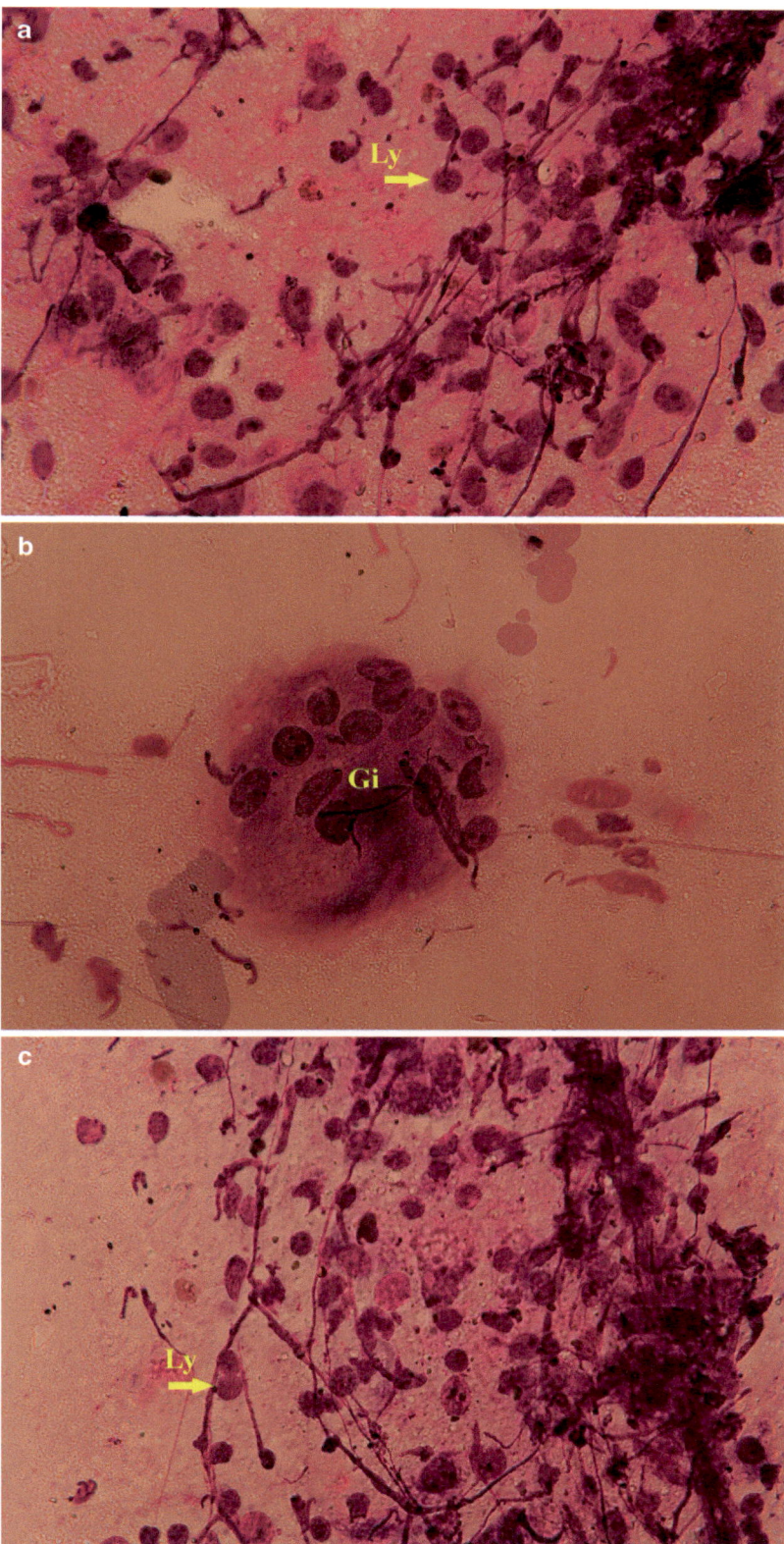

Fig. 5.62 (continued)

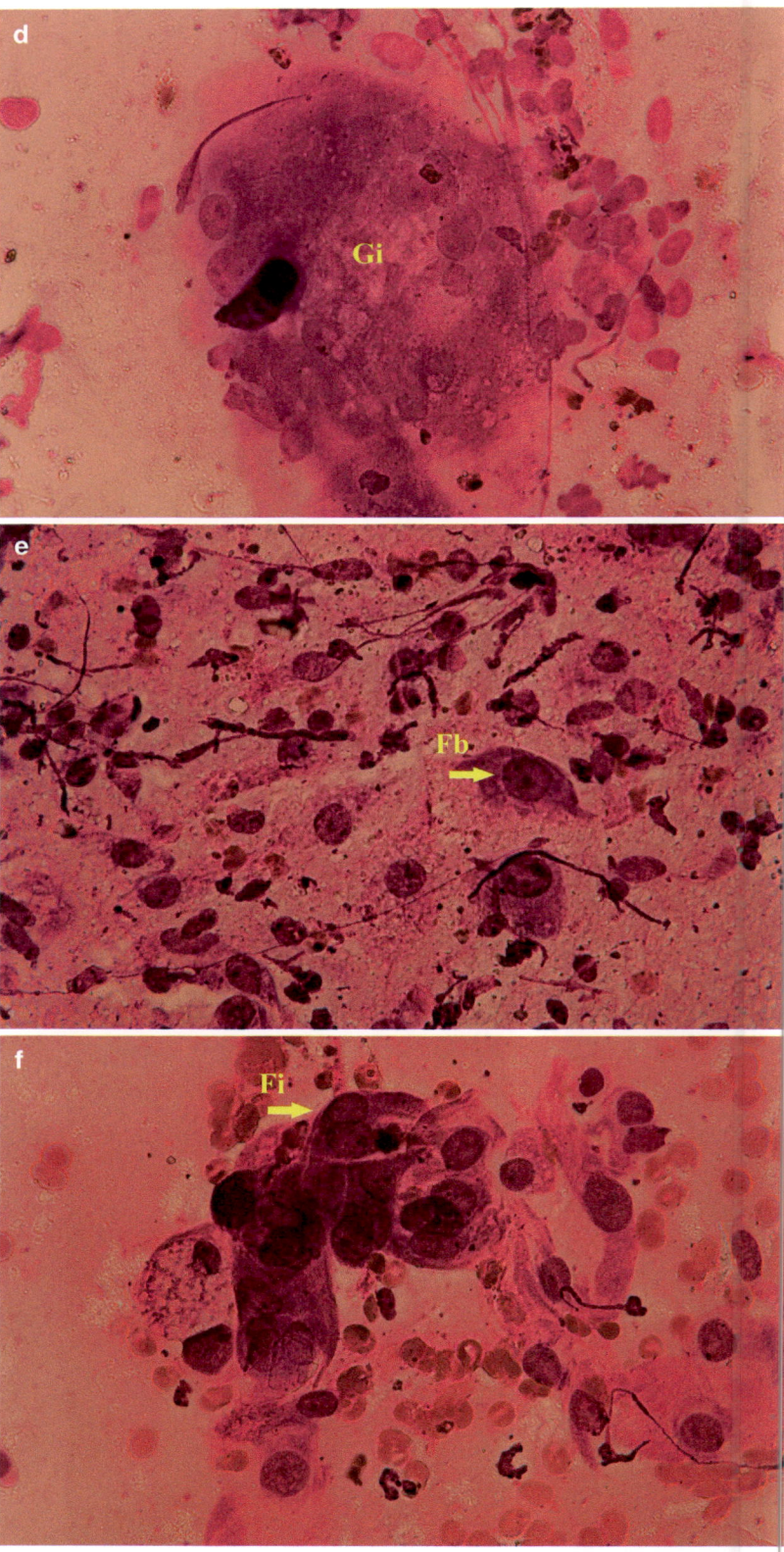

ROSE Cytopathology Cases of Organizing Pneumonia

Jing Feng and Jingyu Chen

6.1 Organizing Pneumonia Case 1

Brief history: Coughing with mild shortness of breath for 1 week, clinically diagnosed as organizing pneumonia.

Technology to obtain the target lesions: Transbronchial lung biopsy (TBLB).

The preparation of cytological slides for ROSE: Imprinting (rolling).

Clustering (categorizing) analysis in ROSE interpretation:

- "Inflammatory changes".
- May conform to organization.

J. Feng
Pulmonary and Critical Care Medicine, Tianjin Medical University General Hospital, Tianjin, China
e-mail: zyyhxkfj@126.com

J. Chen (✉)
Lung Transplantation Group, Nanjing Medical University, Wuxi, China
e-mail: chenjy@wuxiph.com

© Springer Nature Singapore Pte Ltd. 2020
J. Feng et al. (eds.), *Rapid On-Site Evaluation (ROSE) in Diagnostic Interventional Pulmonology*,
https://doi.org/10.1007/978-981-15-0939-1_6

Fig. 6.1 (a–c) A large area of confluent consolidation and exudation in the left lung

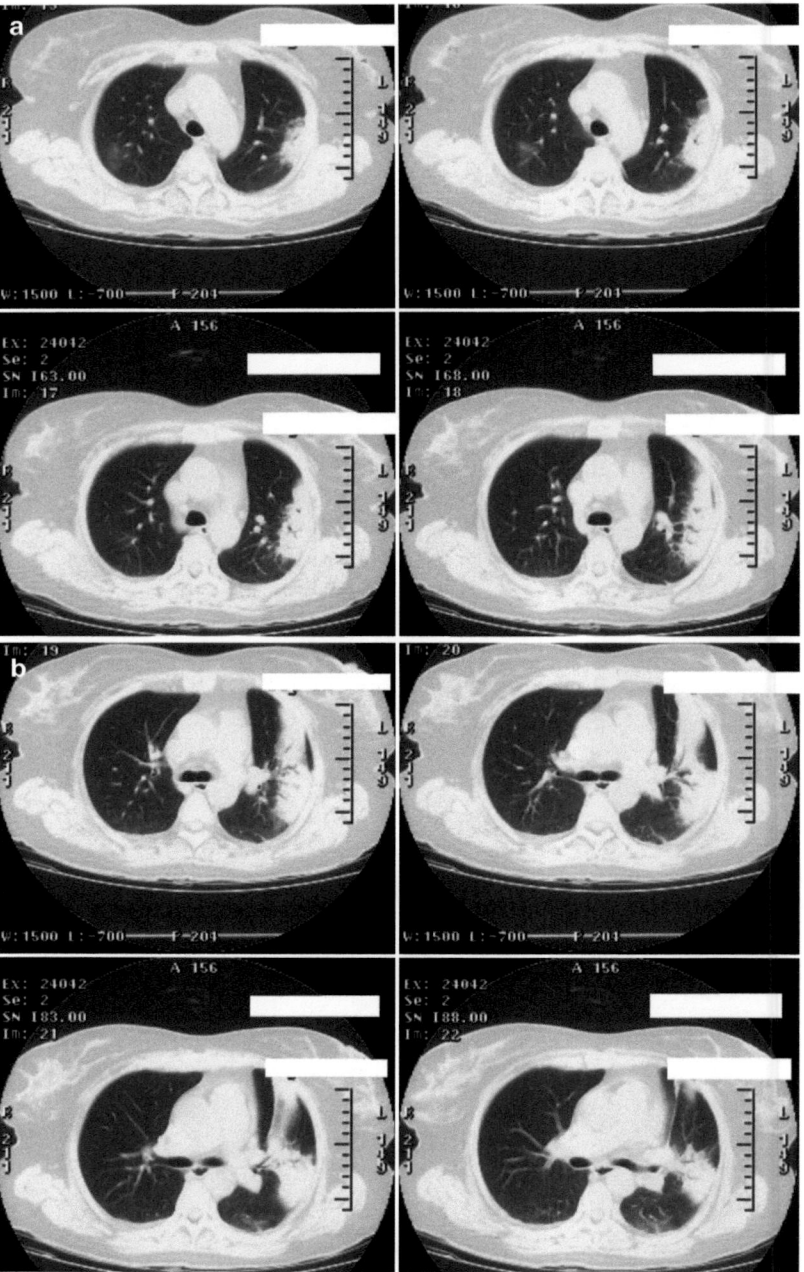

Fig. 6.1 (continued)

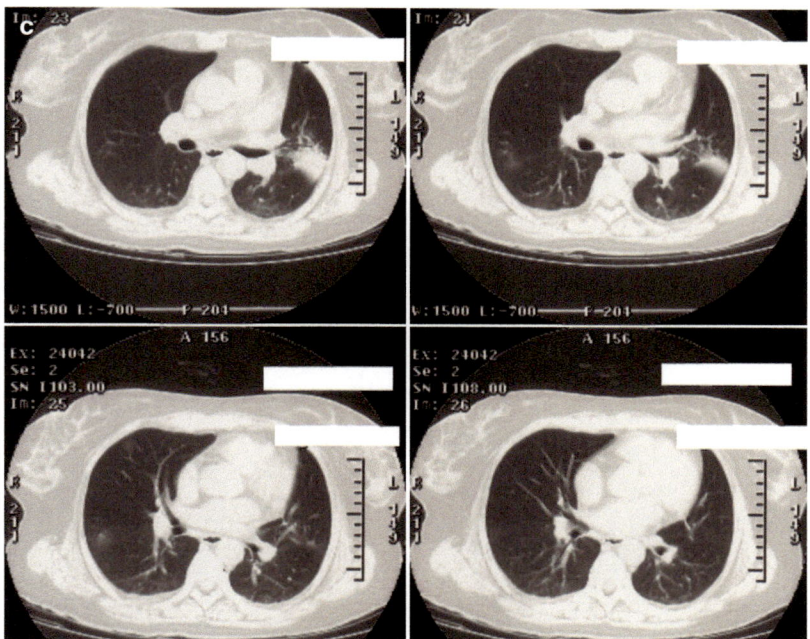

Fig. 6.2 (a–e)
Annotated at the figure
(yellow arrow)

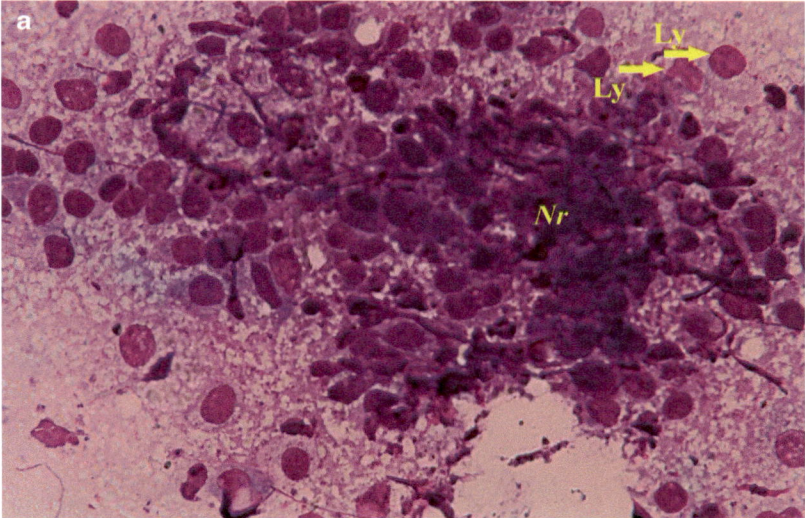

Fig. 6.2 (continued)

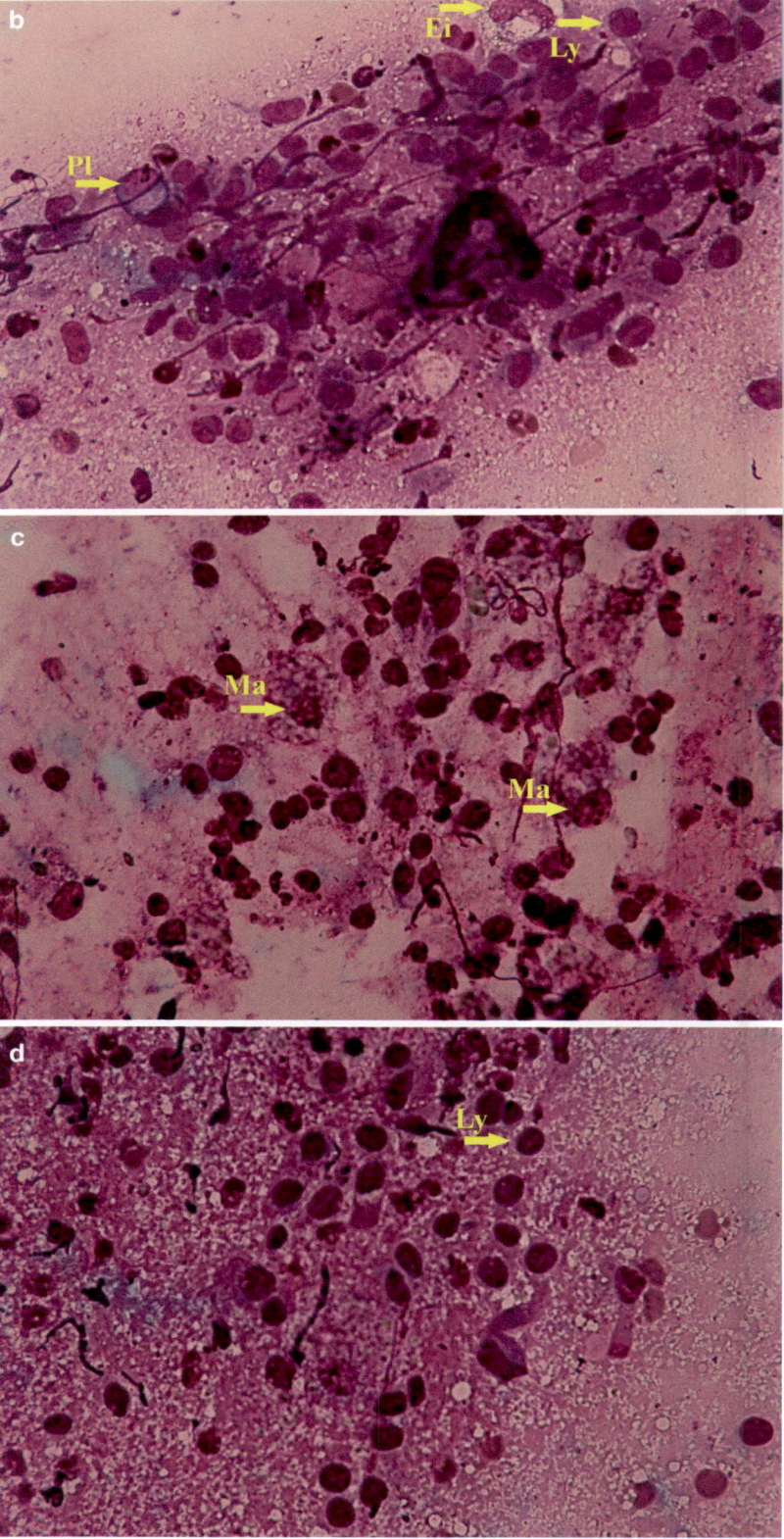

Fig. 6.2 (continued)

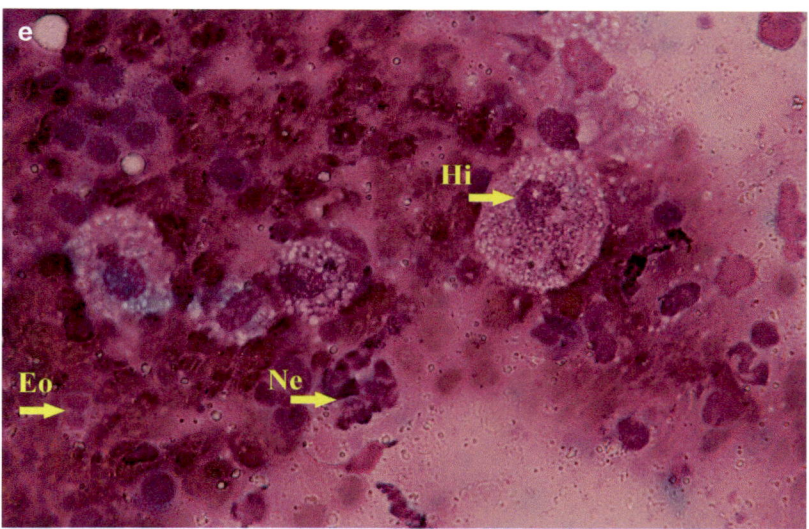

6.2   Cryptogenic Organizing Pneumonia (COP)

Brief history: Coughing for 2 months, running a fever for 1 week, diagnosed as cryptogenic organizing pneumonia clinically.

Technology to obtain the target lesions: Transbronchial lung biopsy (TBLB).

The preparation of cytological slides for ROSE: Imprinting (rolling).

Clustering (categorizing) analysis in ROSE interpretation:

- May conform to organization.

Fig. 6.3 (a–c) Multiple ground-glass opacities and consolidation at the subpleural areas and obvious interstitial thickening

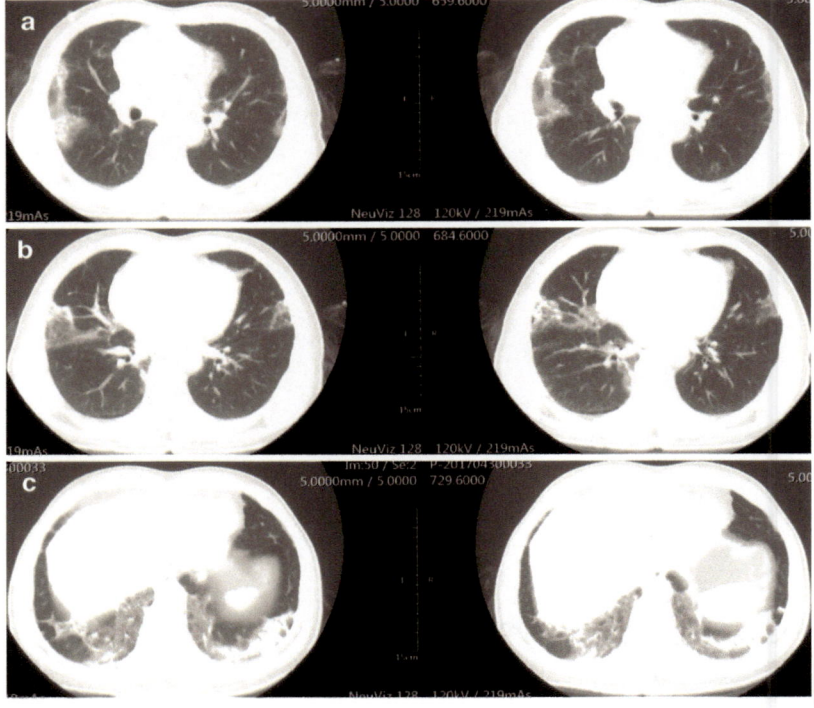

Fig. 6.4 Aggregation of foamy macrophages (yellow arrow), a typical ROSE feature of Masson bodies and alveolar septal thickening, histiocytes (red arrow), some evolving into epithelioid cells (green arrow), fibroblasts (blue arrow), lymphocytes (pink arrow), and scattered neutrophils (brown arrow), all these cells constituting Masson bodies

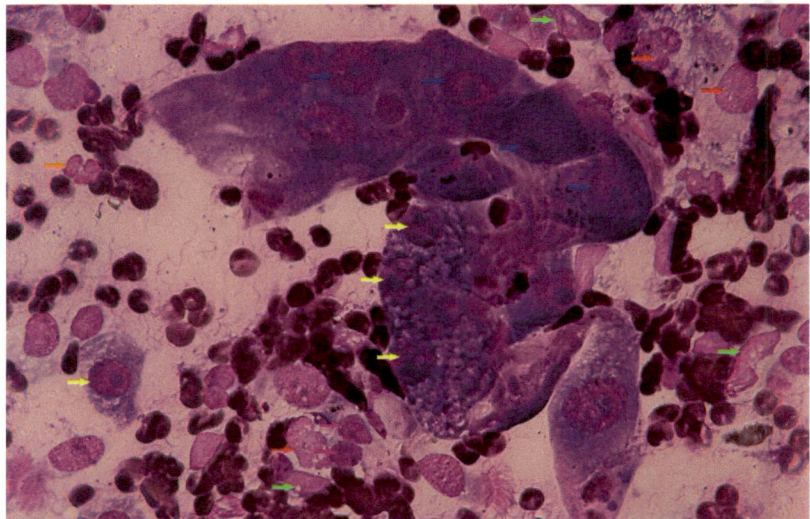

Fig. 6.5 (a, b)
Aggregation of foamy
macrophages (yellow
arrow), a typical ROSE
feature of Masson
bodies and alveolar
septal thickening,
histiocytes (red arrow),
some evolving into
epithelioid cells (green
arrow), fibroblasts (blue
arrow), and lymphocytes
(pink arrow), all these
cells constituting
Masson bodies

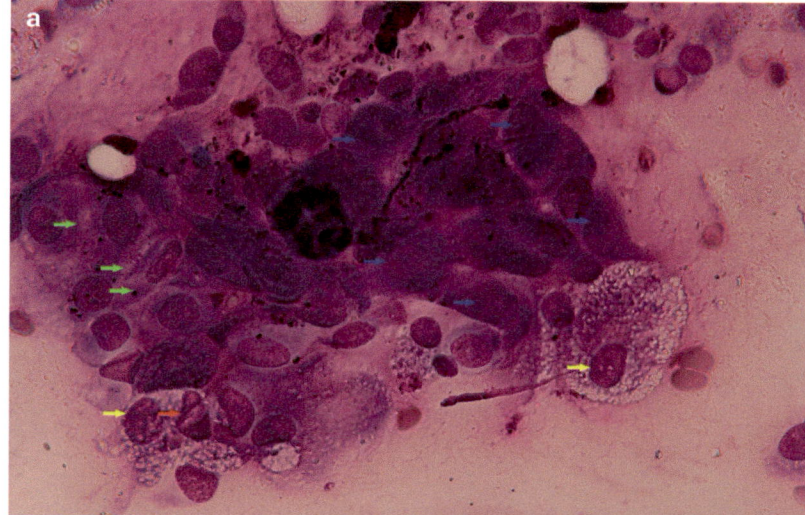

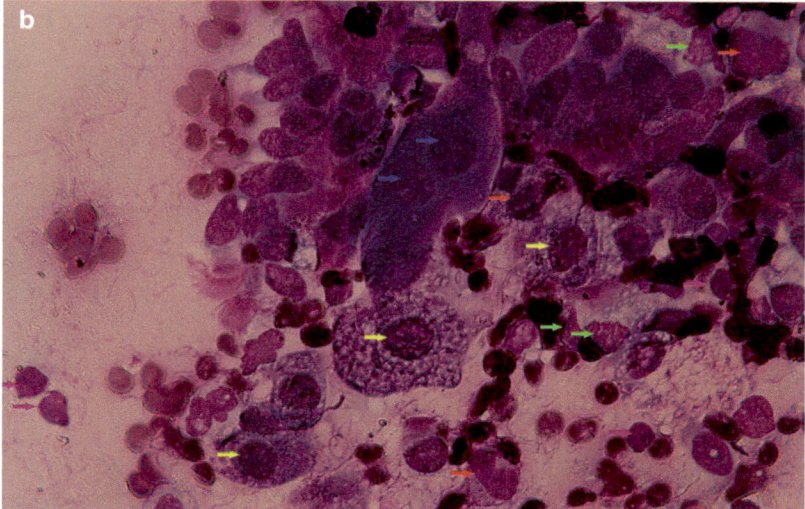

Fig. 6.6 Aggregation of
foamy macrophages
(yellow arrow), a typical
ROSE feature of Masson
bodies and alveolar
septal thickening,
histiocytes (red arrow),
some evolving into
epithelioid cells (green
arrow), and fibroblasts
(blue arrow), all these
cells constituting
Masson bodies

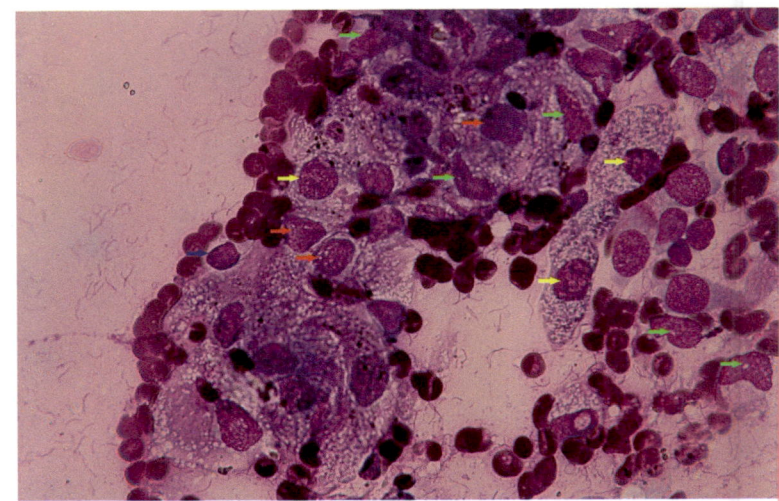

Fig. 6.7 Aggregation of
foamy macrophages
(yellow arrow), a typical
ROSE feature of Masson
bodies and alveolar
septal thickening,
histiocytes (red arrow),
some evolving into
epithelioid cells (green
arrow), lymphocytes
(blue arrow), and
scattered neutrophils
(pink arrow), all these
cells constituting
Masson bodies

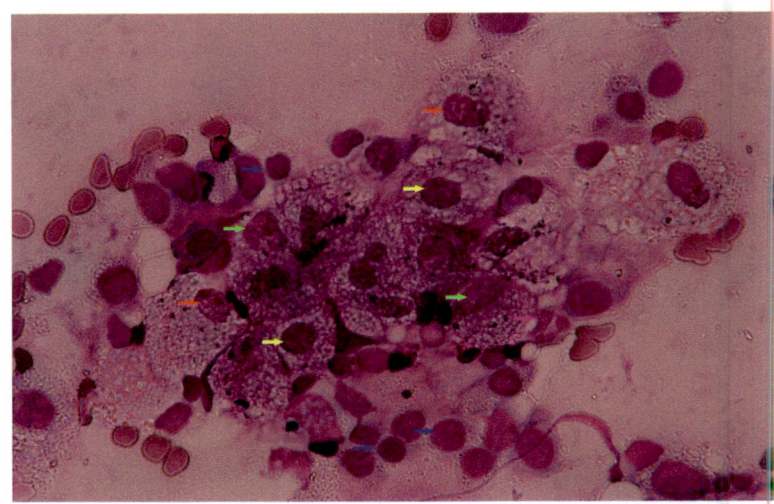

Fig. 6.8 Aggregation of
foamy macrophages
(yellow arrow), a typical
ROSE feature of Masson
bodies and alveolar
septal thickening,
histiocytes (red arrow),
some evolving into
epithelioid cells (green
arrow), fibroblasts (blue
arrow), lymphocytes
(pink arrow), and
scattered neutrophils
(brown arrow), all these
cells constituting
Masson bodies

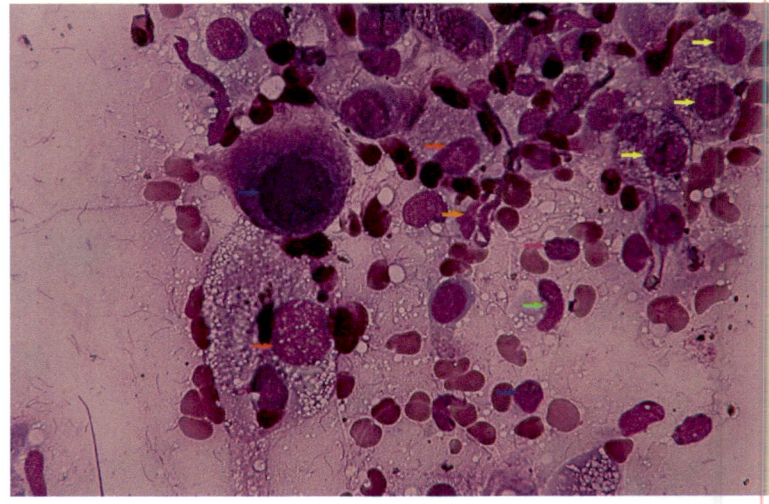

6.3 Acute Fibrinous and Organizing Pneumonia

Brief history: Coughing and running a fever for 2 weeks, with obvious dyspnea.

Technology to obtain the target lesions: Transbronchial lung biopsy (TBLB).

The preparation of cytological slides for ROSE: Imprinting (rolling).

Clustering (categorizing) analysis in ROSE interpretation:

- Granulomatous inflammation.
- May conform to organization.
- Necrotic "inflammatory changes".

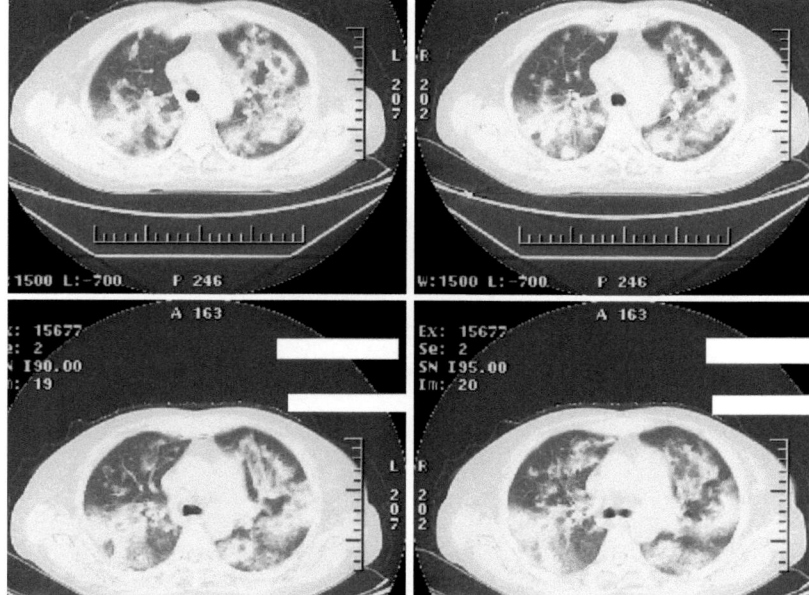

Fig. 6.9 Multiple consolidation, patches, ground-glass opacities, and nodules in both lungs, especially in both upper lungs

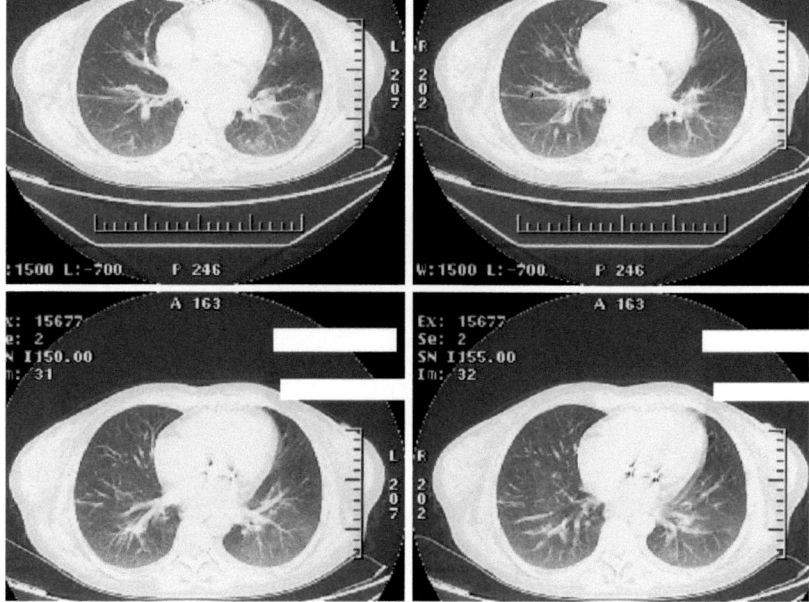

Fig. 6.10 Bronchovascular bundles thickening and interstitial thickening in both lower lungs

Fig. 6.11 Aggregation of foamy macrophages (yellow arrow), some evolving into epithelioid cells (red arrow)

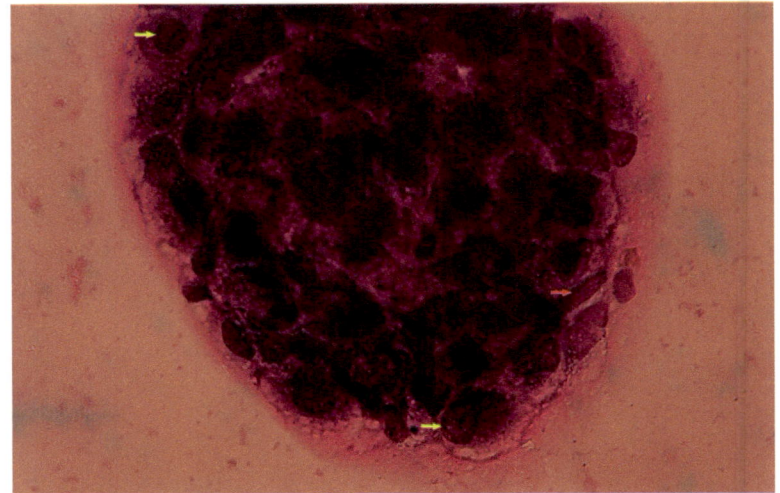

Fig. 6.12 Aggregation of foamy macrophages, some evolving into histiocytes (yellow arrow), and lymphocytes (red arrow)

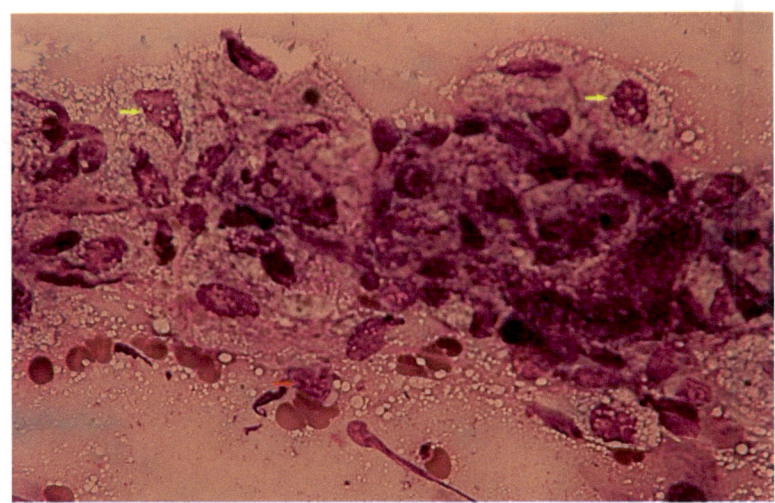

Fig. 6.13 Aggregation of foamy macrophages, some evolving into histiocytes (yellow arrow), lymphocytes (red arrow), and ciliated columnar epithelial cells (green arrow)

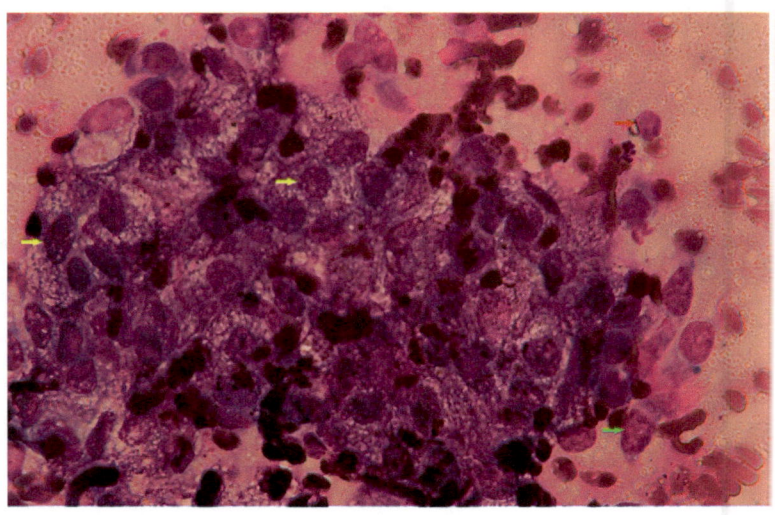

Fig. 6.14 Aggregation of foamy macrophages, some evolving into histiocytes (yellow arrow), and lymphocytes (red arrow)

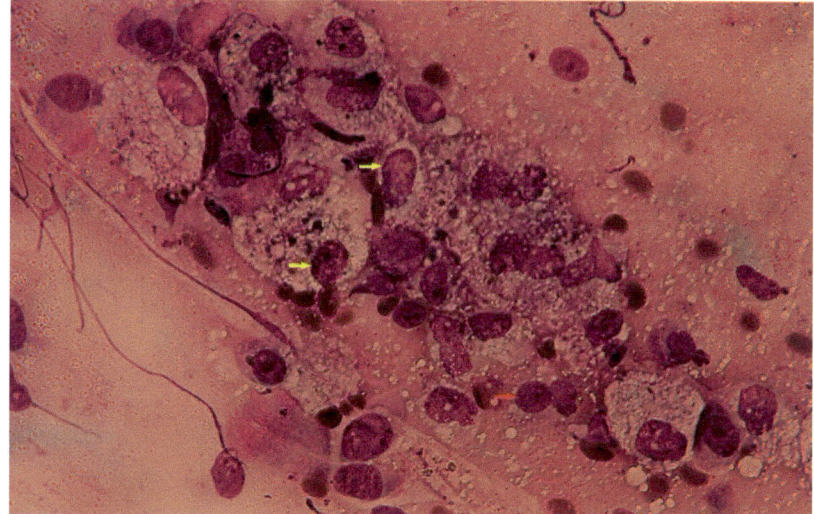

Fig. 6.15 Aggregation of foamy macrophages, some evolving into histiocytes (yellow arrow), lymphocytes (red arrow), and obvious amorphous hyperchromatic fibrin

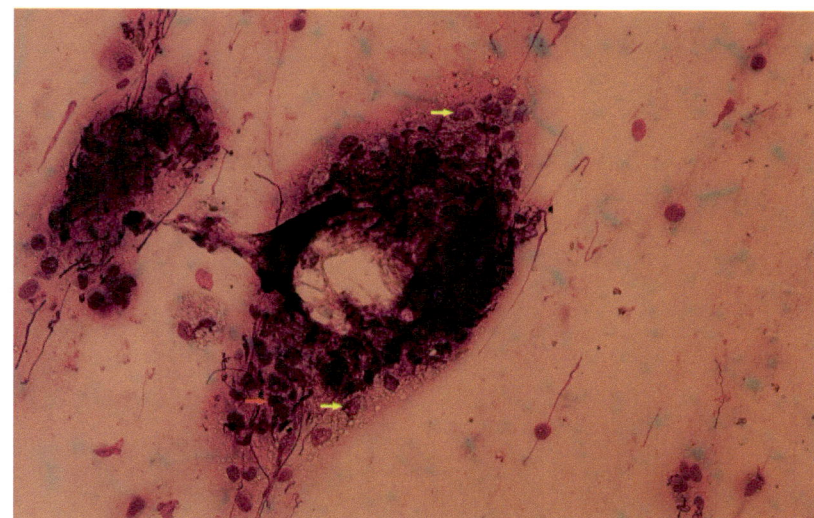

6.4 Organizing Pneumonia Case 2

Brief history: Coughing for more than 1 month, clinically diagnosed as organizing pneumonia.

Technology to obtain the target lesions: Transbronchial lung biopsy (TBLB).

The preparation of cytological slides for ROSE: Imprinting (rolling).

Clustering (categorizing) analysis in ROSE interpretation:

- Granulomatous inflammation.
- May conform to organization.

Fig. 6.16 (a, b)
Multiple patches,
consolidation, and
exudation in both lungs,
distributed along the
bronchial vascular
bundles

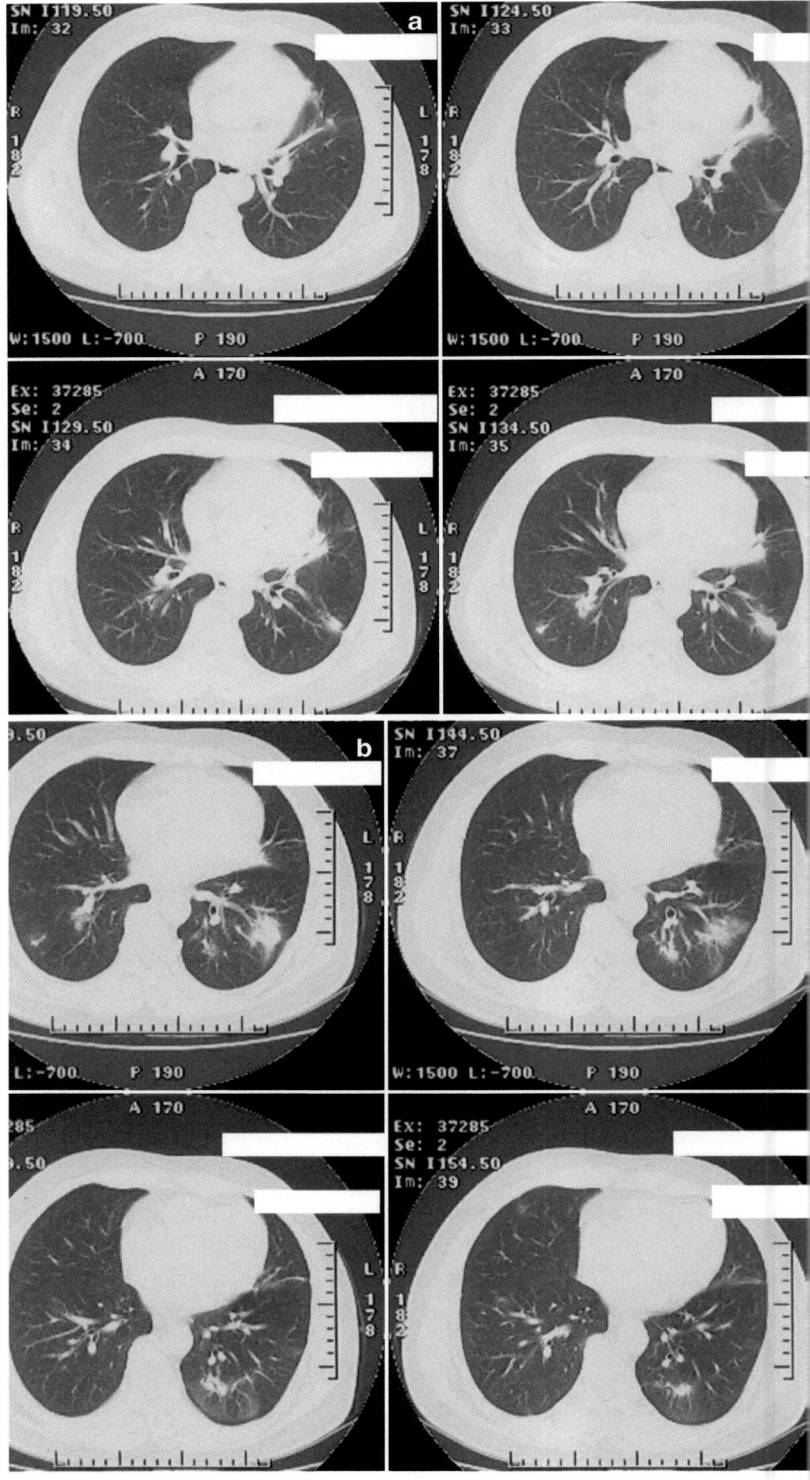

Fig. 6.17 (a–e)
Annotated at the
figure (yellow arrow)

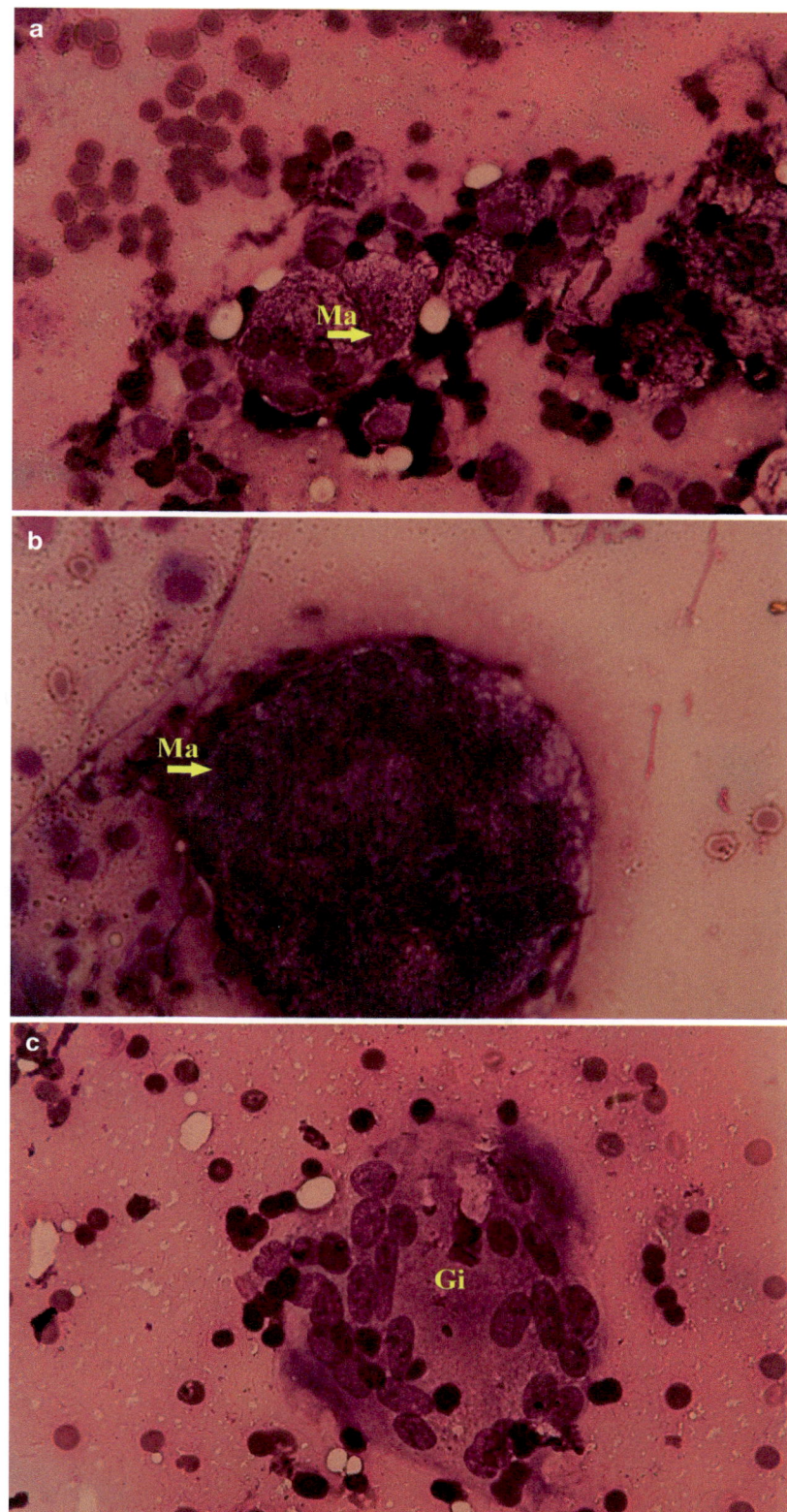

Fig. 6.17 (continued)

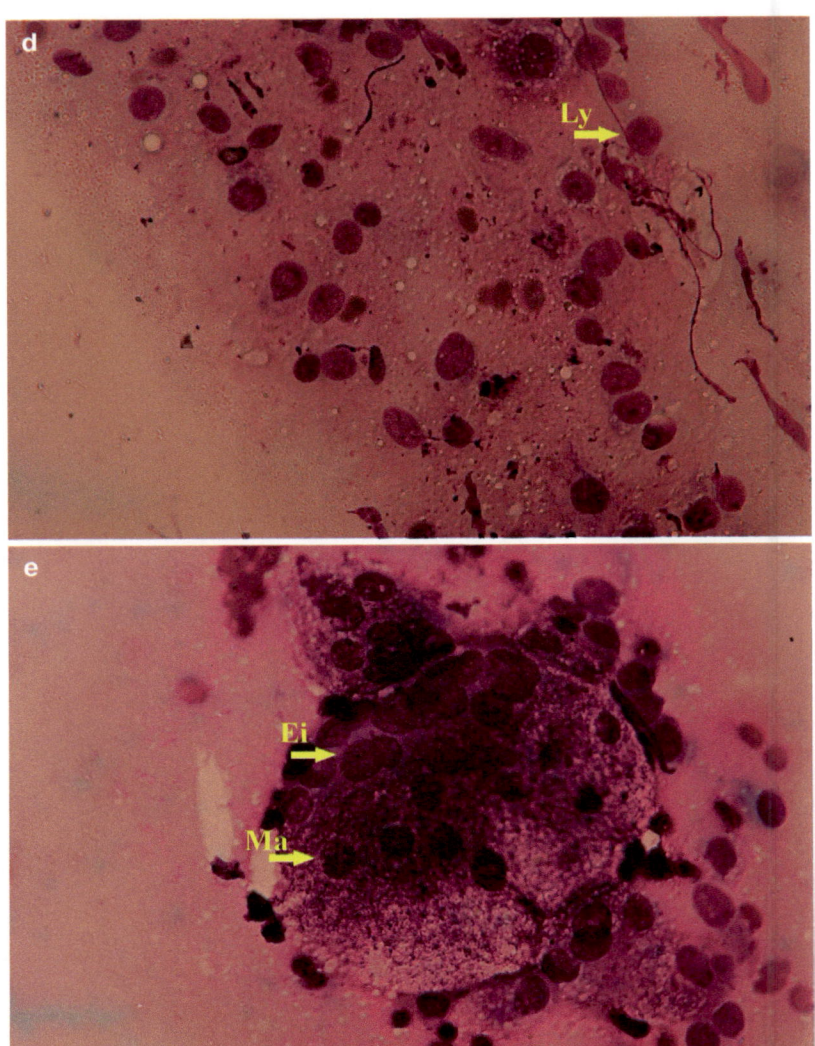

6.5   Organizing Pneumonia Case 3

Brief history: Coughing for more than 1 month with obvious shortness of breath, pectoralgia at the right side, running a fever, progressing rapidly, clinically diagnosed as organizing pneumonia.

Technology to obtain the target lesions: Transbronchial lung biopsy (TBLB).

The preparation of cytological slides for ROSE: Imprinting (rolling).

Clustering (categorizing) analysis in ROSE interpretation:

- "Inflammatory changes".
- May conform to organization.

Fig. 6.18 (**a**, **b**) Initial CT, multiple patches, consolidation, and air bronchogram in both lungs and slight interstitial thickening distributed along the bronchovascular bundle or subpleural areas

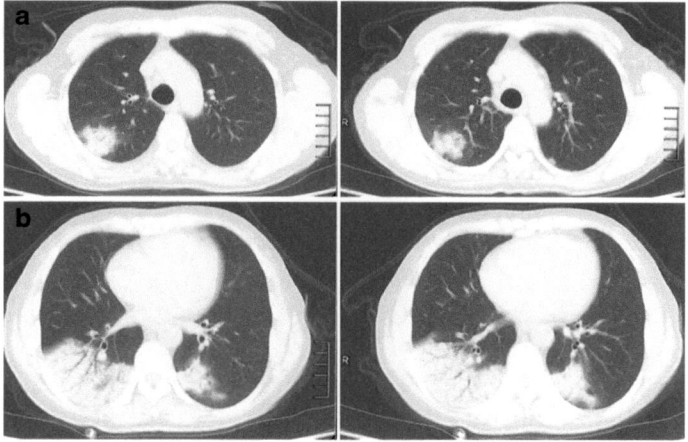

Fig. 6.19 (**a**, **b**) CT taken 20 days later, progressing rapidly, large subpleural areas of confluent consolidation and exudation in both lungs

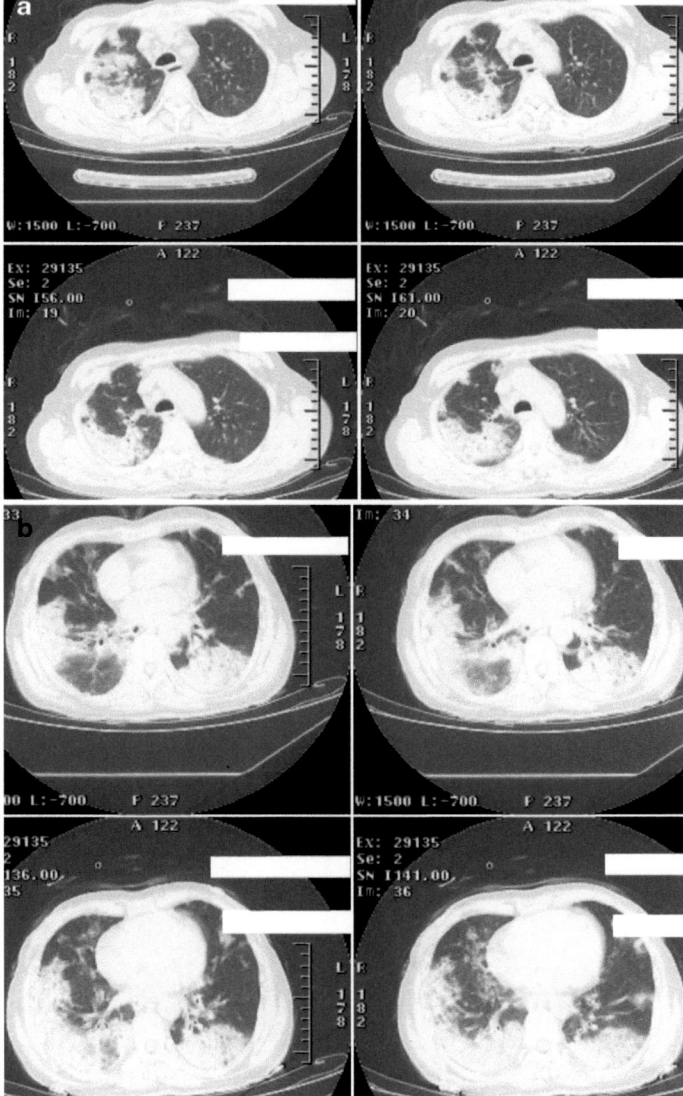

Fig. 6.20 (a–e)
Annotated at the figure
(yellow arrow)

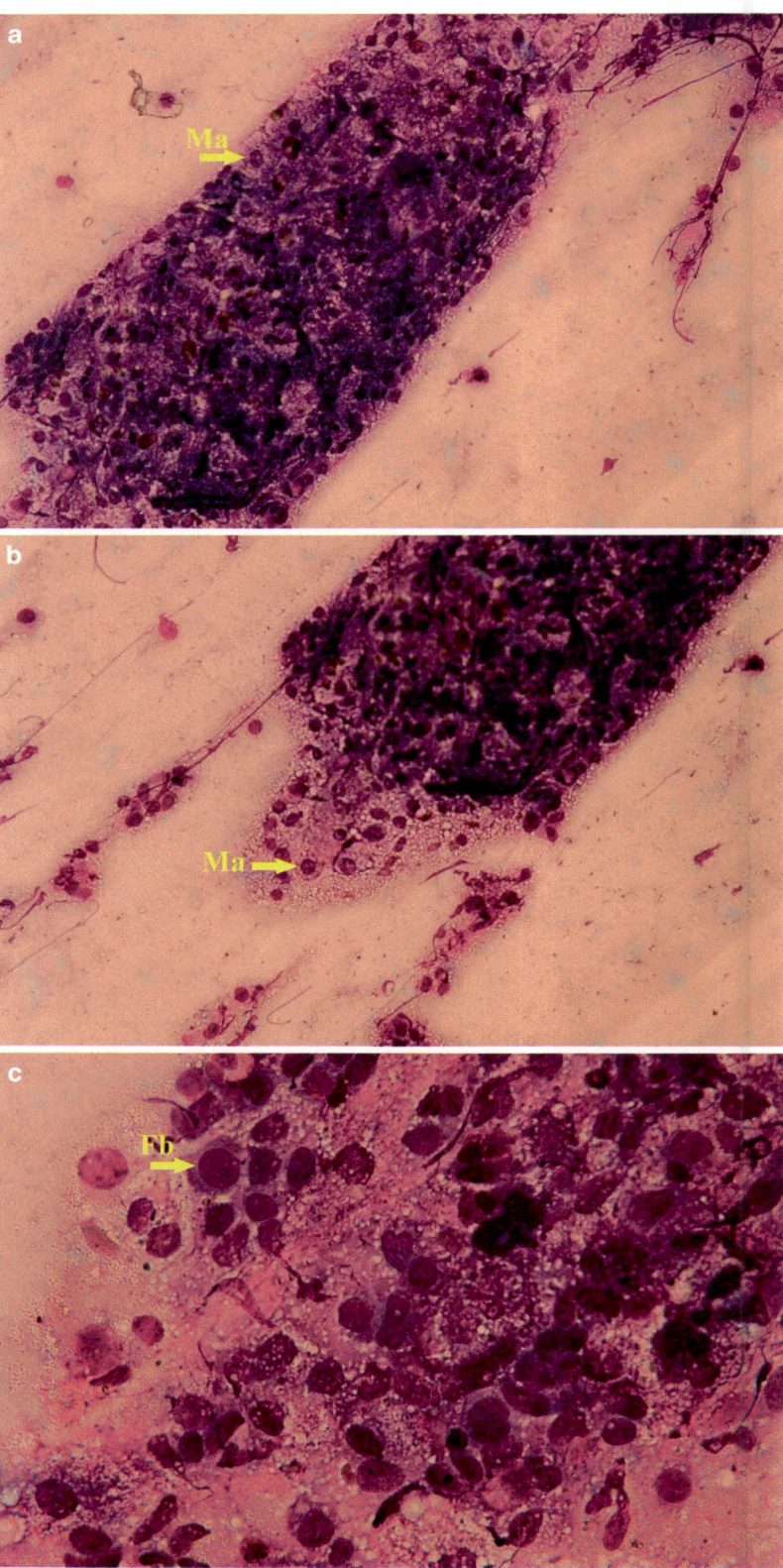

Fig. 6.20 (continued)

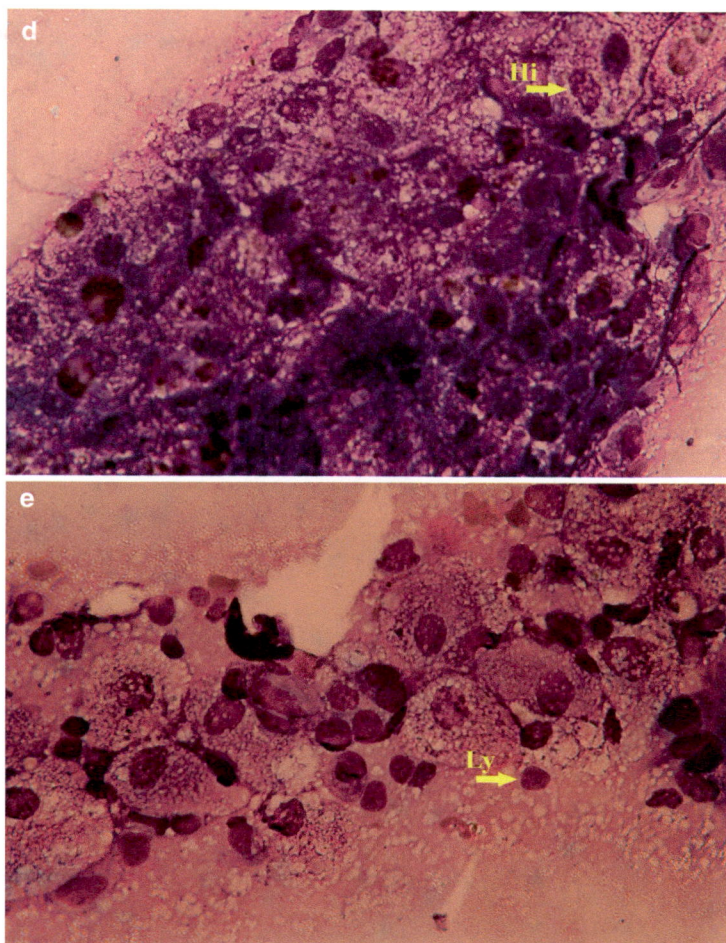

6.6 Organizing Pneumonia Case 4

Brief history: Female, 31 years old, coughing for 2 weeks, running a low fever, clinically diagnosed as organizing pneumonia.

Technology to obtain the target lesions: Transbronchial lung biopsy (TBLB).

The preparation of cytological slides for ROSE: Imprinting (rolling).

Clustering (categorizing) analysis in ROSE interpretation:

- "Inflammatory changes".
- Granulomatous inflammation.
- May conform to organization.

Fig. 6.21 (a–c) Multiple
patches, consolidation, and air
bronchogram in both lungs and
slight interstitial thickening

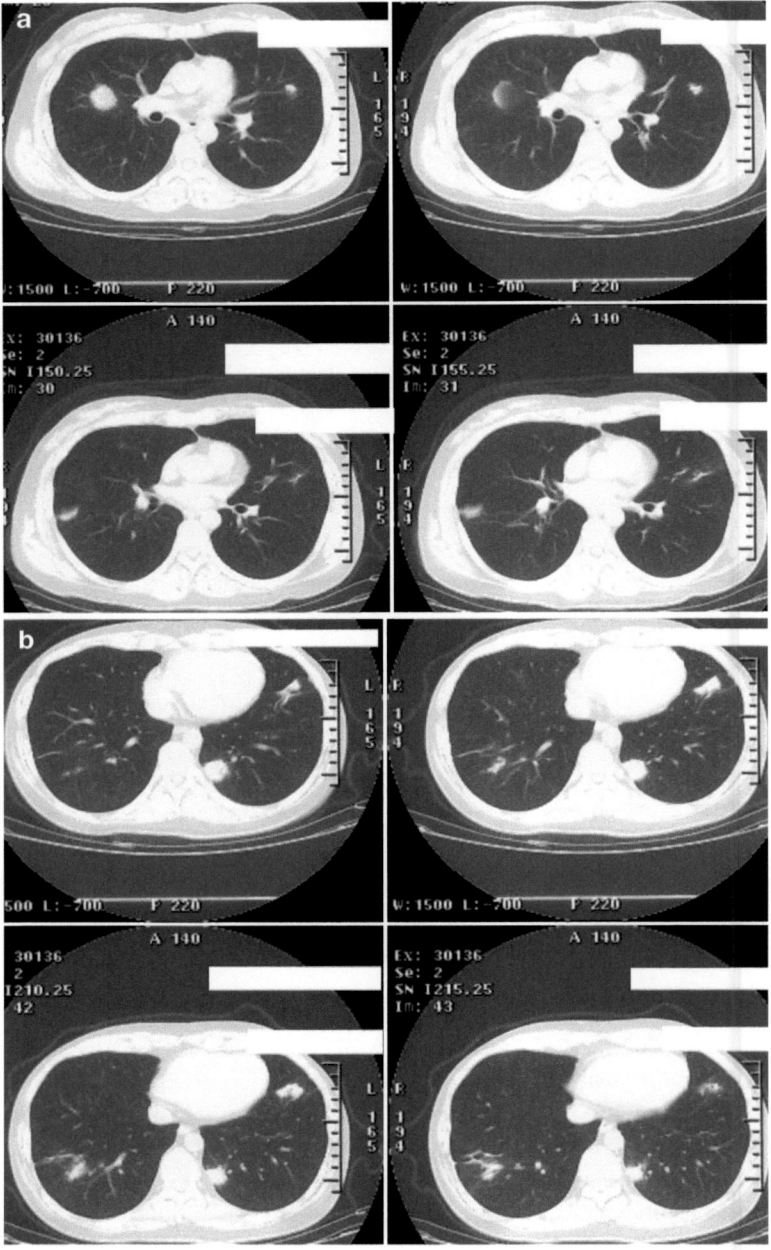

Fig. 6.21 (continued)

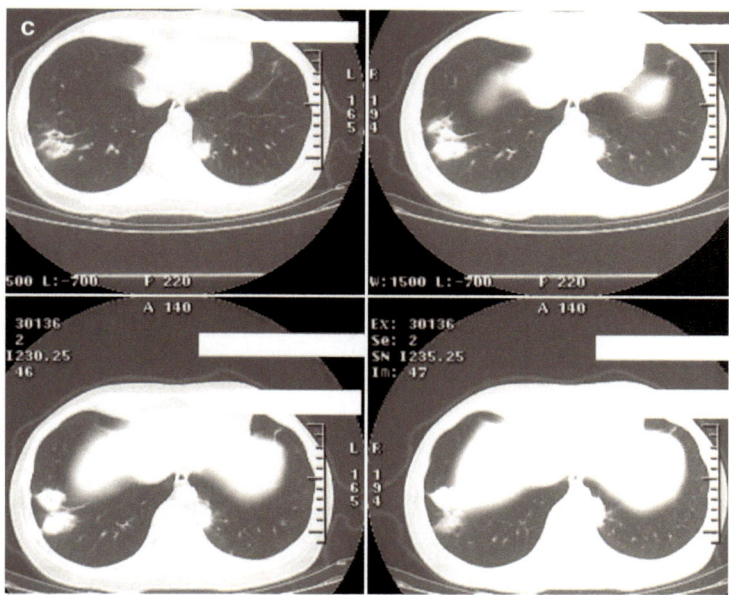

Fig. 6.22 (a–e)
Annotated at the figure
(yellow arrow)

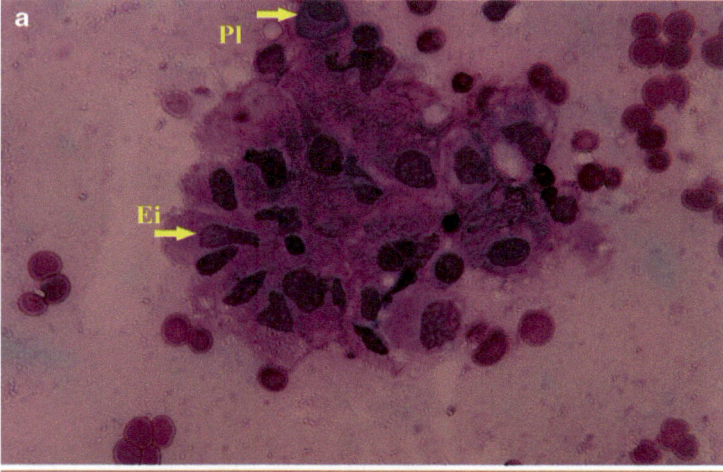

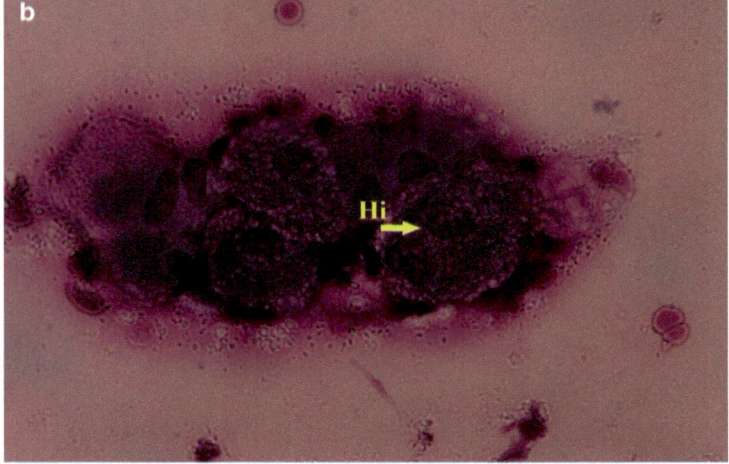

Fig. 6.22 (continued)

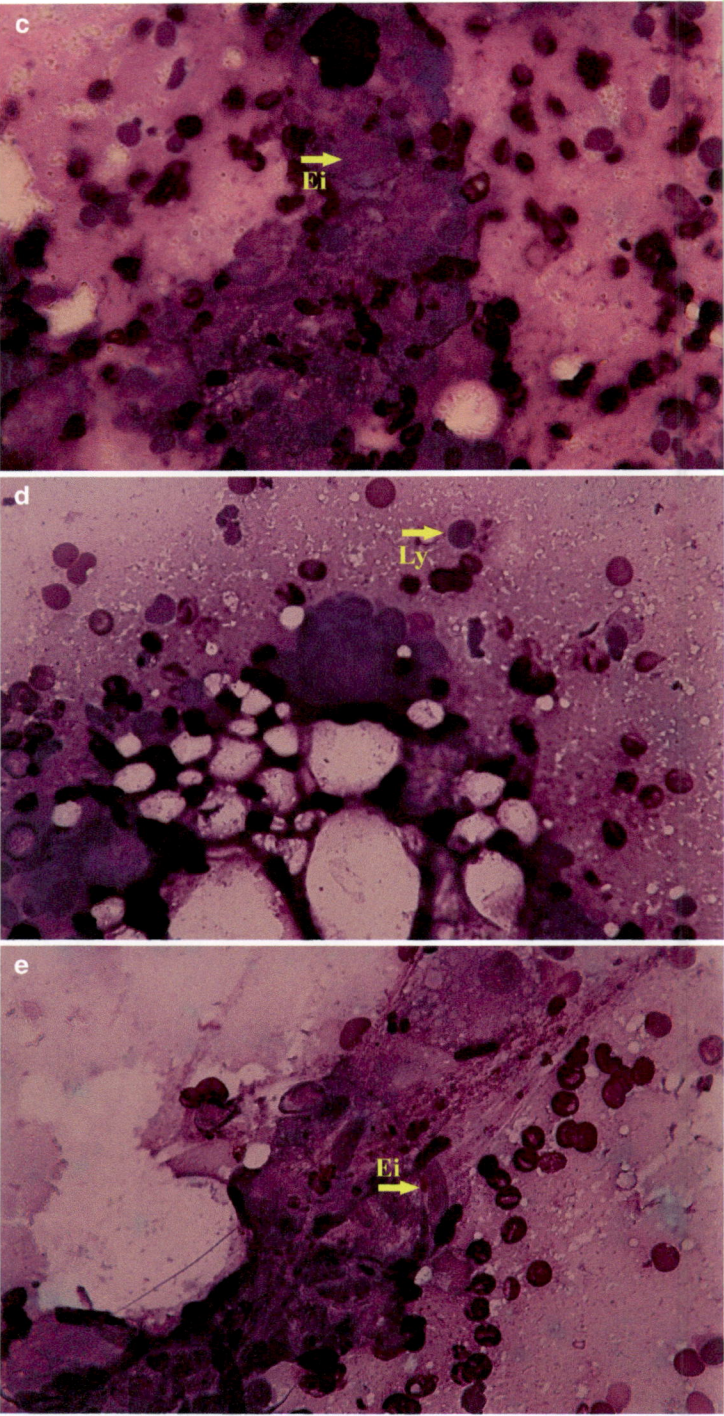

6.7   Organizing Pneumonia Secondary to Myositis

Brief history: Clinically diagnosed as myositis, running a low fever with coughing for more than 2 weeks.

Technology to obtain the target lesions: Transbronchial lung biopsy (TBLB).

The preparation of cytological slides for ROSE: Imprinting (rolling).

Clustering (categorizing) analysis in ROSE interpretation:

• May conform to organization.

Fig. 6.23 (a, b) Consolidation, exudation, and interstitial thickening in the right lower lobe

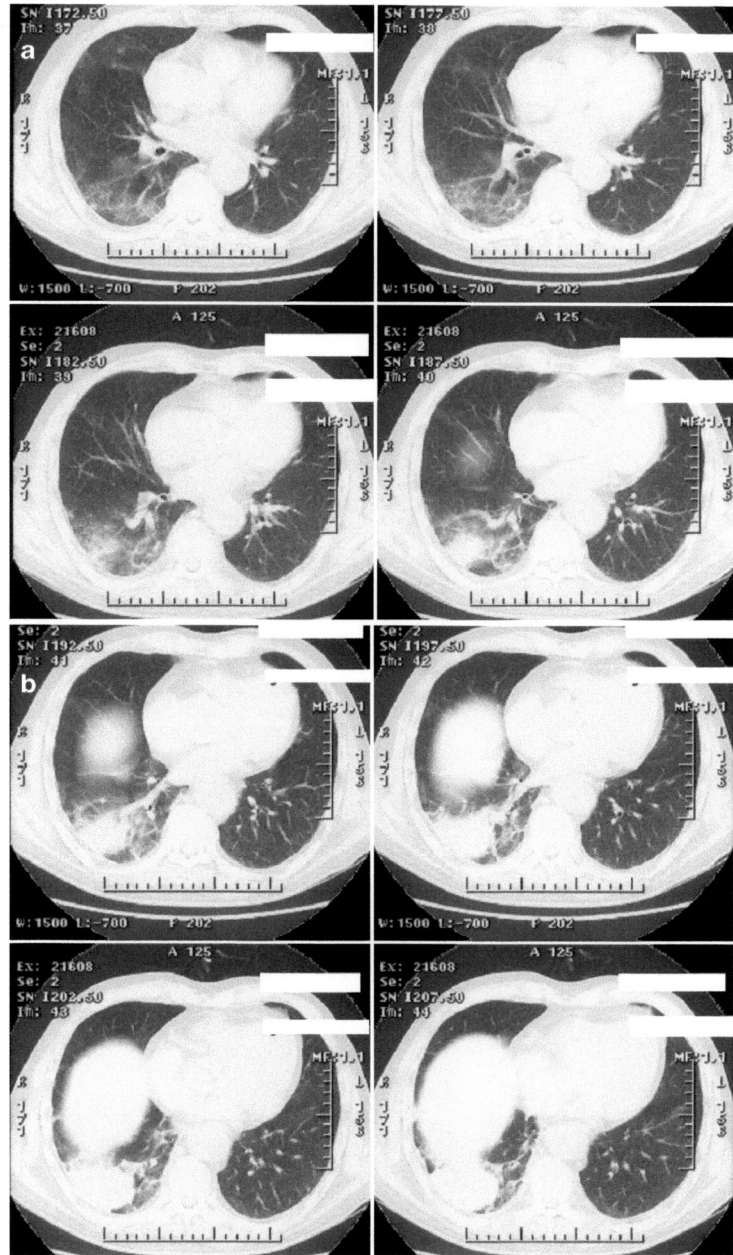

Fig. 6.24 (**a–e**)
Annotated at the
figure (yellow arrow)

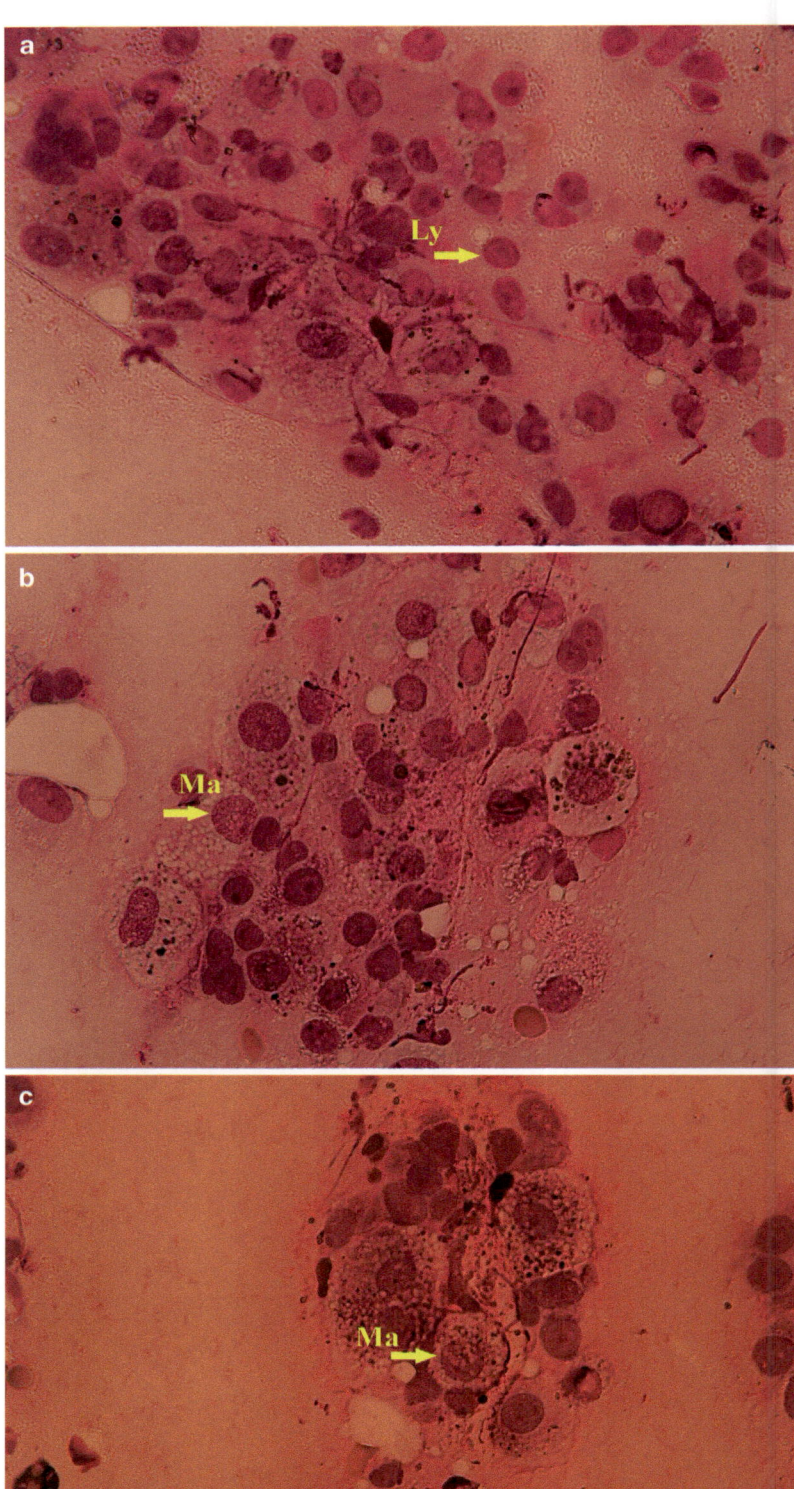

Fig. 6.24 (continued)

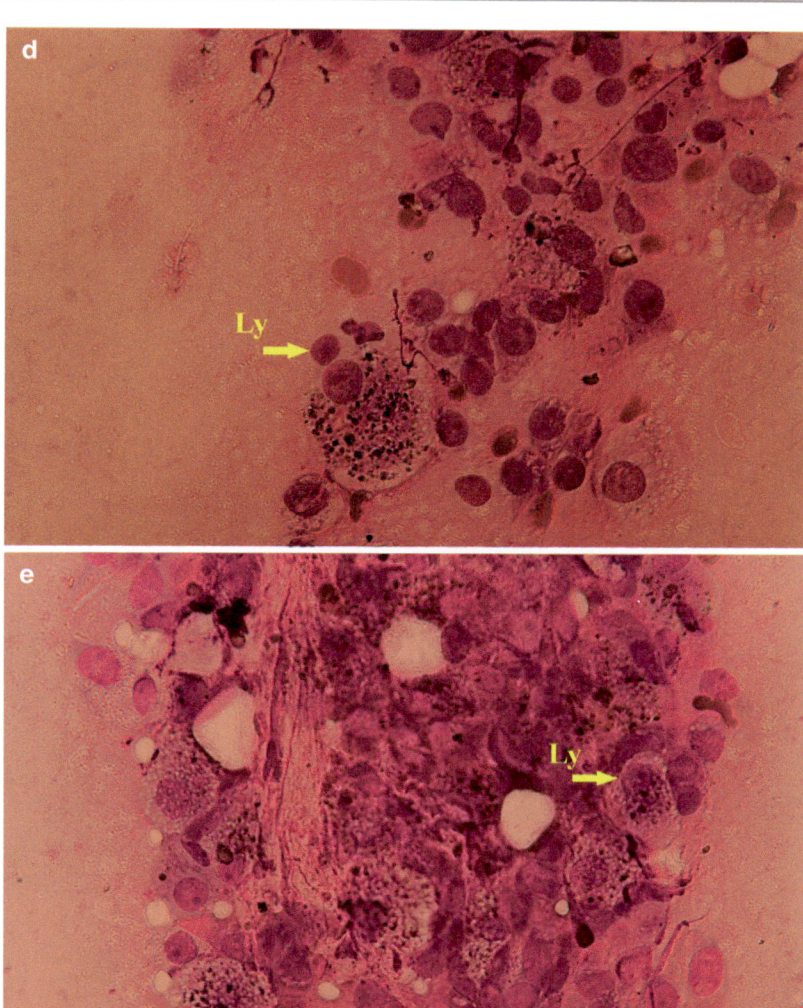

ROSE Cytopathology Cases of Pulmonary Infiltration with Eosinophilia

7

Jing Feng and Bo Wu

7.1 Pulmonary Infiltration with Eosinophilia (PIE) Case 1

Brief history: Male, 50 years old, coughing with mild shortness of breath for nearly a week, clinically diagnosed as pulmonary infiltration with eosinophilia (PIE).

Technology to obtain the target lesions: Transbronchial lung biopsy (TBLB).

The preparation of cytological slides for ROSE: Imprinting (rolling).

Clustering (categorizing) analysis in ROSE interpretation:

- "Inflammatory changes".
- May conform to organization.
- Lymphocyte-based immune inflammatory response.
- Eosinophil-based immune inflammatory response.

J. Feng
Pulmonary and Critical Care Medicine, Tianjin Medical University General Hospital, Tianjin, China
e-mail: zyyhxkfj@126.com

B. Wu (✉)
Lung Transplantation Group, Nanjing Medical University, Wuxi, China
e-mail: fyz333@126.com

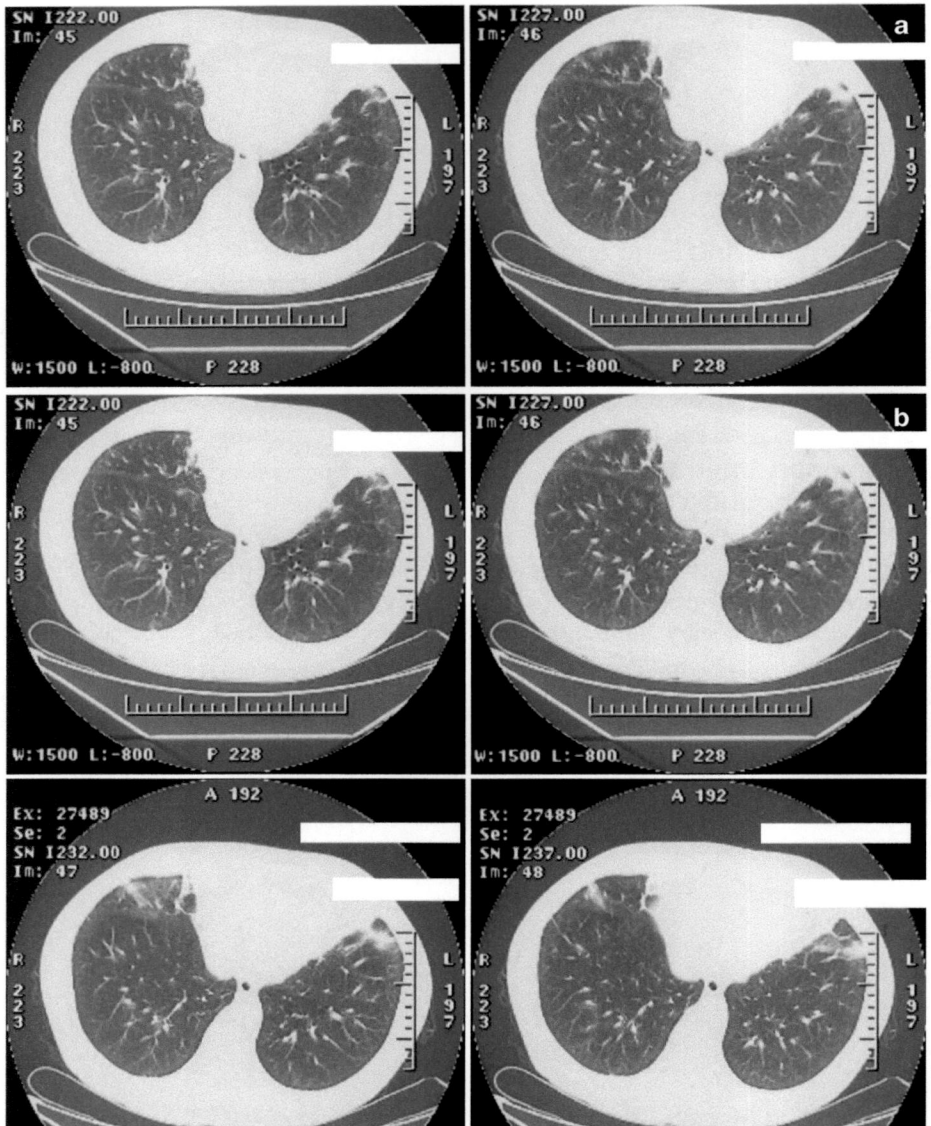

Fig. 7.1 (**a–c**) Multiple patches, consolidation, tree-in-bud sign, exudation, and extensive ground-glass opacities in both lungs

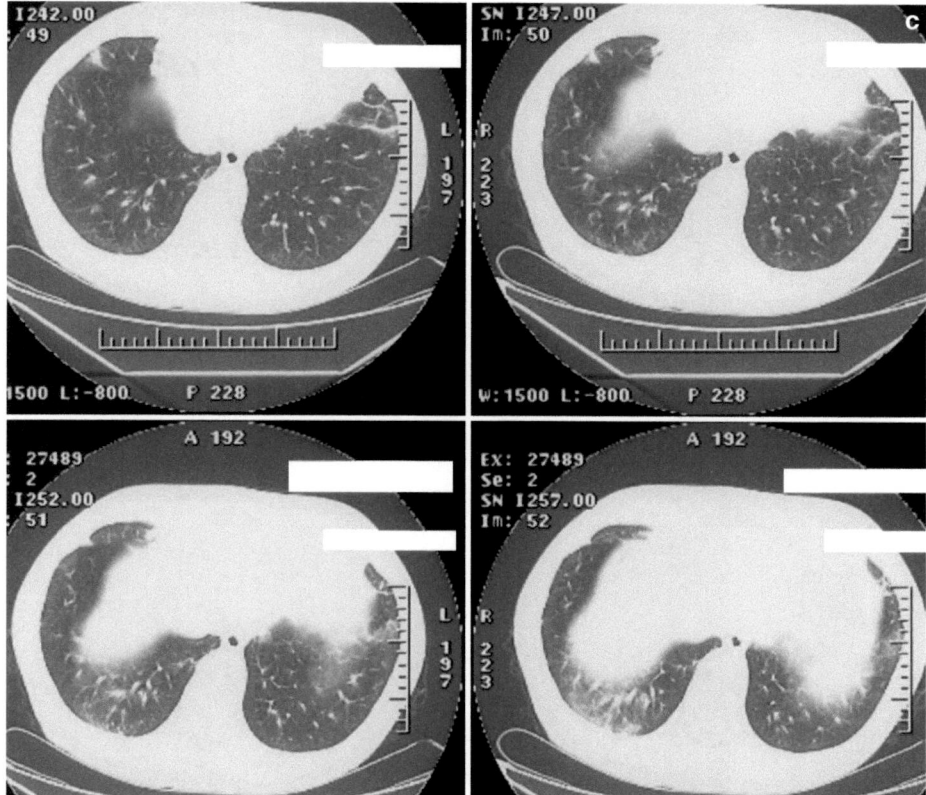

Fig. 7.1 (continued)

Fig. 7.2 (a–e)
Annotated at the figure
(yellow arrow)

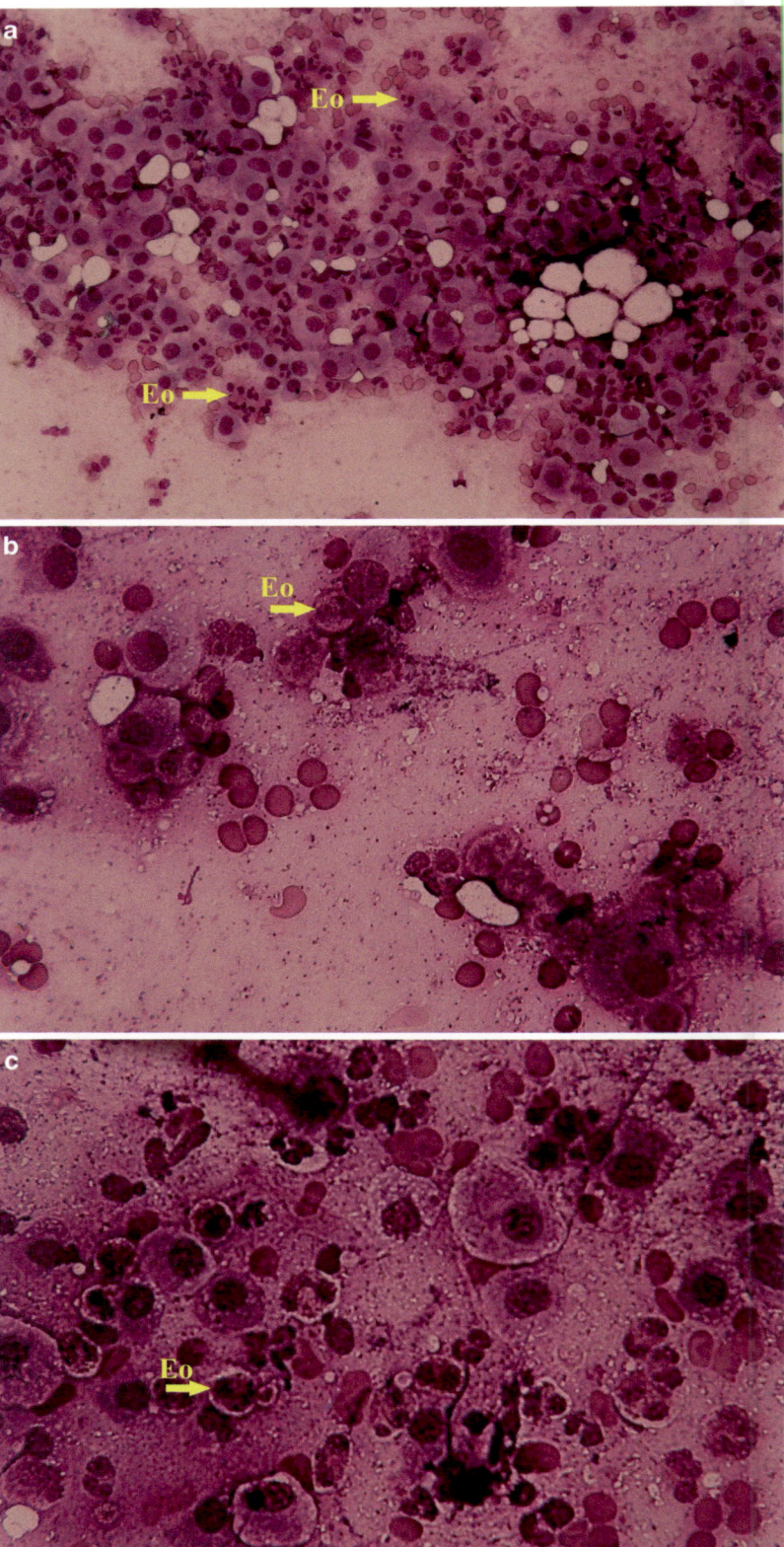

Fig. 7.2 (continued)

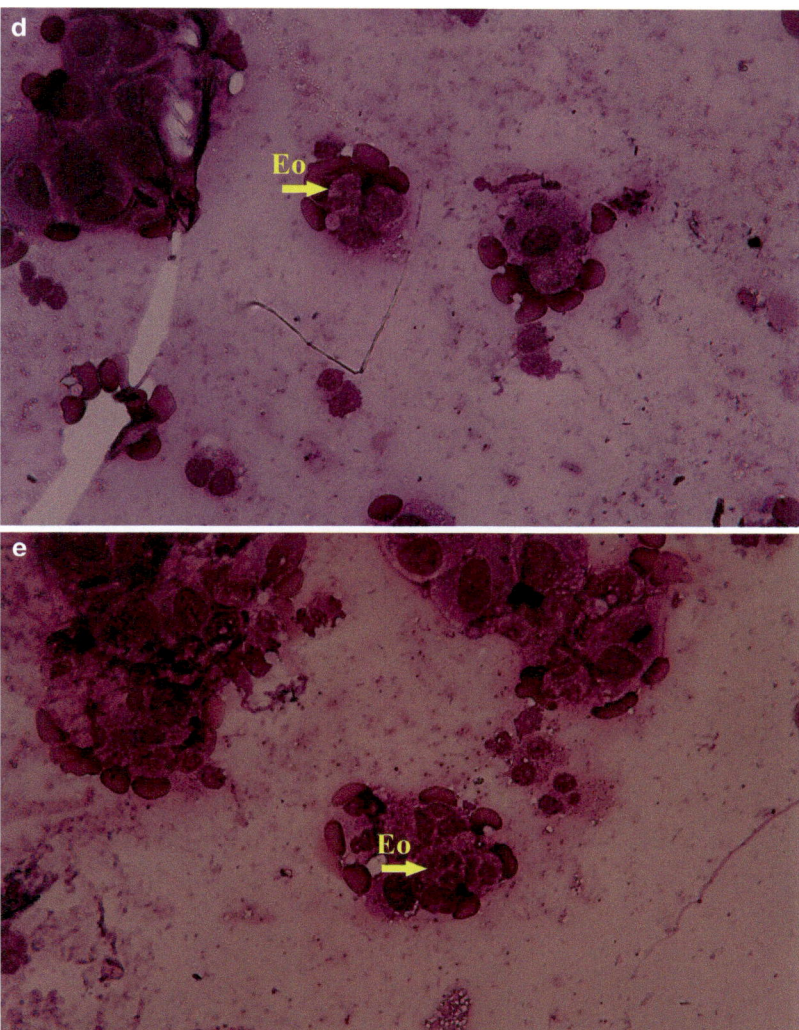

7.2   Pulmonary Infiltration with Eosinophilia (PIE) Case 2

Brief history: Male, 61 years old, coughing with mild shortness of breath for more than 2 weeks, clinically diagnosed as pulmonary infiltration with eosinophilia (PIE).

Technology to obtain the target lesions: Transbronchial lung biopsy (TBLB).

The preparation of cytological slides for ROSE: Imprinting (rolling).

Clustering (categorizing) analysis in ROSE interpretation:

- "Inflammatory changes".
- May conform to organization.
- Eosinophil-based immune inflammatory response.

Fig. 7.3 (**a**, **b**) Multiple
patches, tree-in-bud
sign, exudation, and
extensive ground-glass
opacities in both lungs

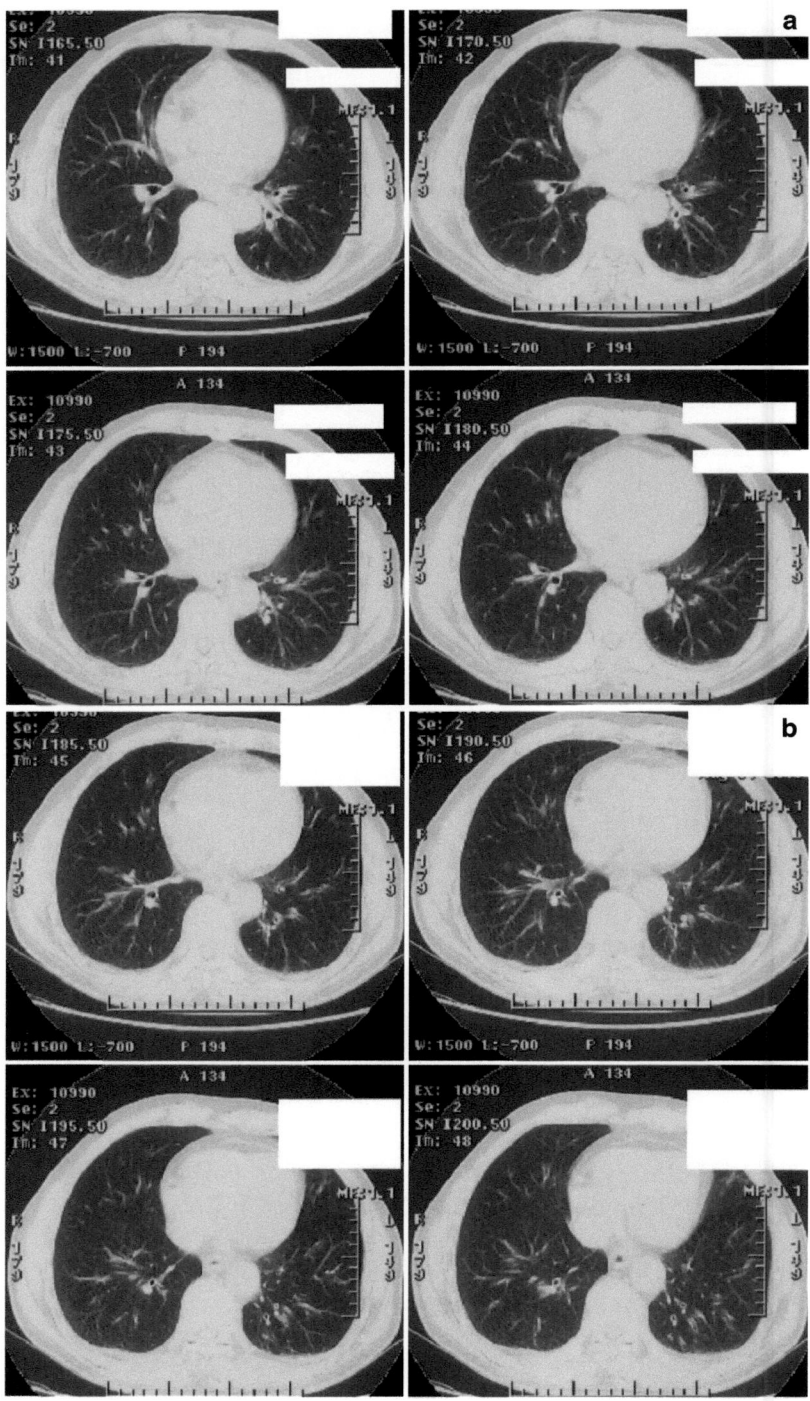

Fig. 7.4 (a–e)
Annotated at the figure
(yellow arrow)

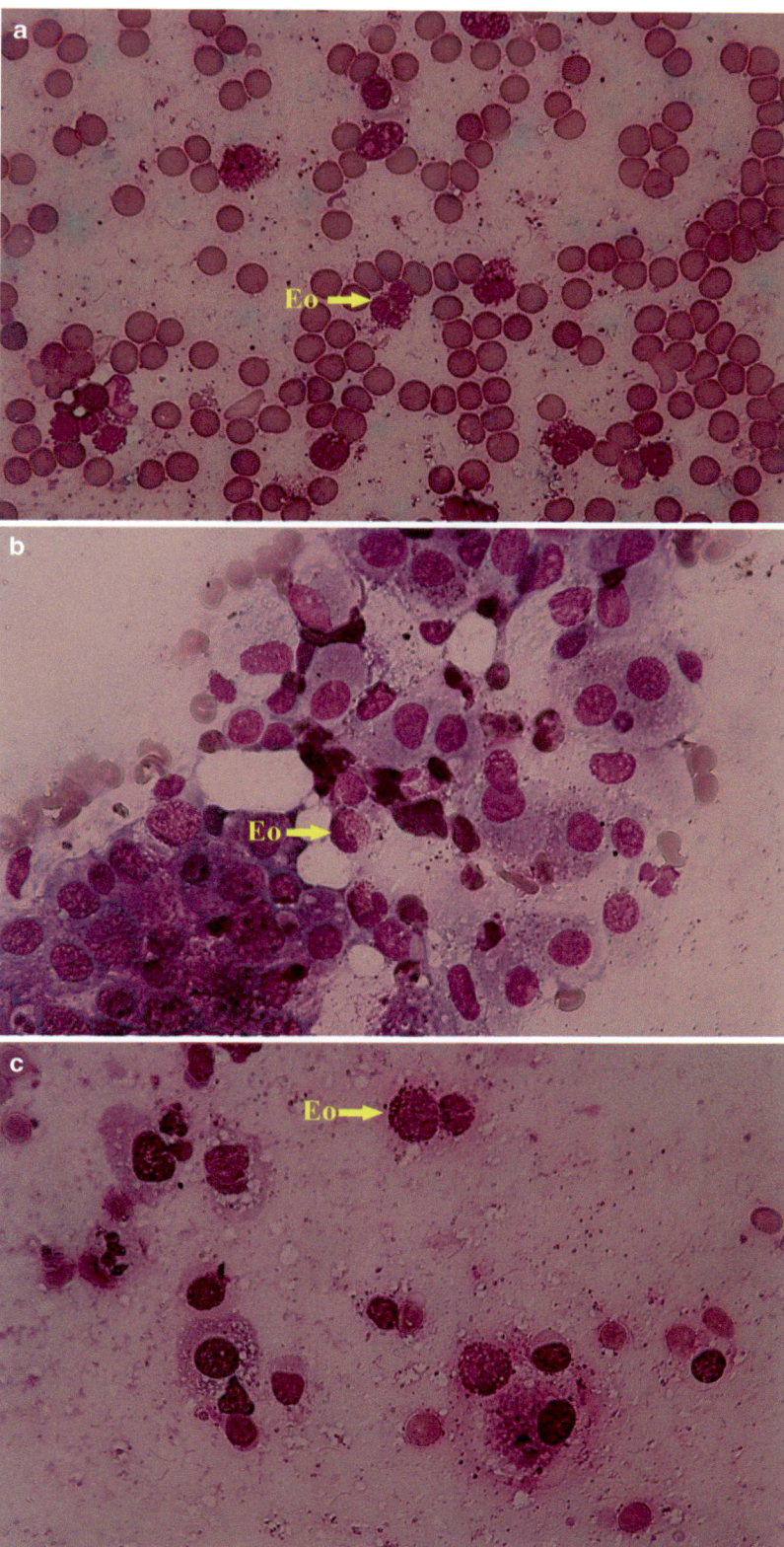

Fig. 7.4 (continued)

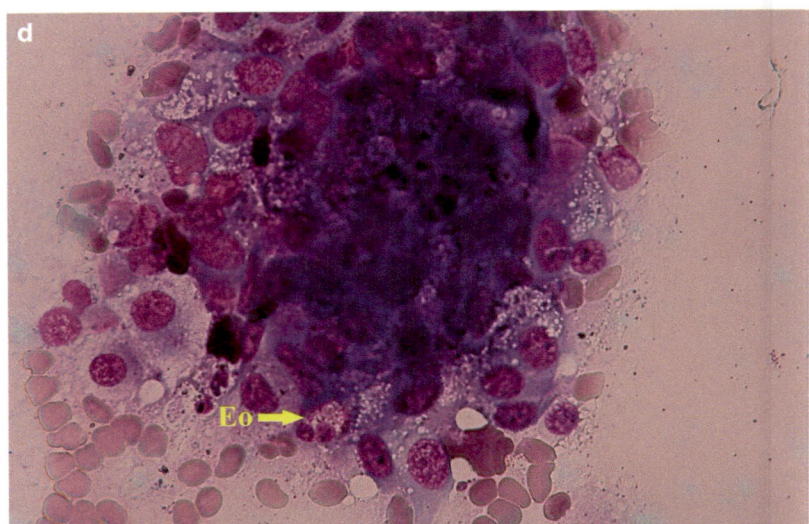

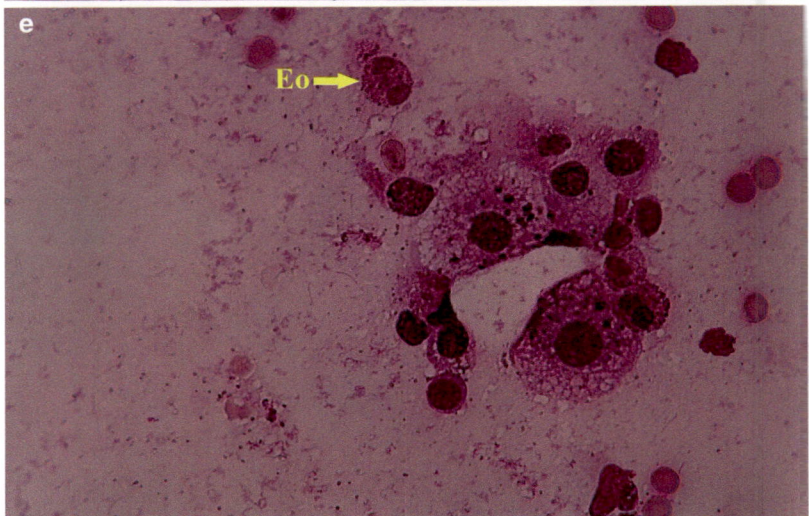

7.3 Pulmonary Infiltration with Eosinophilia (PIE) Case 3

Brief history: Male, 54 years old, persistent coughing with low fever, clinically diagnosed as pulmonary infiltration with eosinophilia (PIE).

Technology to obtain the target lesions: Transbronchial lung biopsy (TBLB).

The preparation of cytological slides for ROSE: Imprinting (rolling).

Clustering (categorizing) analysis in ROSE interpretation:

- "Inflammatory changes".
- Eosinophil-based immune inflammatory response.

Fig. 7.5 (**a**, **b**) Multiple patches, ground-glass opacities, tree-in-bud sign, and slight interstitial thickening in both lungs

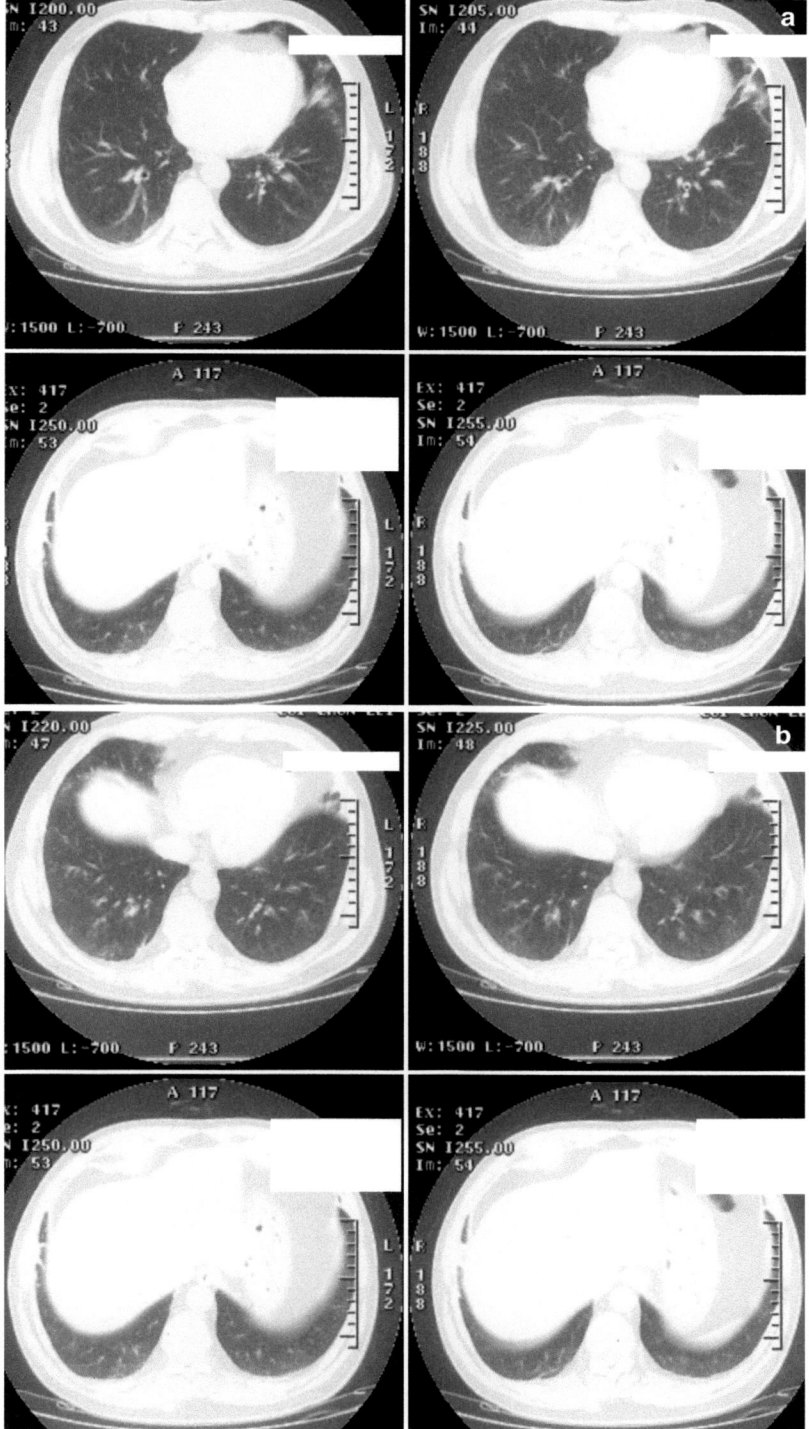

Fig. 7.6 (a–e)
Annotated at the figure
(yellow arrow)

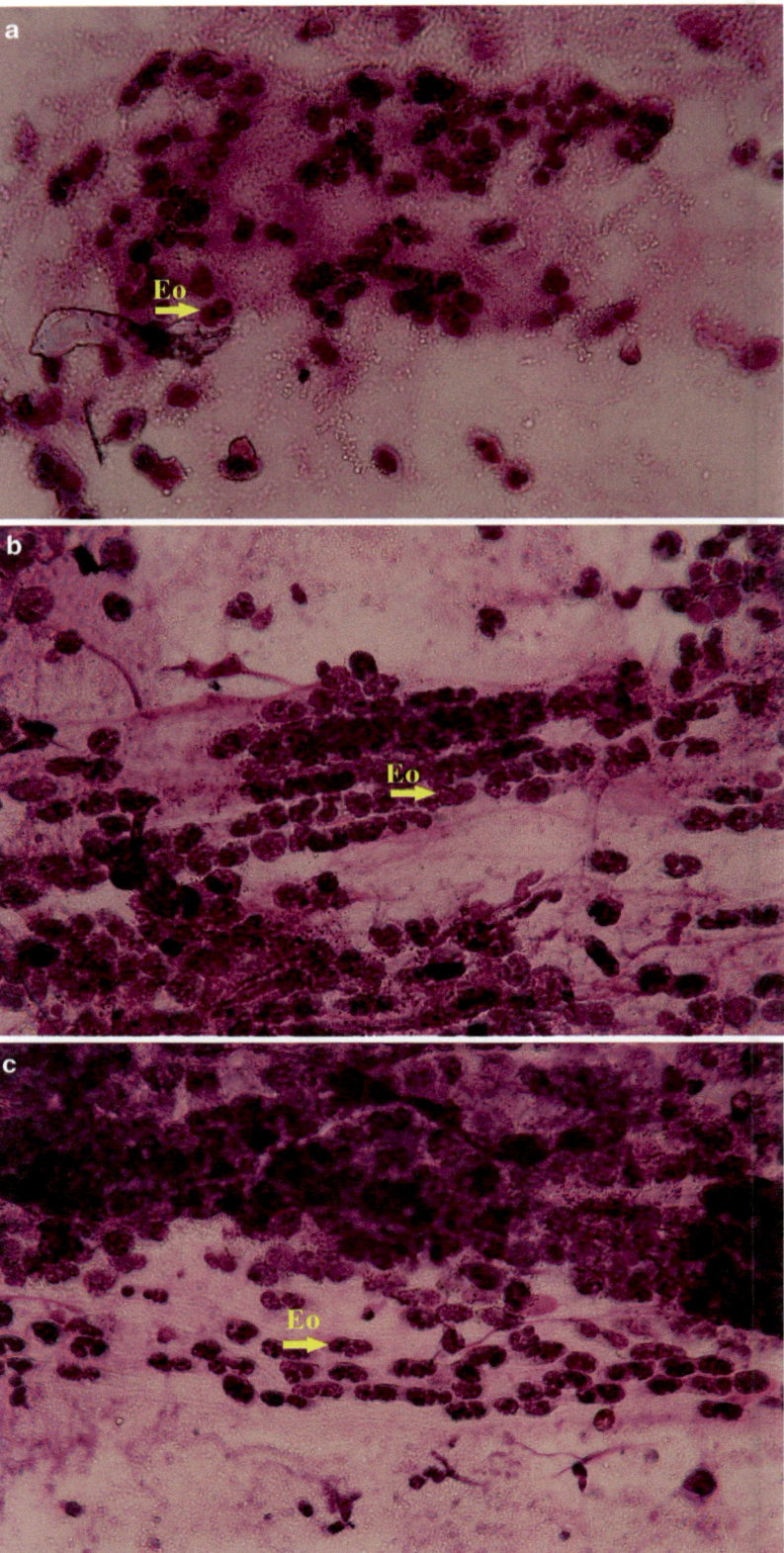

Fig. 7.6 (continued)

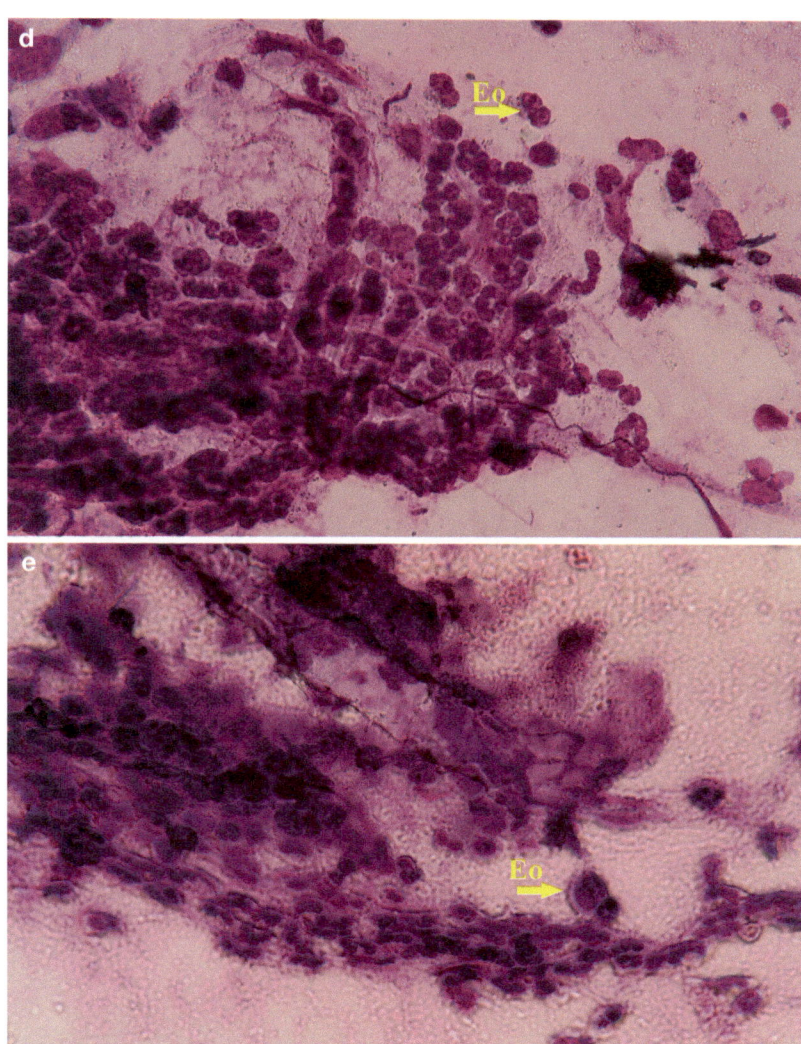

7.4 Hypersensitivity Pneumonitis

Brief history: Coughing for more than 2 months.

Technology to obtain the target lesions: Transbronchial lung biopsy (TBLB).

The preparation of cytological slides for ROSE: Imprinting (rolling).

Lymphocyte-based immune inflammatory response.

Eosinophil-based immune inflammatory response.

Fig. 7.7 (a, b) Interstitial thickening, interlobular septal thickening, scattered ground-glass opacities, patches, and consolidation, mainly in subpleural areas

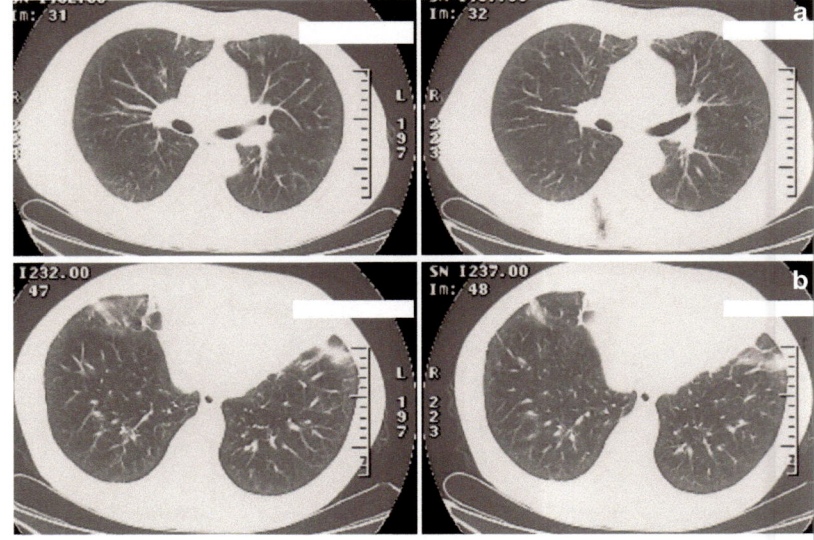

Fig. 7.8 (a, b) Eosinophils (yellow arrow); scattered neutrophils (red arrow); foamy macrophages, some evolving into histiocytes (green arrow); and lymphocytes (blue arrow)

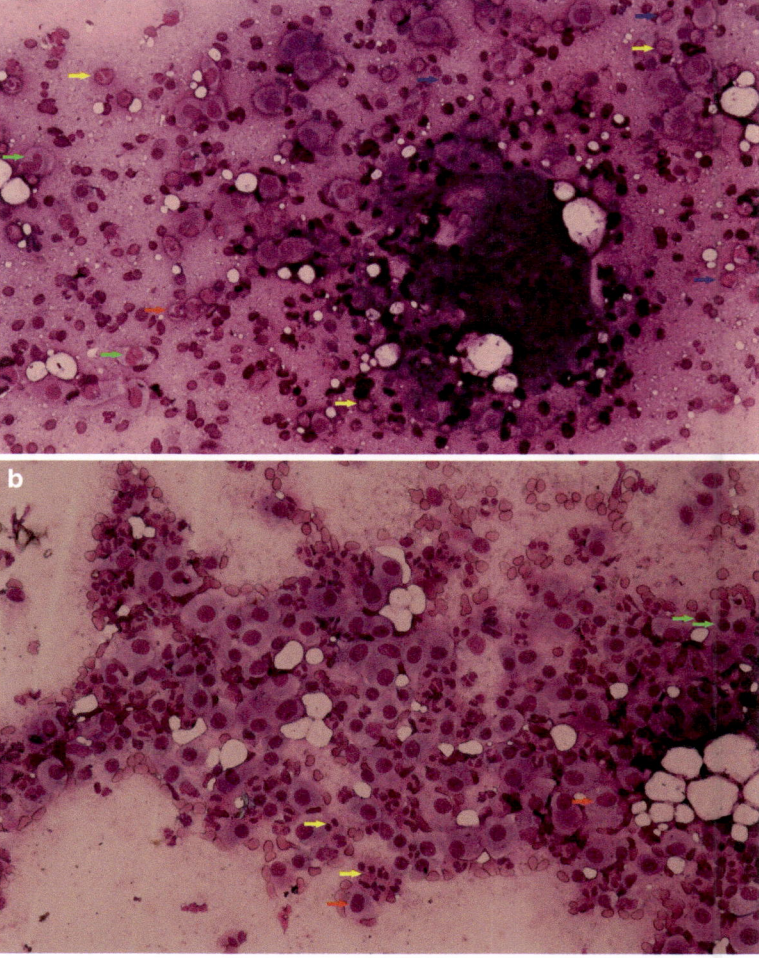

Fig. 7.9 Eosinophils (yellow arrow), histiocytes (red arrow), and lymphocytes (green arrow)

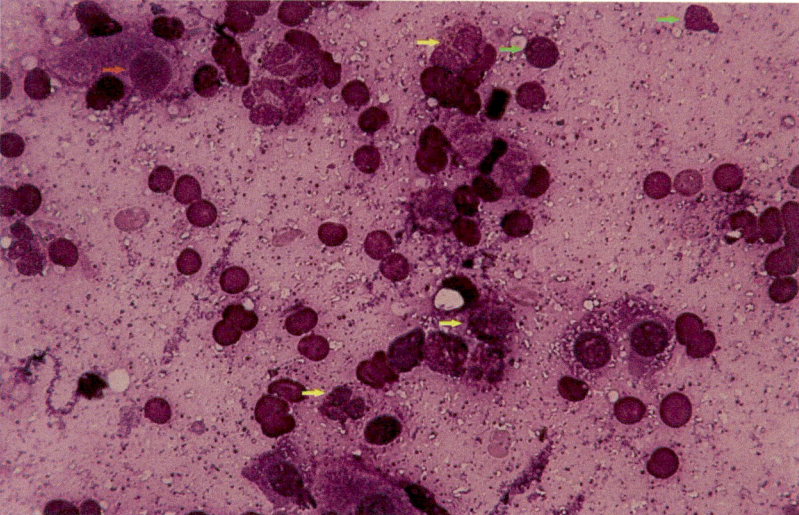

Fig. 7.10 Eosinophils (yellow arrow); foamy macrophages, some evolving into histiocytes (red arrow); and type II alveolar epithelial cell hyperplasia (green arrow)

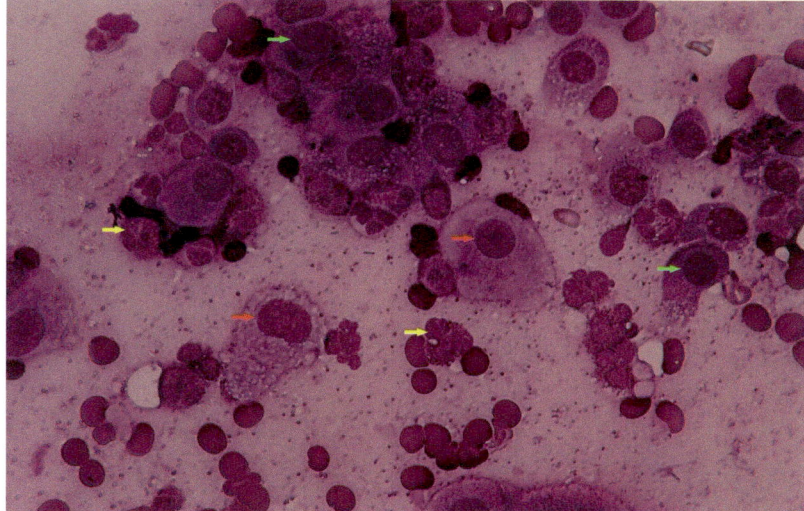

Fig. 7.11 Eosinophils
(yellow arrow), scattered
neutrophils (red arrow),
and foamy macrophages,
some evolving into
histiocytes (green arrow)

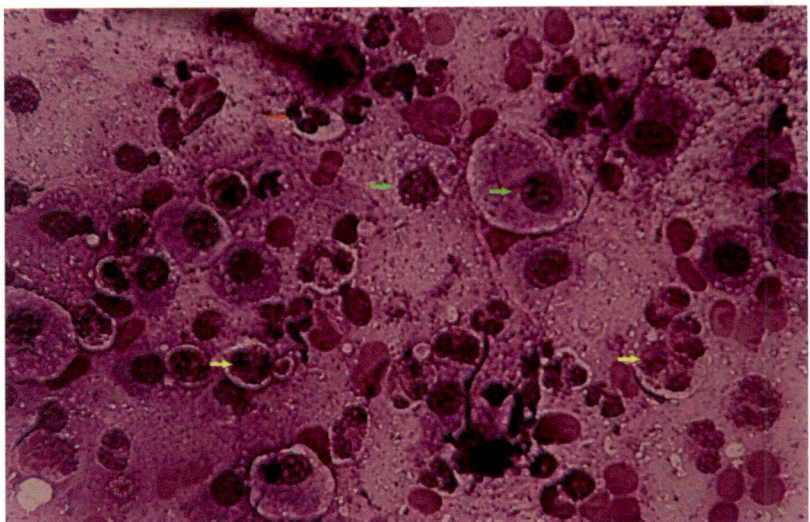

Fig. 7.12 Eosinophils
(yellow arrow), scattered
neutrophils (red arrow),
and lymphocytes (green
arrow)

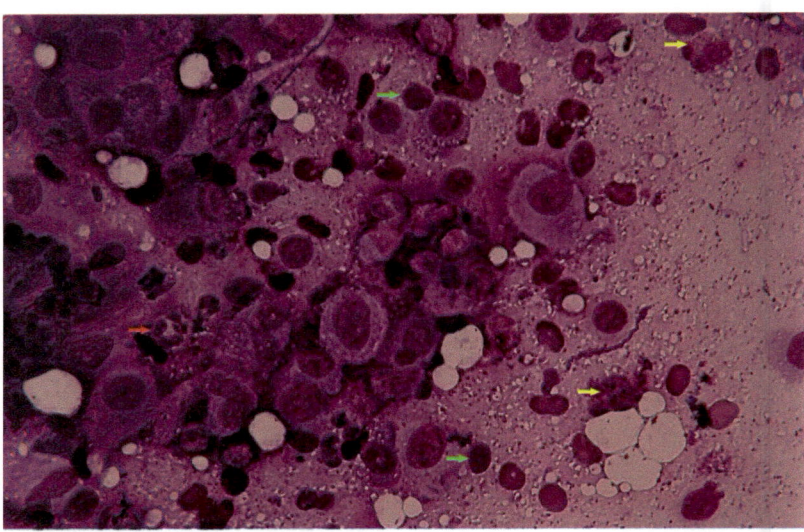

ROSE Cytopathology Cases of Connective Tissue Disease/ Interstitial Lung Diseases

8

Jing Feng, Jingyu Chen, and Wen Ning

8.1 Pulmonary Involvement from Connective Tissue Disease (Myositis)

Brief history: Coughing, shorting of breath after activity, clinically diagnosed as myositis.

Technology to obtain the target lesions: Transbronchial lung biopsy (TBLB).

The preparation of cytological slides for ROSE: Imprinting (rolling).

Clustering (categorizing) analysis in ROSE interpretation:

- "Inflammatory changes".
- May conform to fibrosis (fibroblast dominant or fibrocyte dominant).
- Lymphocyte-based immune inflammatory response.
- Necrotic "Inflammatory changes".

J. Feng
Pulmonary and Critical Care Medicine, Tianjin
Medical University General Hospital, Tianjin, China
e-mail: zyyhxkfj@126.com

J. Chen
Lung Transplantation Group, Nanjing Medical
University, Wuxi, China
e-mail: chenjy@wuxiph.com

W. Ning (✉)
College of Life Sciences, Nankai University
Tianjin, China
e-mail: ningwen108@nankai.edu.cn

© Springer Nature Singapore Pte Ltd. 2020
J. Feng et al. (eds.), *Rapid On-Site Evaluation (ROSE) in Diagnostic Interventional Pulmonology*,
https://doi.org/10.1007/978-981-15-0939-1_8

Fig. 8.1 Subpleural interstitial thickening in both upper lungs and interlobular septal thickening

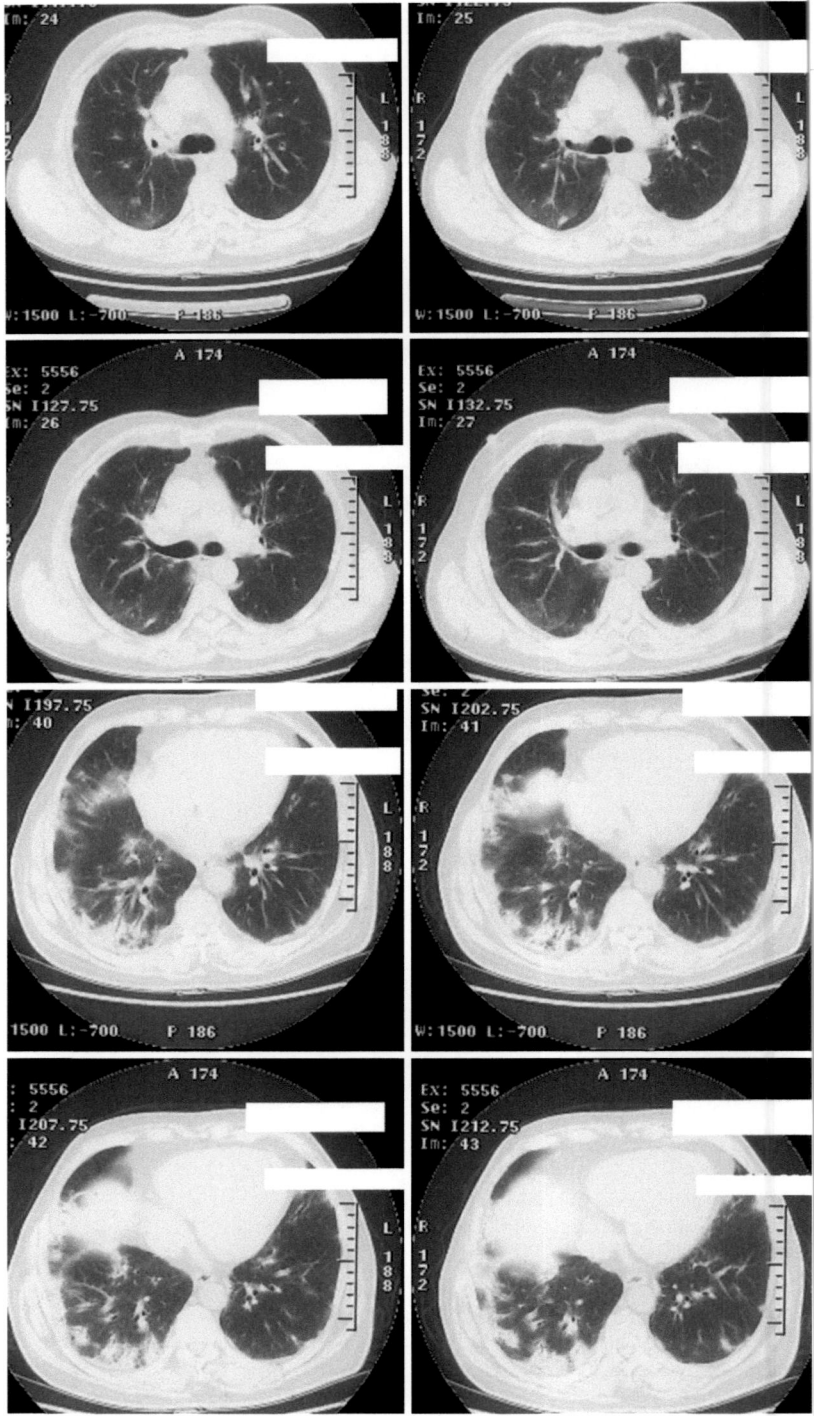

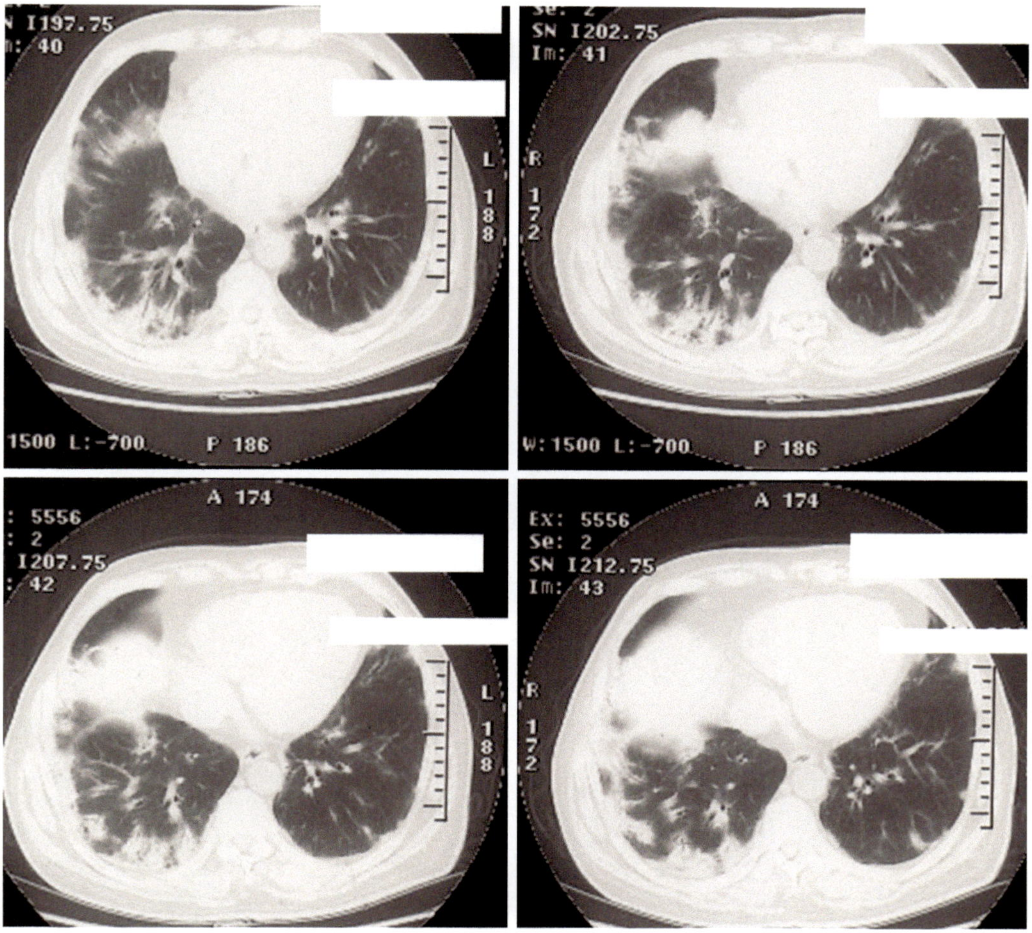

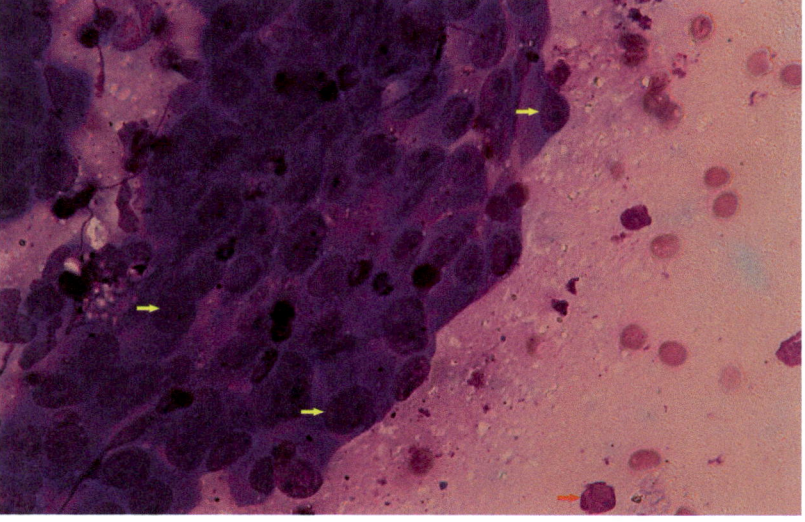

Fig. 8.2 Subpleural interstitial thickening in both upper lungs with interlobular septal thickening, patches, and consolidation and air bronchograms more severe than those in both upper lungs

Fig. 8.3 Fibroblasts (yellow arrow), serial arrangement, forming sheets (red arrow), and reactive lymphocytes (green arrow)

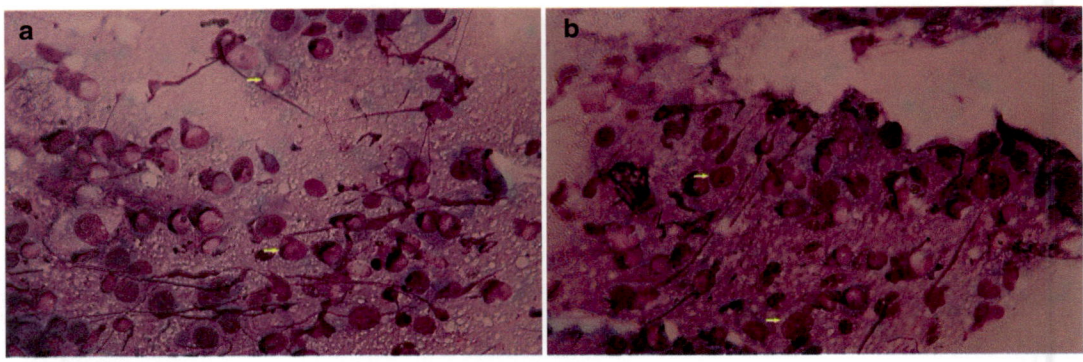

Fig. 8.4 (**a**, **b**) Lots of reactive lymphocytes (yellow arrow)

Fig. 8.5 Lots of reactive lymphocytes (yellow arrow) and necrosis (red arrow)

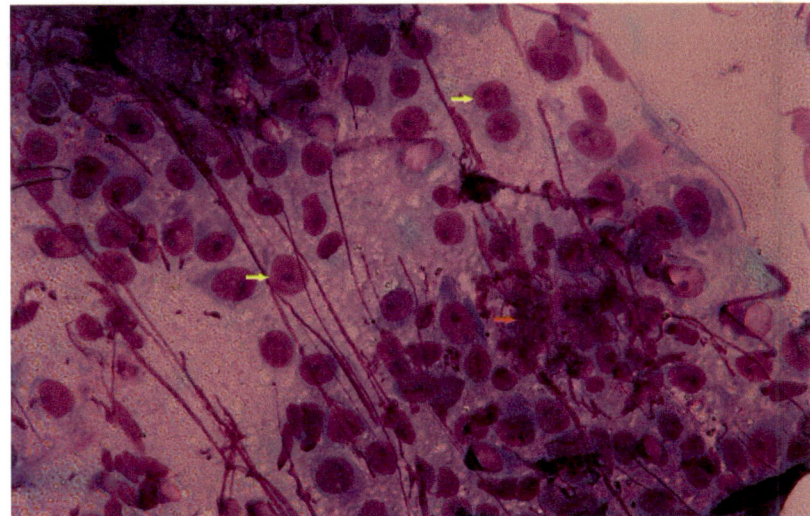

Fig. 8.6 Fibroblasts, serial arrangement, forming sheets (yellow arrow), and reactive lymphocytes (red arrow)

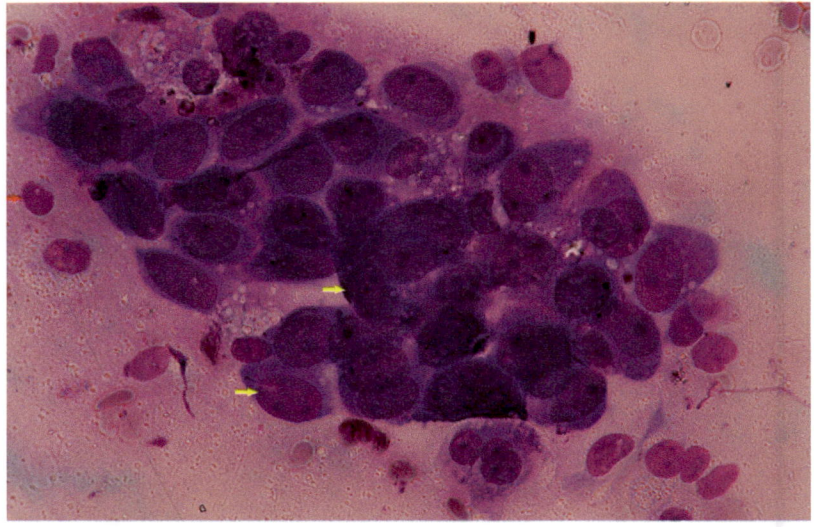

Fig. 8.7 Fibroblasts, serial arrangement, forming sheets (yellow arrow)

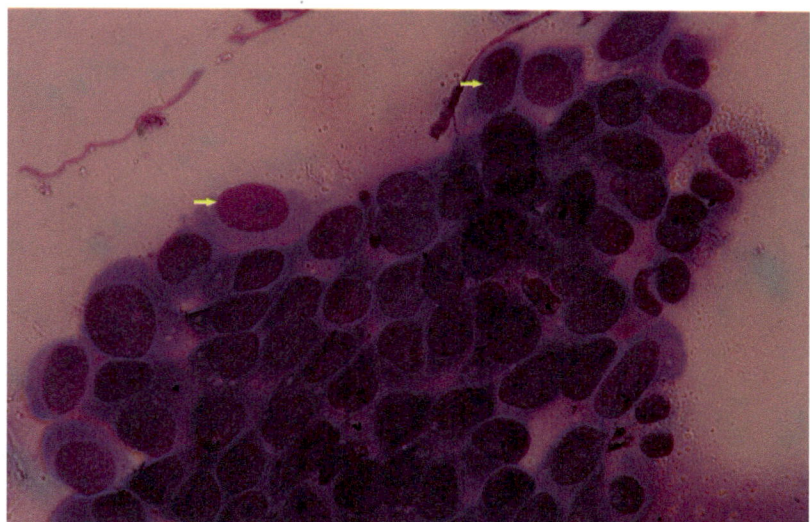

Fig. 8.8 Fibroblasts, serial arrangement, forming sheets (yellow arrow), and reactive lymphocytes (red arrow)

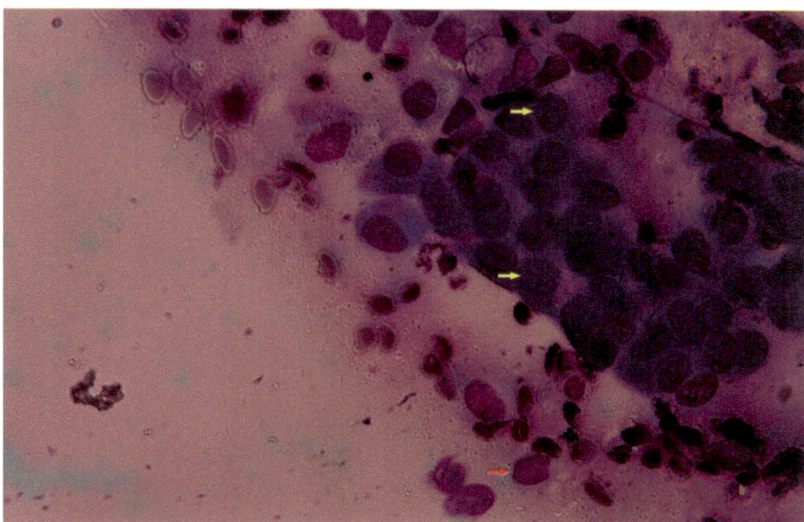

Fig. 8.9 Proliferation, degeneration, necrosis, and denaturation of distal airway epithelial cells (yellow arrow) and reactive lymphocytes (red arrow)

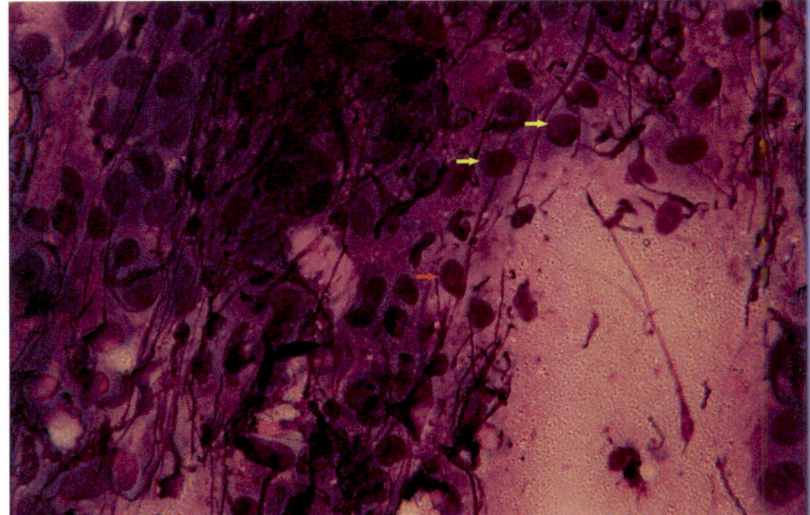

Fig. 8.10 Proliferation, degeneration, necrosis, and denaturation of distal airway epithelial cells (yellow arrow) and obvious necrosis (red arrow)

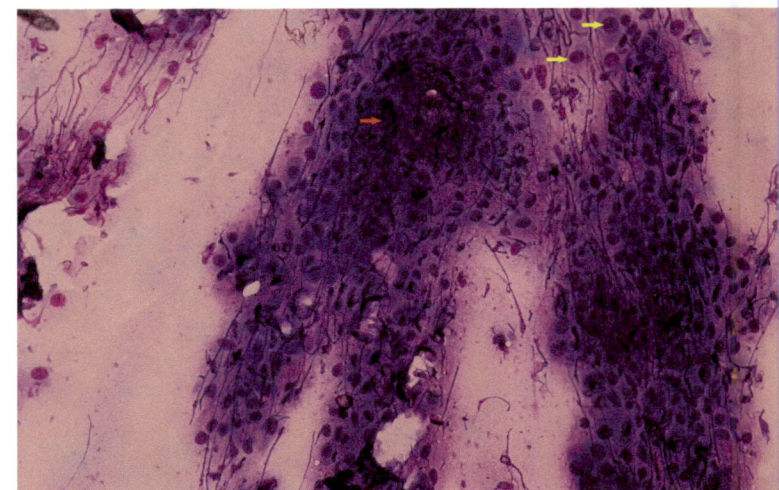

Fig. 8.11 Fibroblasts, serial arrangement, forming sheets (yellow arrow), and reactive lymphocytes (red arrow)

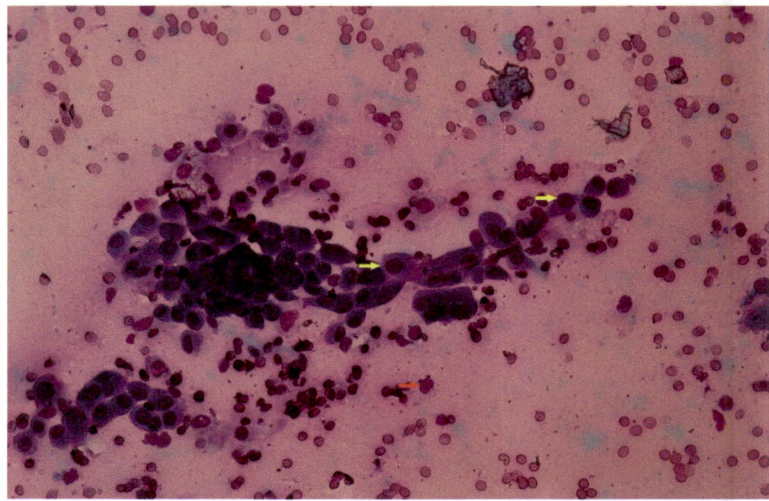

Fig. 8.12 (a, b)
Fibroblasts, serial
arrangement, forming
sheets (yellow arrow)

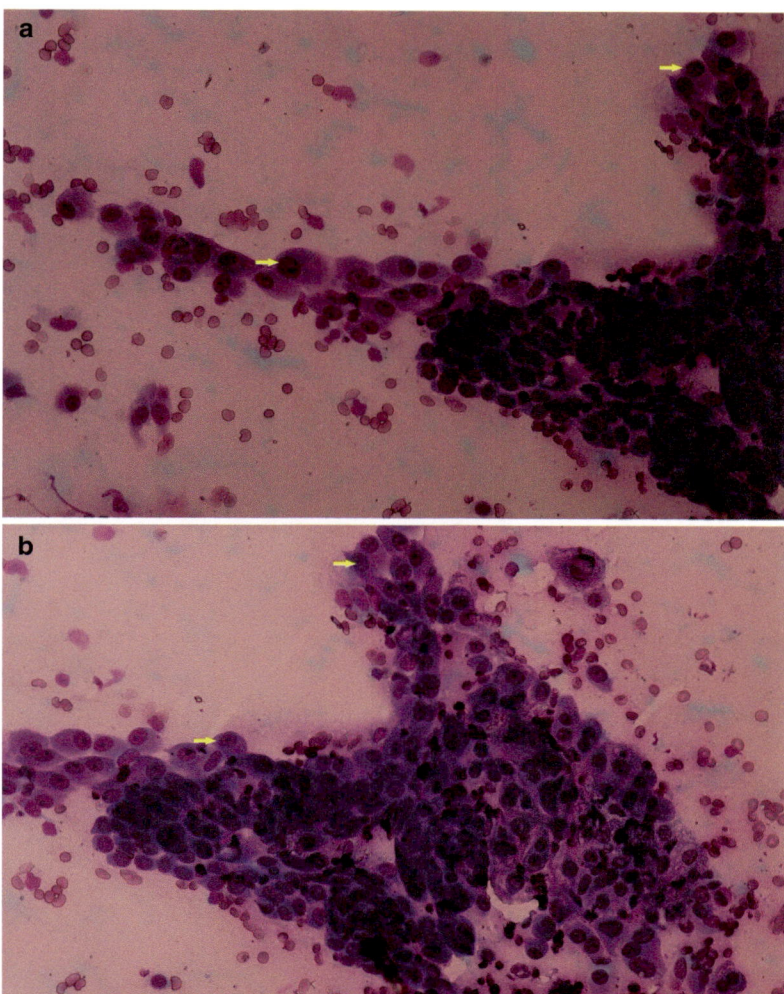

Fig. 8.13 Fibroblasts,
serial arrangement,
forming sheets (yellow
arrow), and reactive
lymphocytes (red arrow)

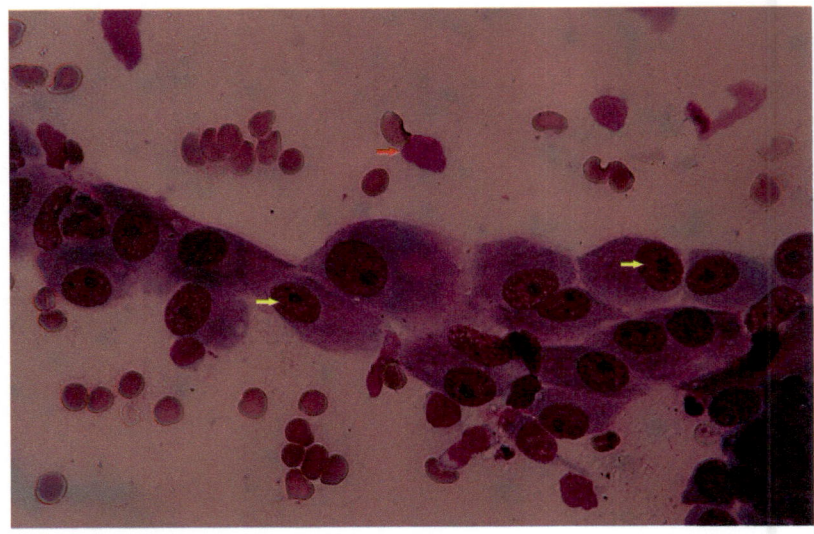

Fig. 8.14 Fibroblasts,
serial arrangement,
forming sheets (yellow
arrow)

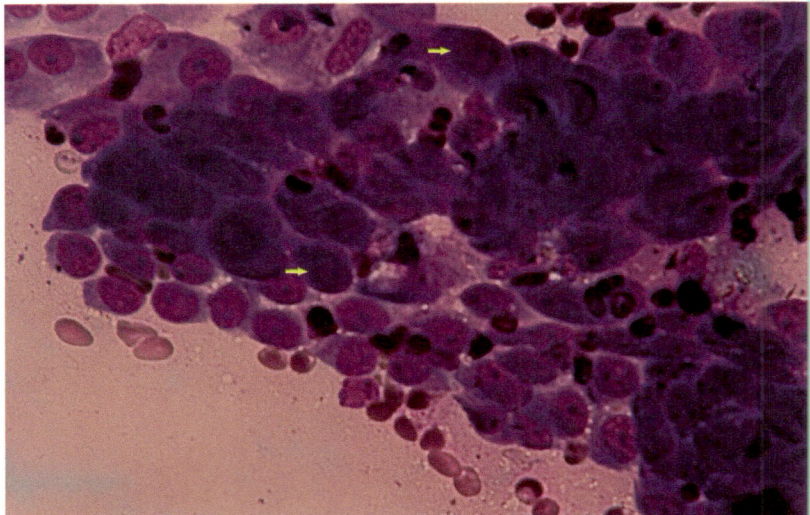

Fig. 8.15 (a–c) Fibroblasts, serial arrangement, forming sheets (yellow arrow), and reactive lymphocytes (red arrow)

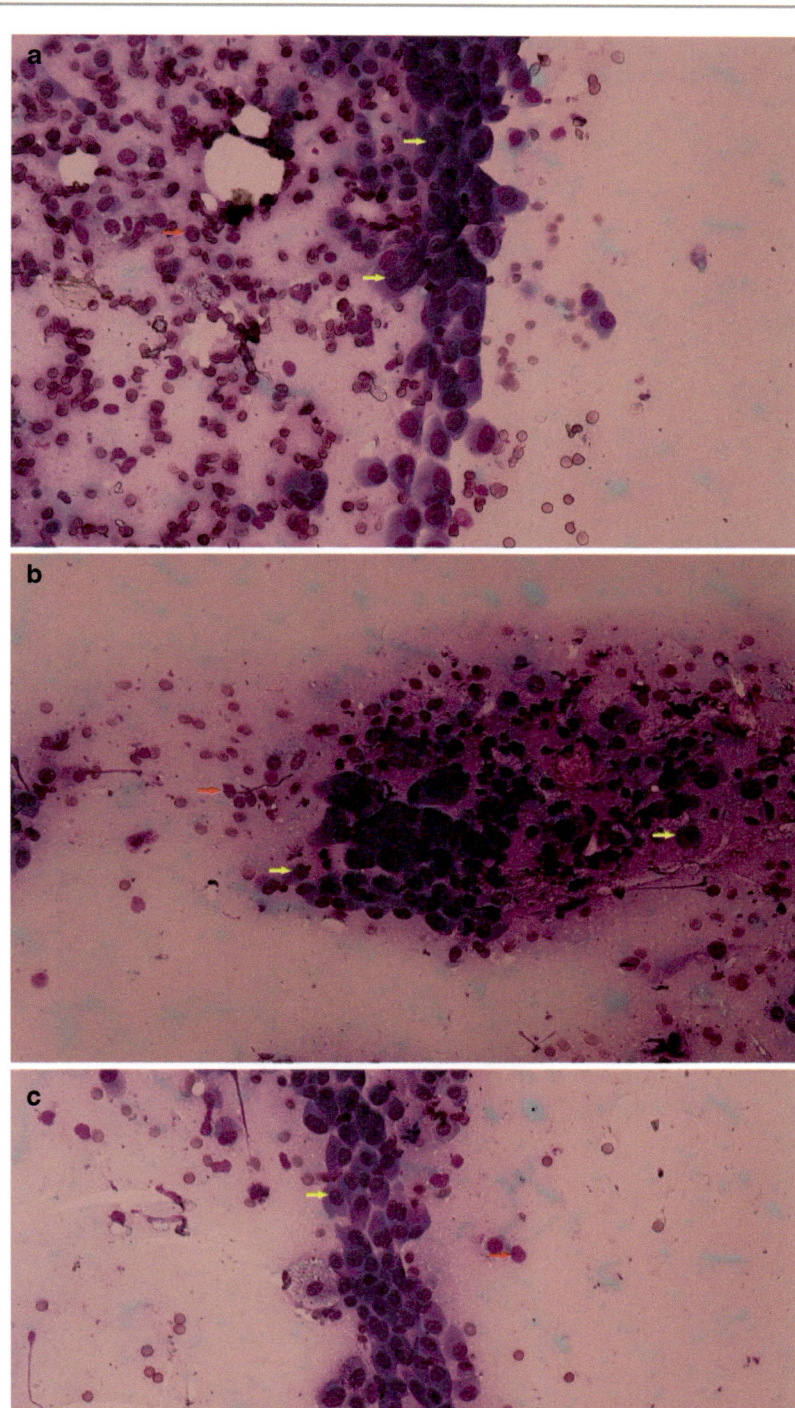

Fig. 8.16 Fibroblasts, serial arrangement, forming sheets (yellow arrow)

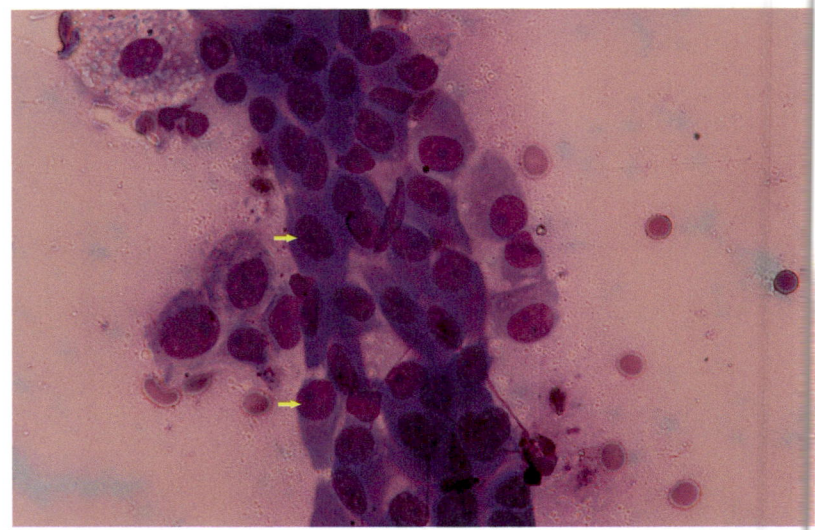

Fig. 8.17 (a–d) Fibroblasts, serial arrangement, forming sheets (yellow arrow), and reactive lymphocytes (red arrow)

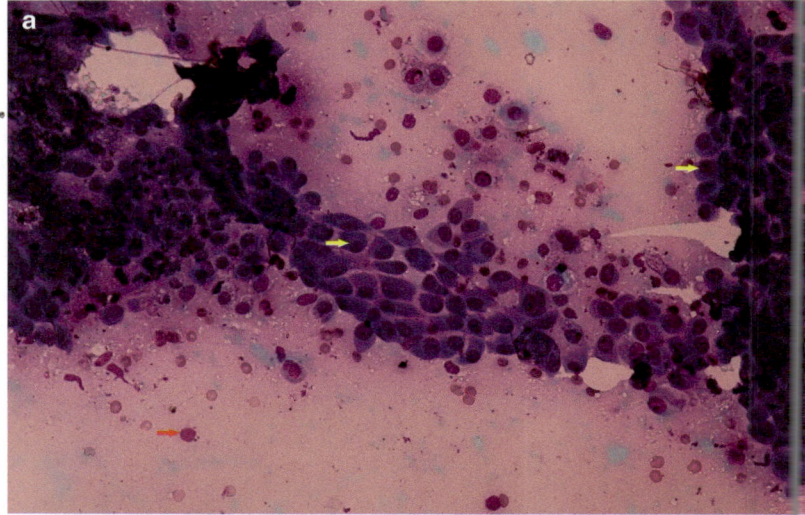

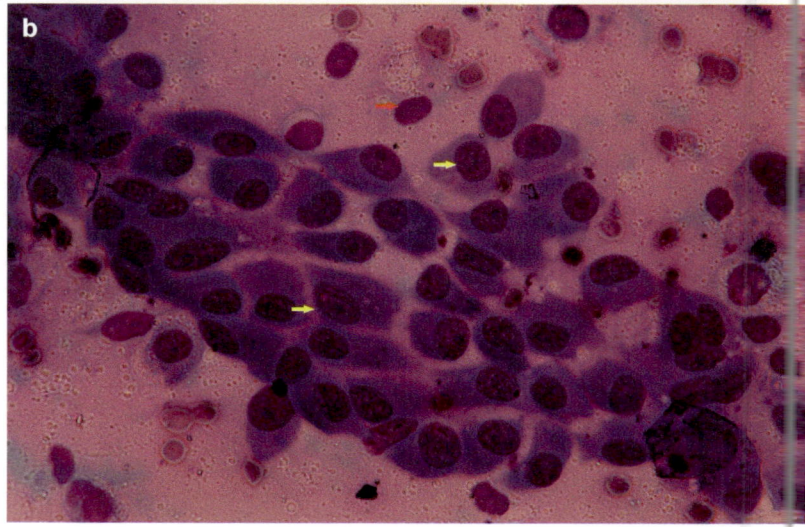

Fig. 8.17 (continued)

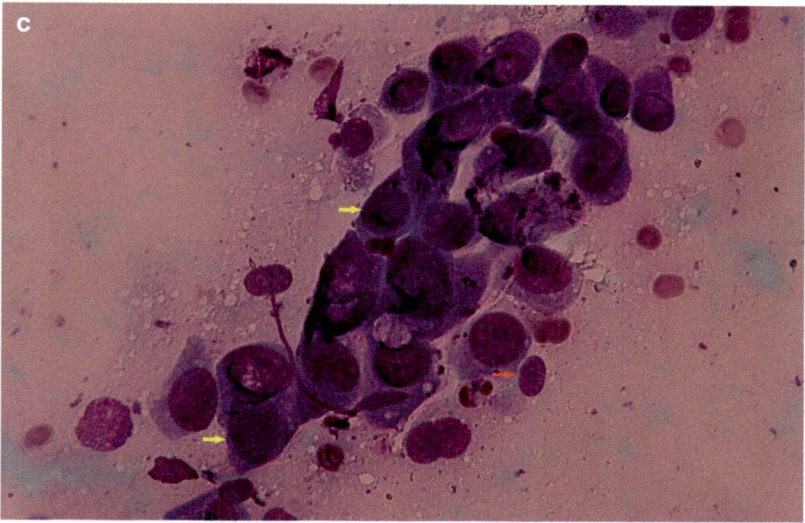

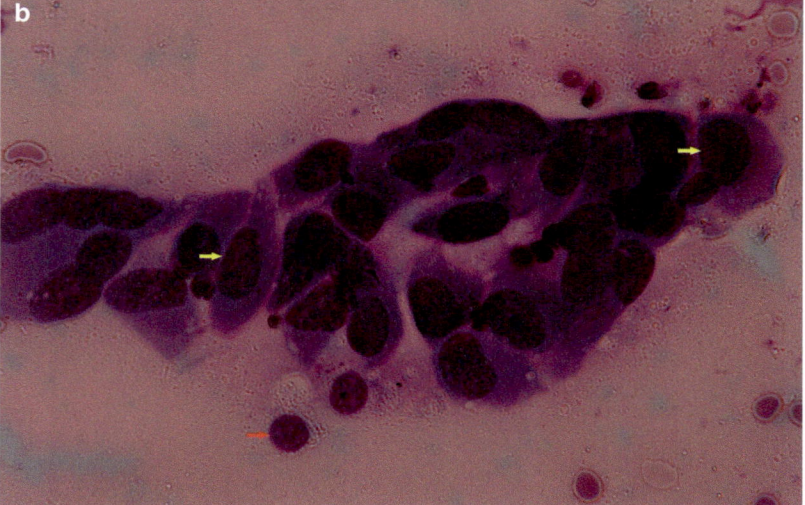

Fig. 8.18 (**a–c**) Lots of reactive lymphocytes (yellow arrow) and proliferation, degeneration, necrosis, and denaturation of distal airway epithelial cells (red arrow)

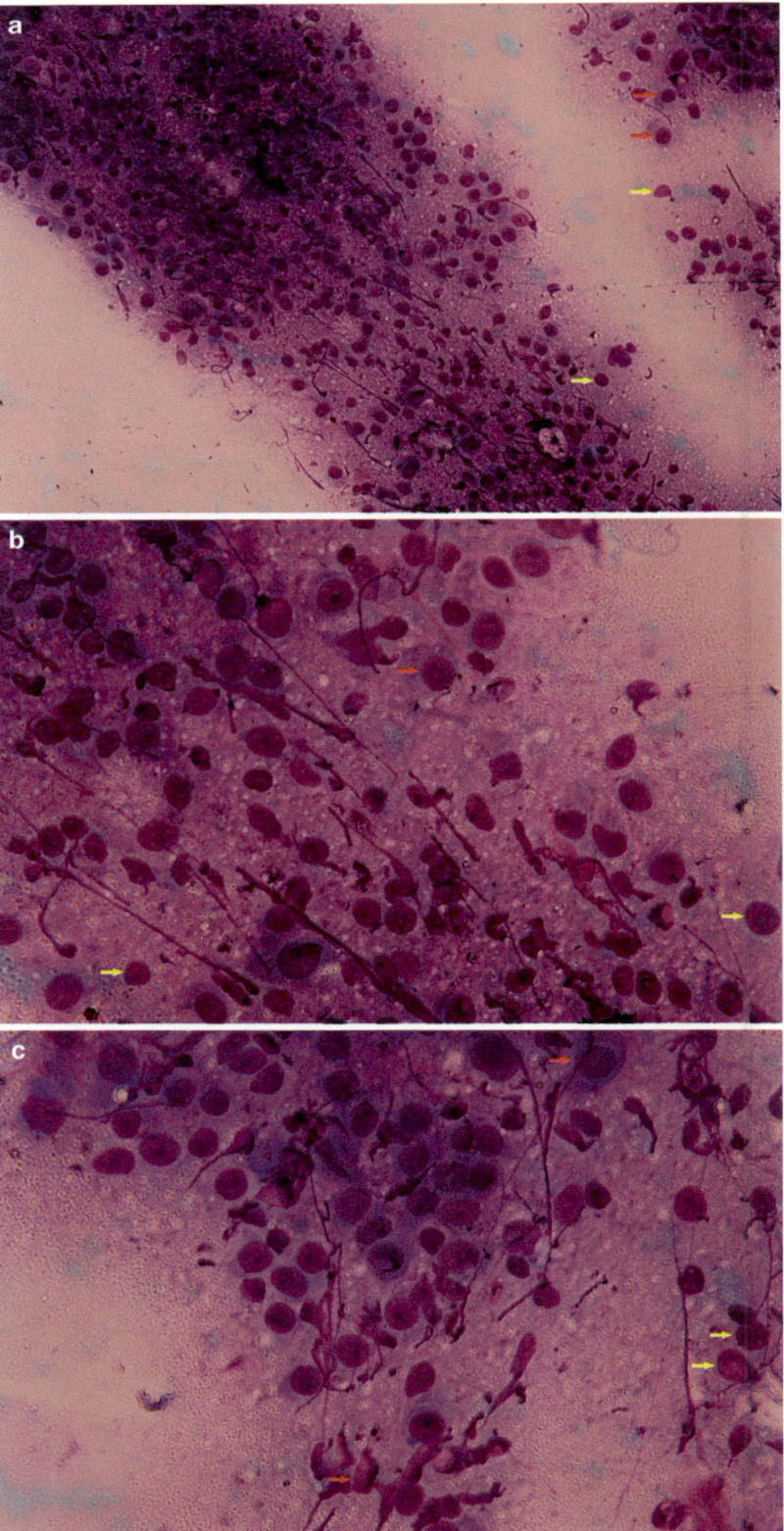

Fig. 8.19 (a, b) Proliferation, degeneration, necrosis, and denaturation of distal airway epithelial cells (yellow arrow)

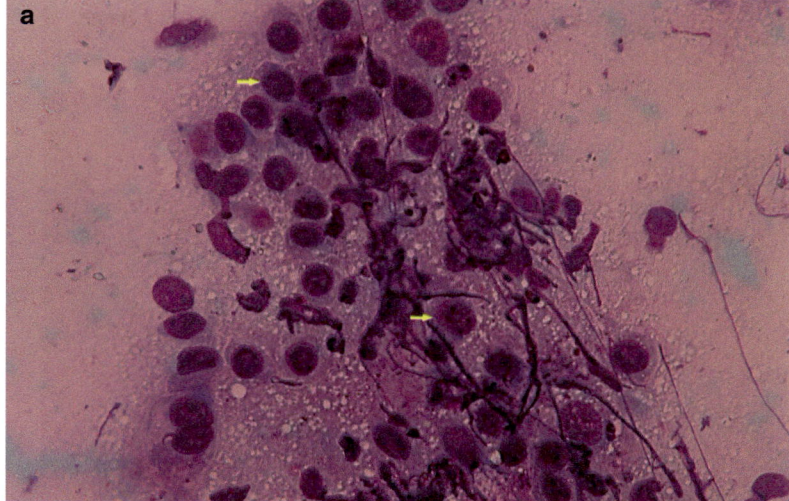

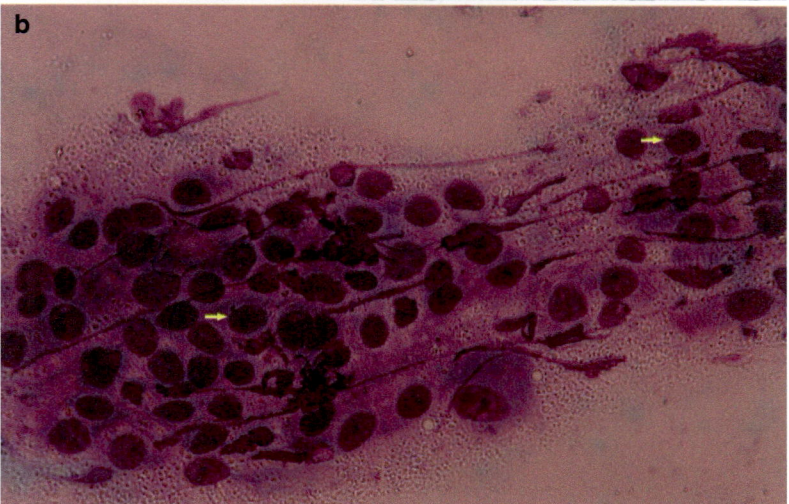

Fig. 8.20 Fibroblasts, serial arrangement, forming sheets (yellow arrow)

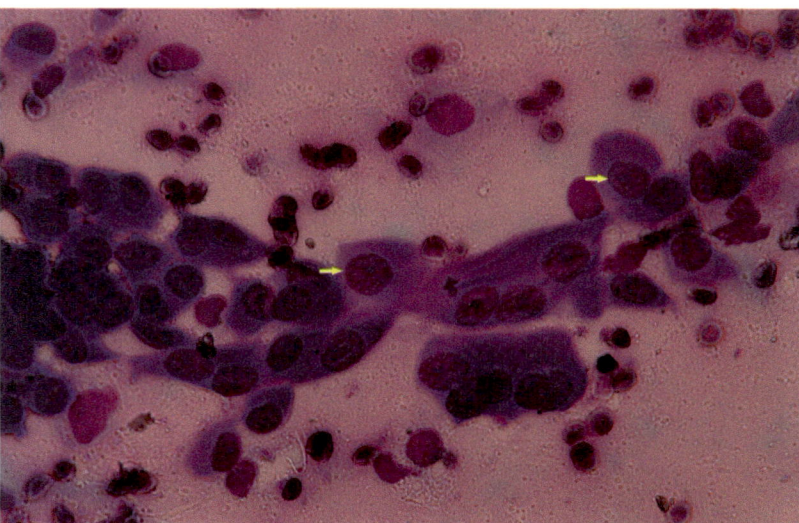

Fig. 8.21 (a, b)
Fibroblasts, serial
arrangement, forming
sheets (yellow arrow),
and proliferation,
degeneration, necrosis,
and denaturation of
distal airway epithelial
cells (red arrow)

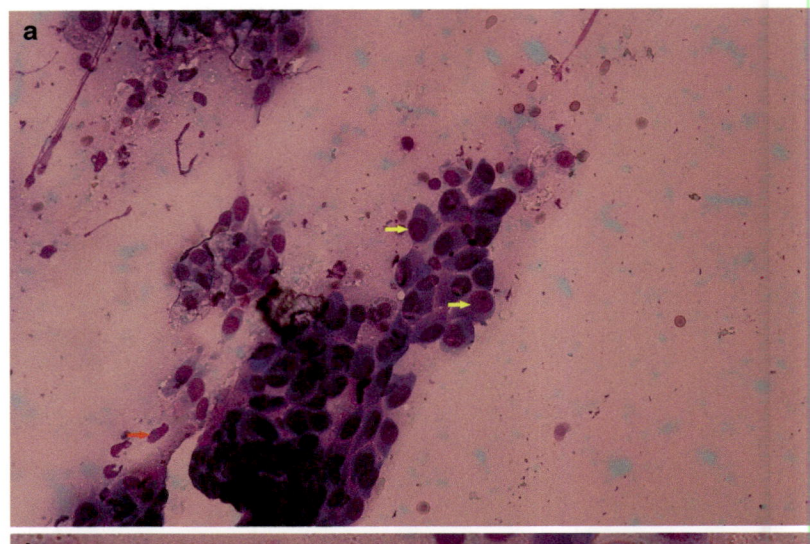

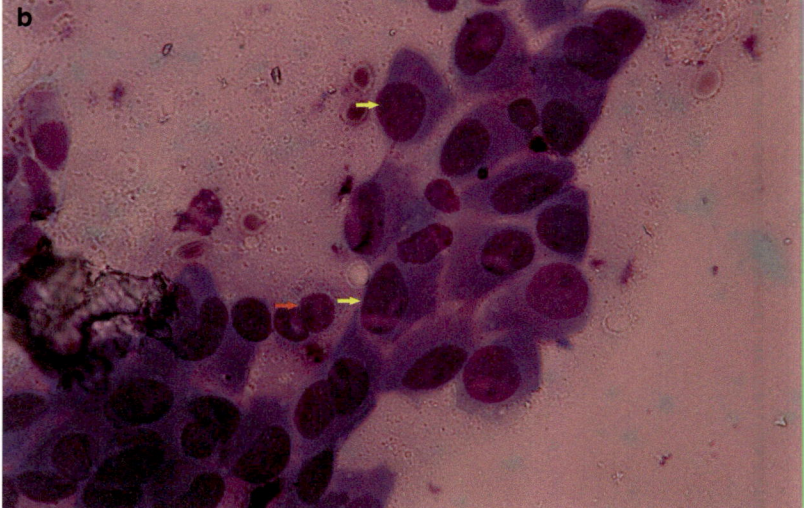

Fig. 8.22 (**a**, **b**) Fibroblasts, serial arrangement, forming sheets (yellow arrow), and reactive lymphocytes (red arrow)

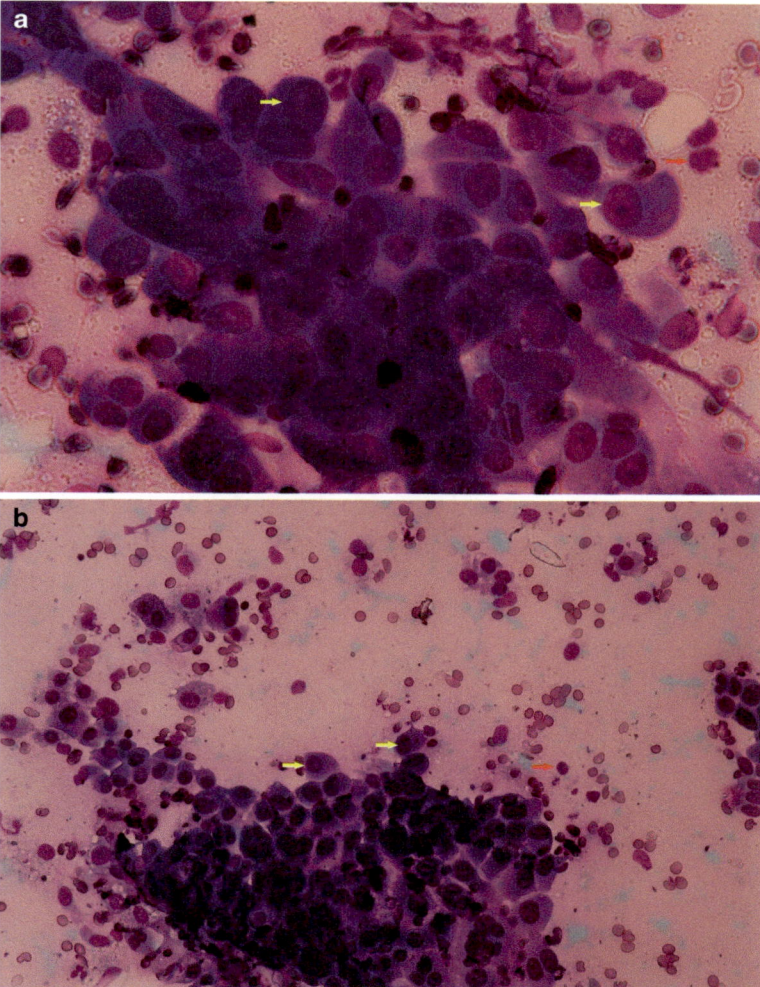

Fig. 8.23 Fibroblasts, serial arrangement, forming sheets (yellow arrow), and proliferation, degeneration, necrosis, and denaturation of distal airway epithelial cells (red arrow)

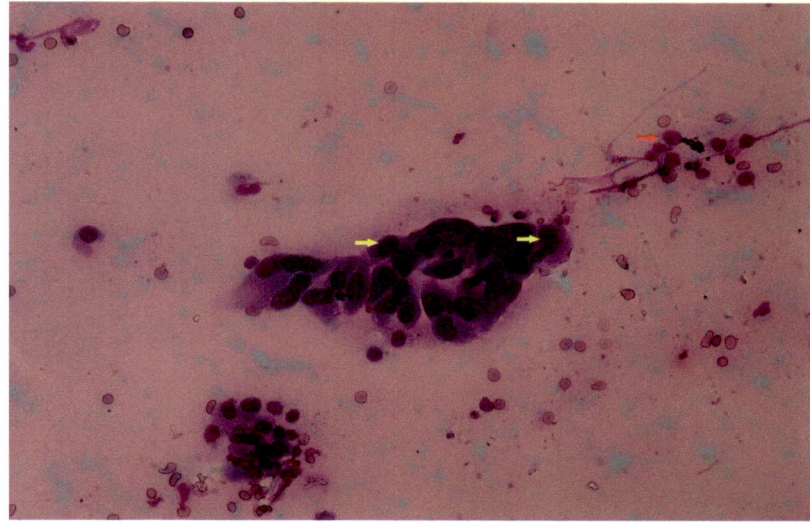

8.2   Pulmonary Involvement from Myositis

Brief history: Female, 59 years old, persistent coughing with shortness of breath for nearly a week, running a fever for 3 days, clinically diagnosed as myositis.

Technology to obtain the target lesions: Transbronchial lung biopsy (TBLB).

The preparation of cytological slides for ROSE: Imprinting (rolling).

Clustering (categorizing) analysis in ROSE interpretation:

- "Inflammatory changes".
- Granulomatous inflammation.
- Lymphocyte-based immune inflammatory response.

Fig. 8.24 (a, b) Multiple patches, consolidation, and air bronchogram in both lungs, slight interstitial thickening distributed along the bronchovascular bundles or subpleural areas, and large area of confluent consolidation and exudation in the left lower lobe

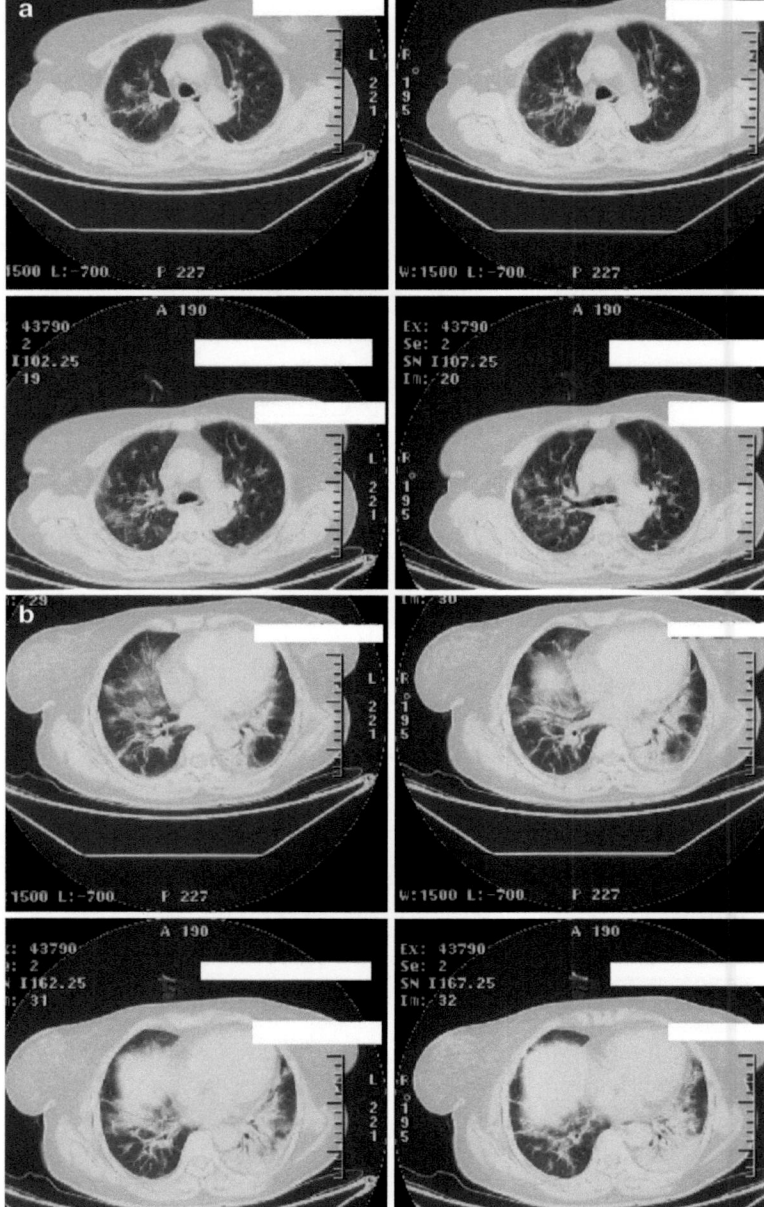

Fig. 8.25 (a–e)
Annotated at the figure
(yellow arrow)

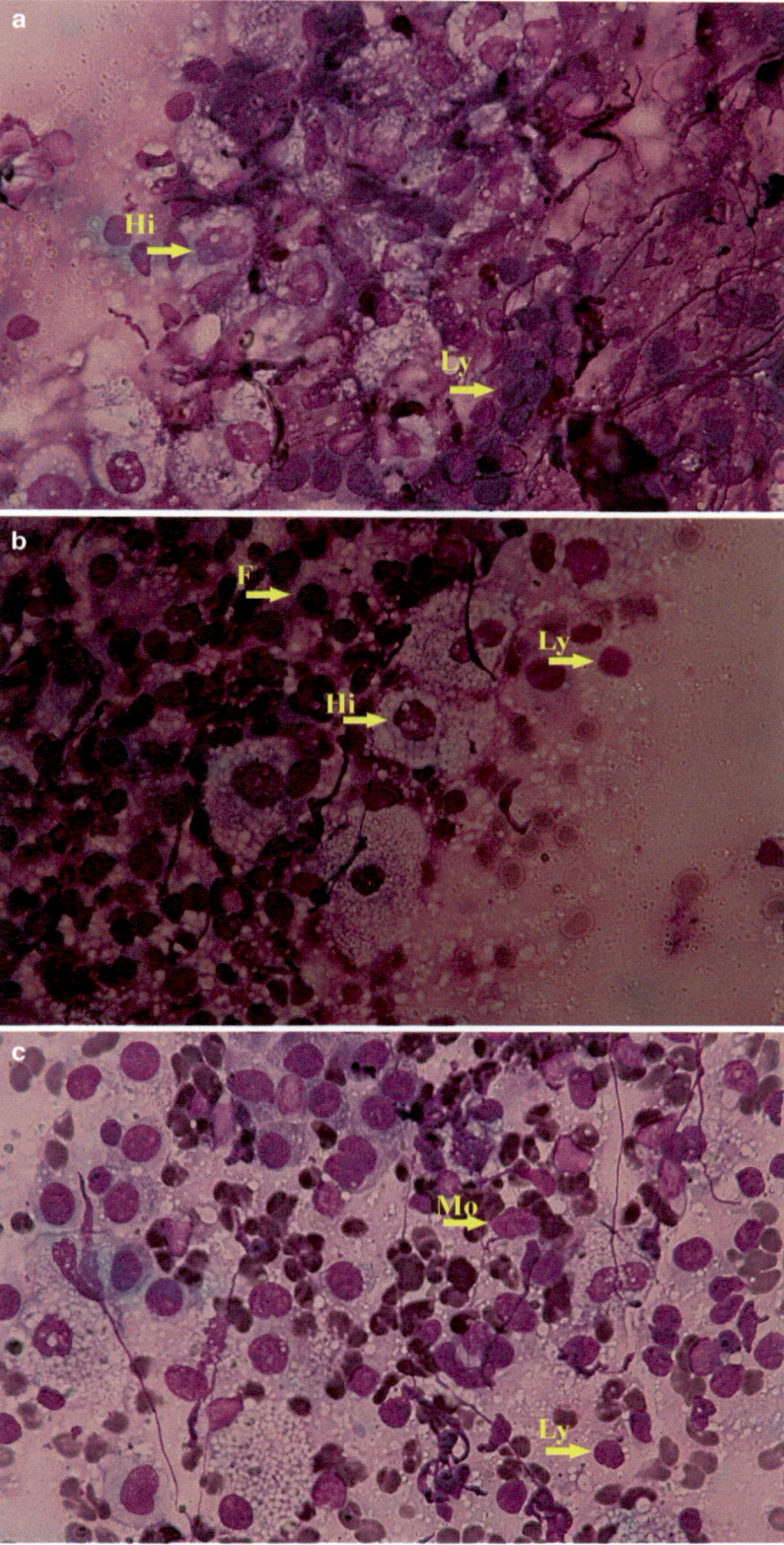

Fig. 8.25 (continued)

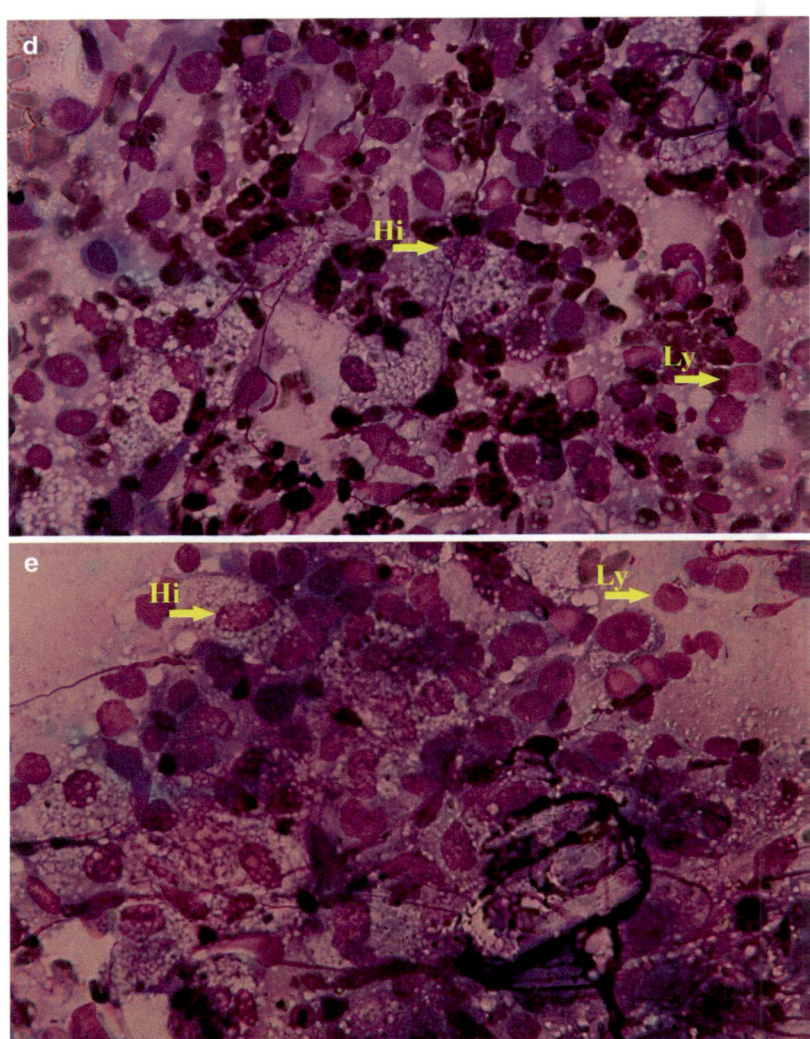

8.3 Pulmonary Involvement from Systemic Lupus Erythematosus (SLE)

Brief history: Coughing with shortness of breath for more than 2 weeks, clinically diagnosed as systemic lupus erythematosus (SLE).

Technology to obtain the target lesions: Transbronchial lung biopsy (TBLB).

The preparation of cytological slides for ROSE: Imprinting (rolling).

Clustering (categorizing) analysis in ROSE interpretation:

- "Inflammatory changes".
- May conform to fibrosis (fibroblast dominant or fibrocyte dominant).
- Lymphocyte-based immune inflammatory response.

Fig. 8.26 (**a, b**) Extensive ground-glass opacities, slight interstitial thickening in both lungs, and large subpleural areas of confluent consolidation and exudation in the left lower lungs

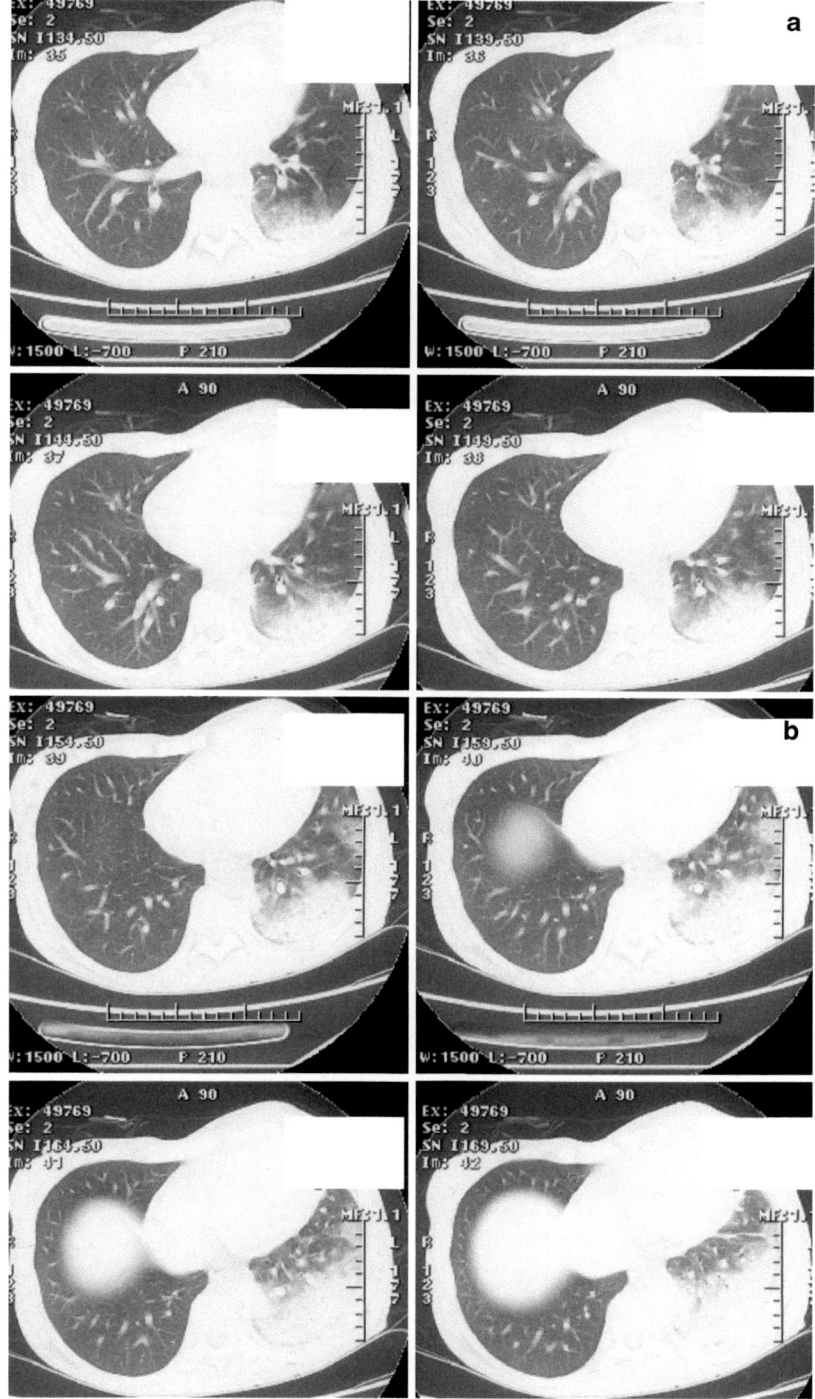

Fig. 8.27 (a–e)
Annotated at the figure
(yellow arrow)

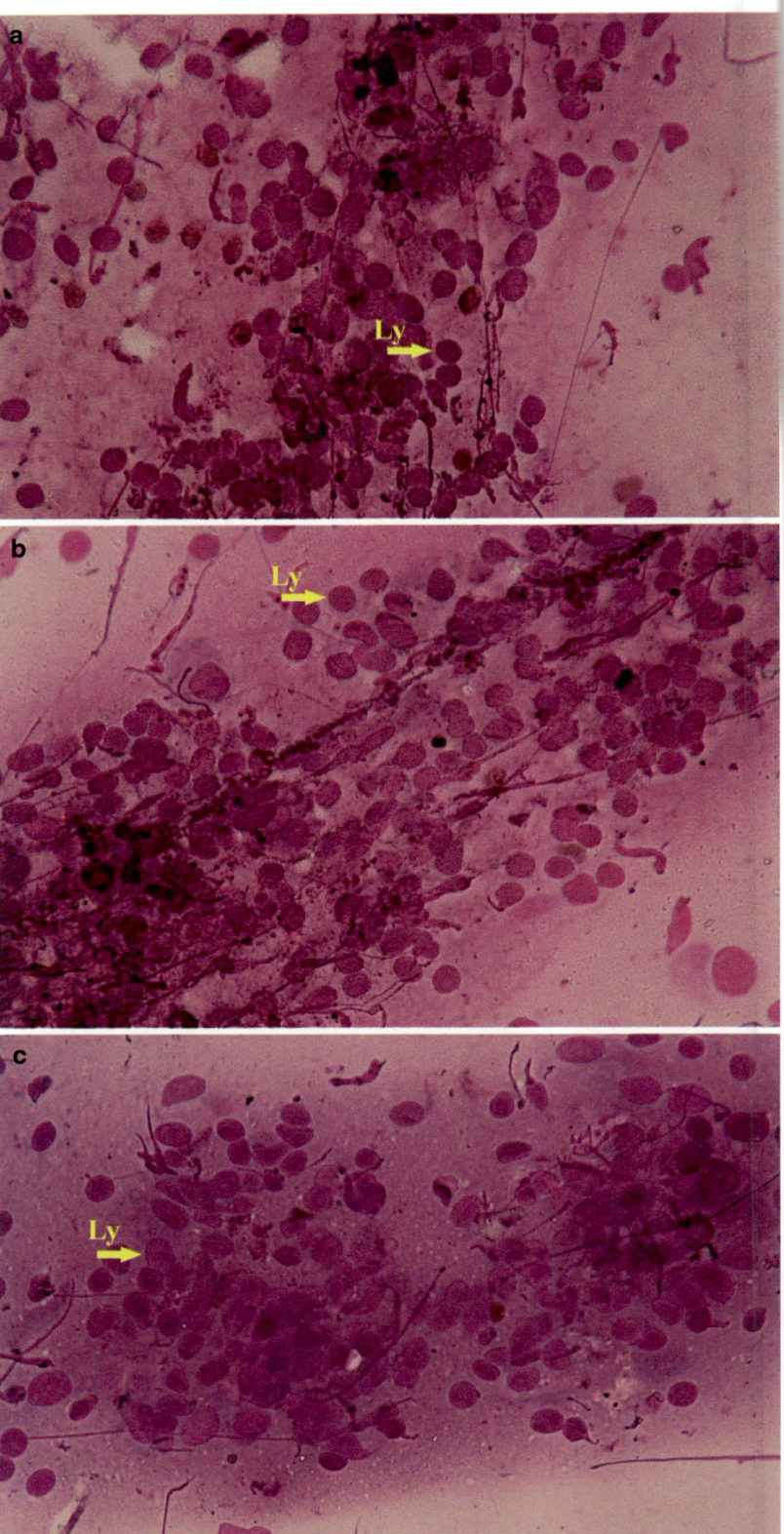

Fig. 8.27 (continued)

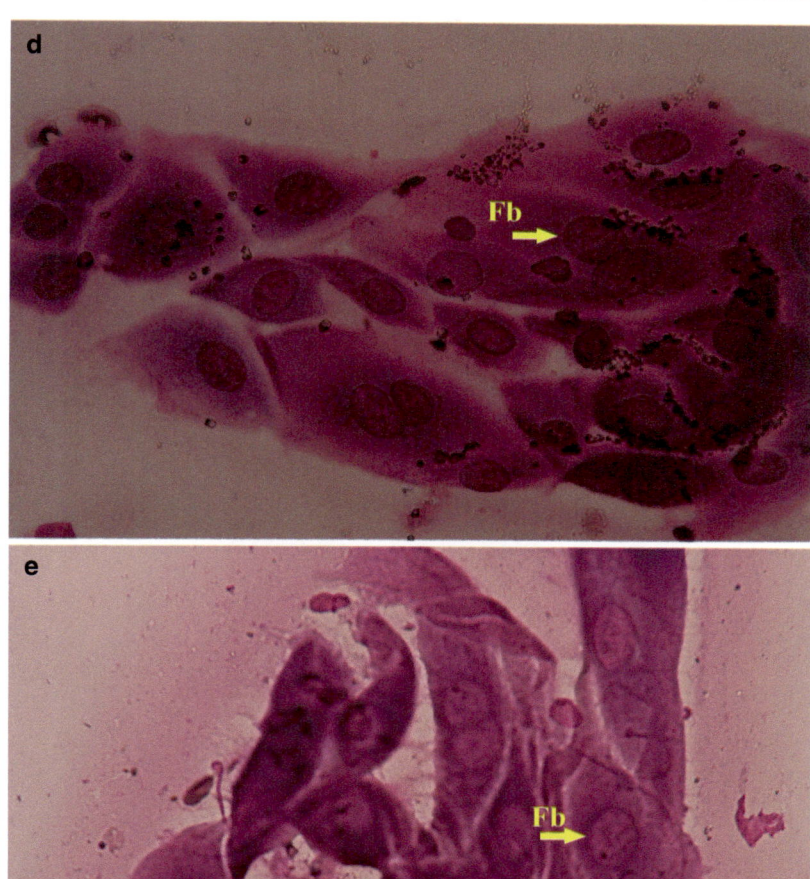

8.4 Pulmonary Involvement from Systemic Lupus Erythematosus (SLE)

Brief history: Coughing with shortness of breath for 1 month, clinically diagnosed as systemic lupus erythematosus.

Technology to obtain the target lesions: Transbronchial lung biopsy (TBLB).

The preparation of cytological slides for ROSE: Imprinting (rolling).

Clustering (categorizing) analysis in ROSE interpretation:

- "Inflammatory changes".
- Granulomatous inflammation.
- Lymphocyte-based immune inflammatory response.

Fig. 8.28 (a, b) Extensive ground-glass opacities in both lungs and slight interstitial thickening

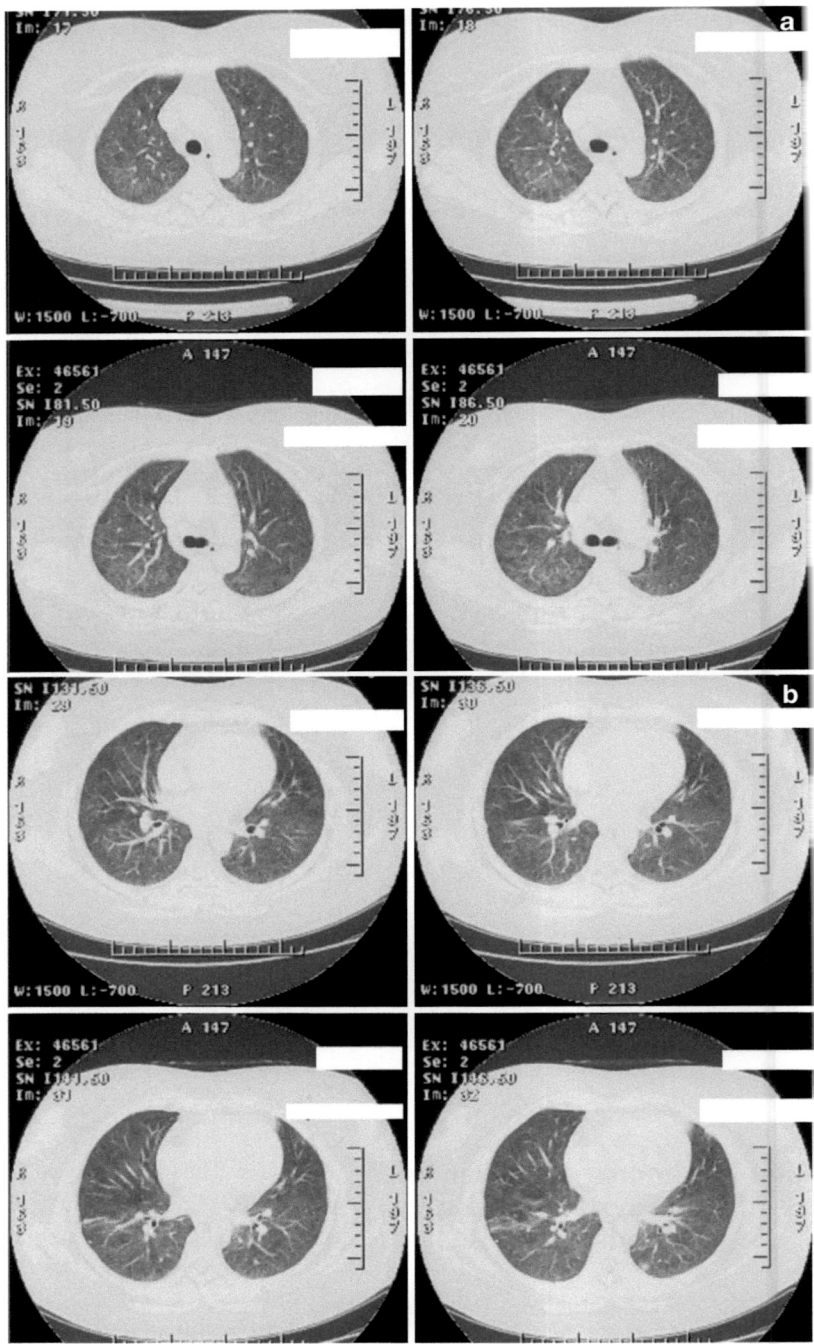

Fig. 8.29 (a–e)
Annotated at the figure
(yellow arrow)

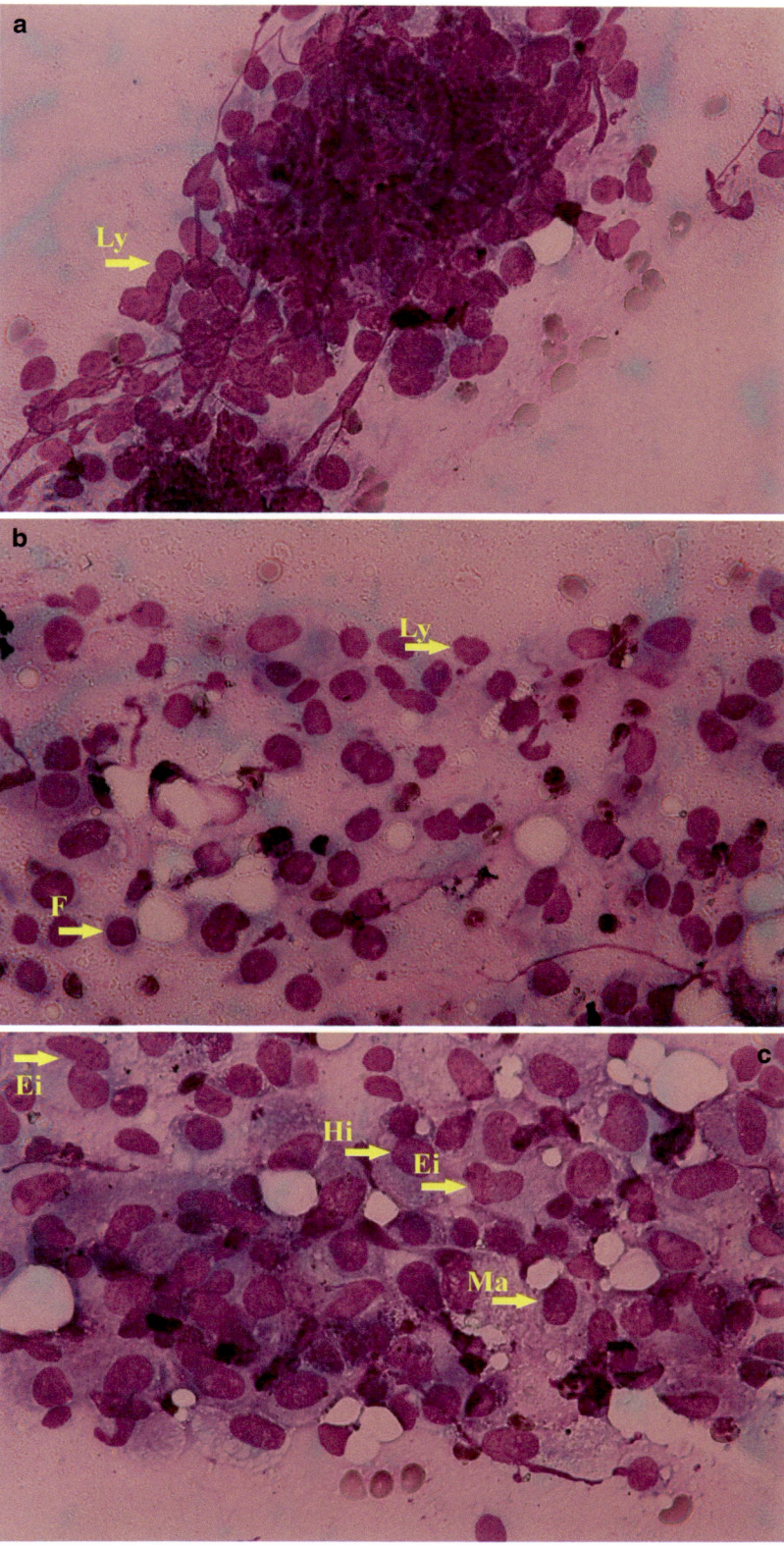

Fig. 8.29 (continued)

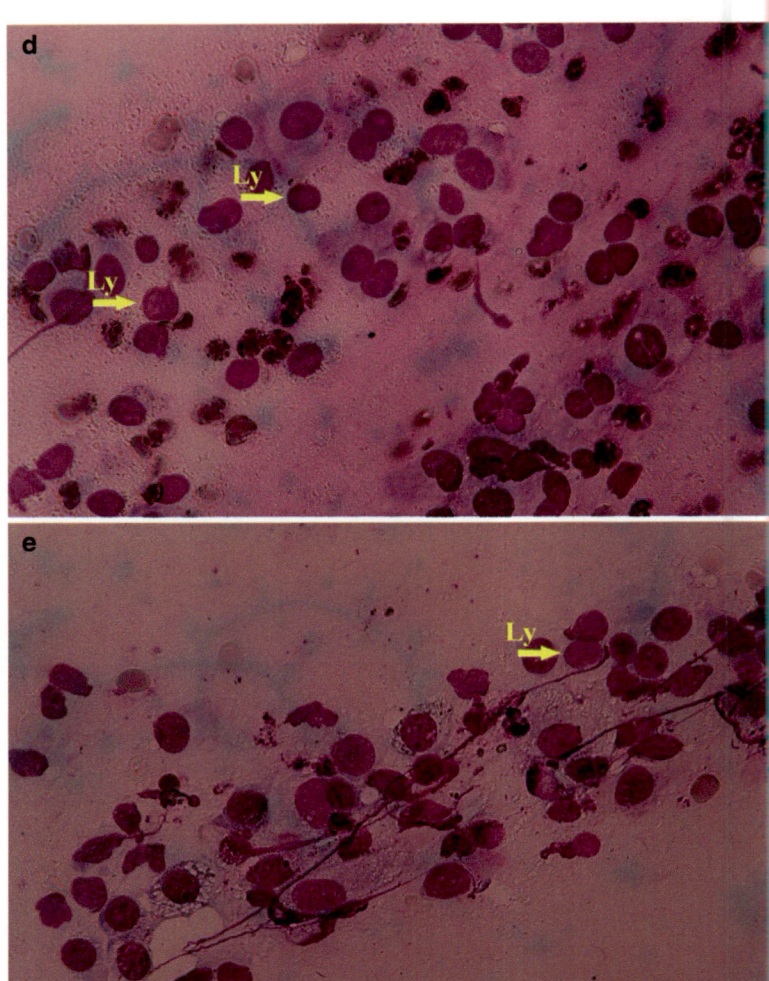

8.5   Pulmonary Involvement from Rheumatoid Arthritis

Brief history: Clinically diagnosed as rheumatoid arthritis, irritable dry cough for 4 weeks.

Technology to obtain the target lesions: Transbronchial lung biopsy (TBLB).

The preparation of cytological slides for ROSE: Imprinting (rolling).

Clustering (categorizing) analysis in ROSE interpretation:

- Approximately normal/mild nonspecific inflammatory response.
- Lymphocyte-based immune inflammatory response.
- Proliferative/reparative inflammatory response.

Fig. 8.30 (**a, b**) Subpleural interstitial thickening in both lungs, especially in both lower lungs, with tiny honeycombs

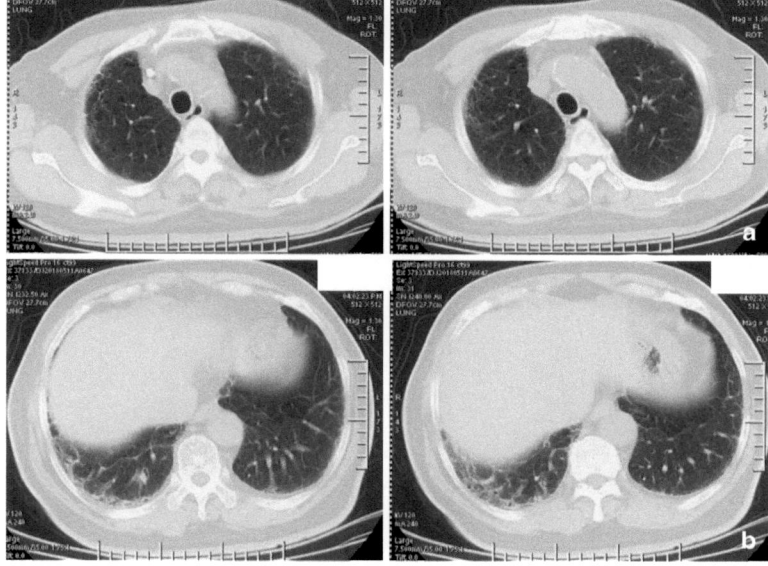

Fig. 8.31 (**a–e**) Annotated at the figure (yellow arrow)

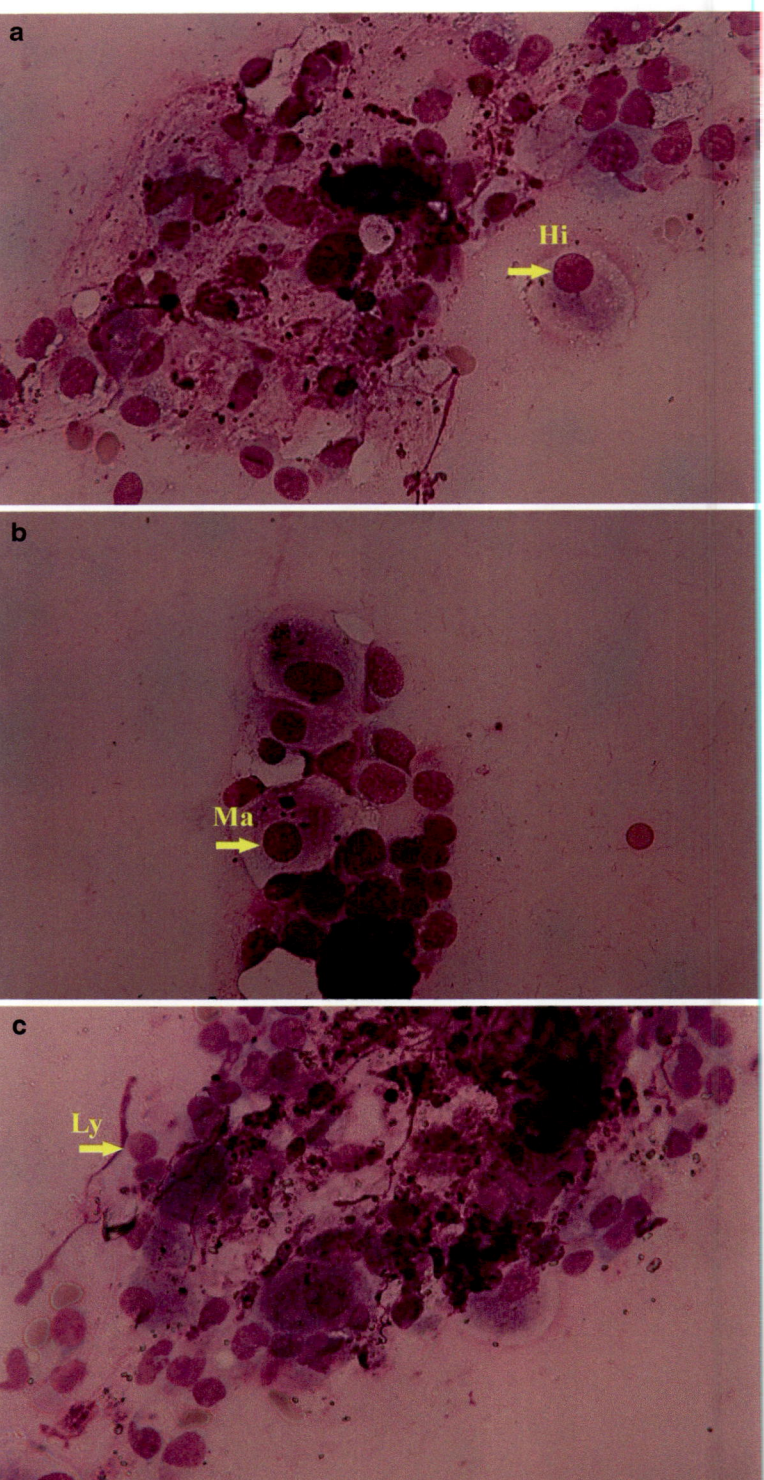

Fig. 8.31   (continued)

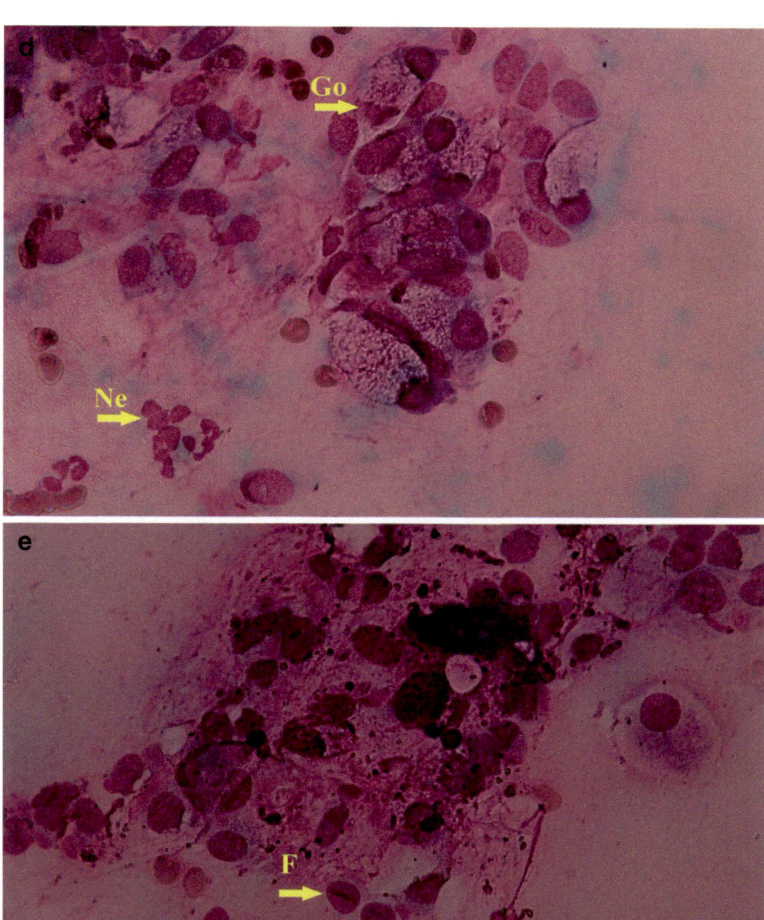

Fig. 8.32 (**a**, **b**) Hyaline
membrane fragments (red
arrow)

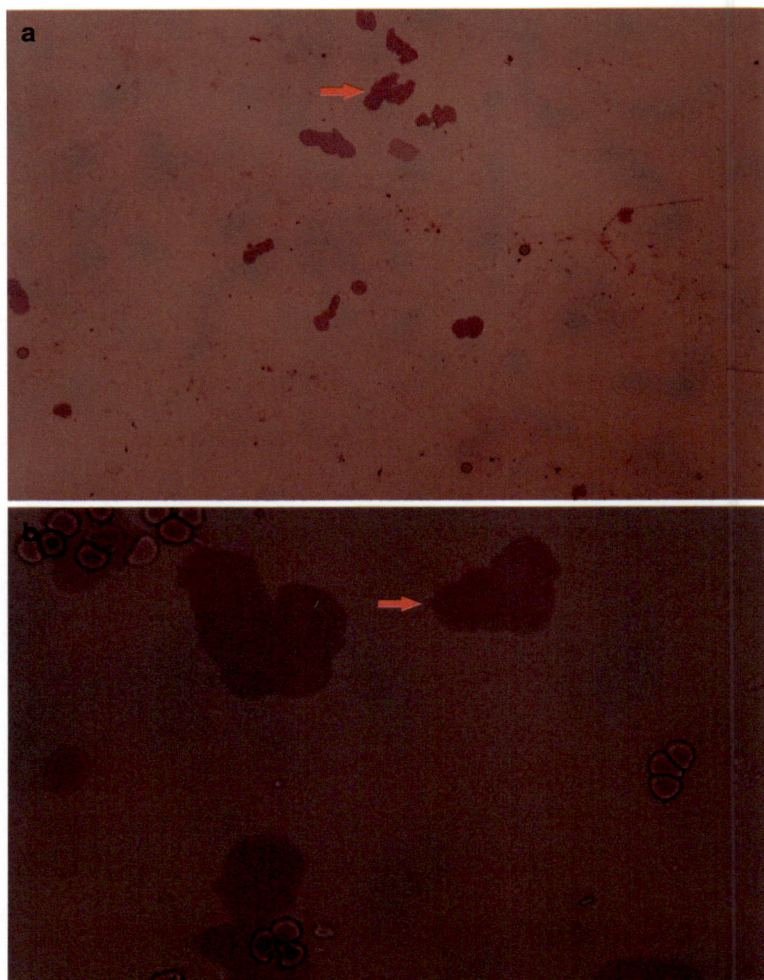

8.6   Pulmonary Involvement from Primary Sjogren's Syndrome (Sicca Syndrome)

Brief history: Male, 59 years old, nonproductive coughing with mild shortness of breath for nearly a week, clinically diagnosed as primary Sjogren's syndrome (sicca syndrome).

Technology to obtain the target lesions: Transbronchial lung biopsy (TBLB).

The preparation of cytological slides for ROSE: Imprinting (rolling).

Clustering (categorizing) analysis in ROSE interpretation:

- "Inflammatory changes".
- May conform to fibrosis (fibroblast dominant or fibrocyte dominant).
- Lymphocyte-based immune inflammatory response.

Fig. 8.33 (a–c)
Multiple patches,
consolidation, and air
bronchogram in both
lungs and interstitial
thickening distributed
along the
bronchovascular bundles
or subpleural areas

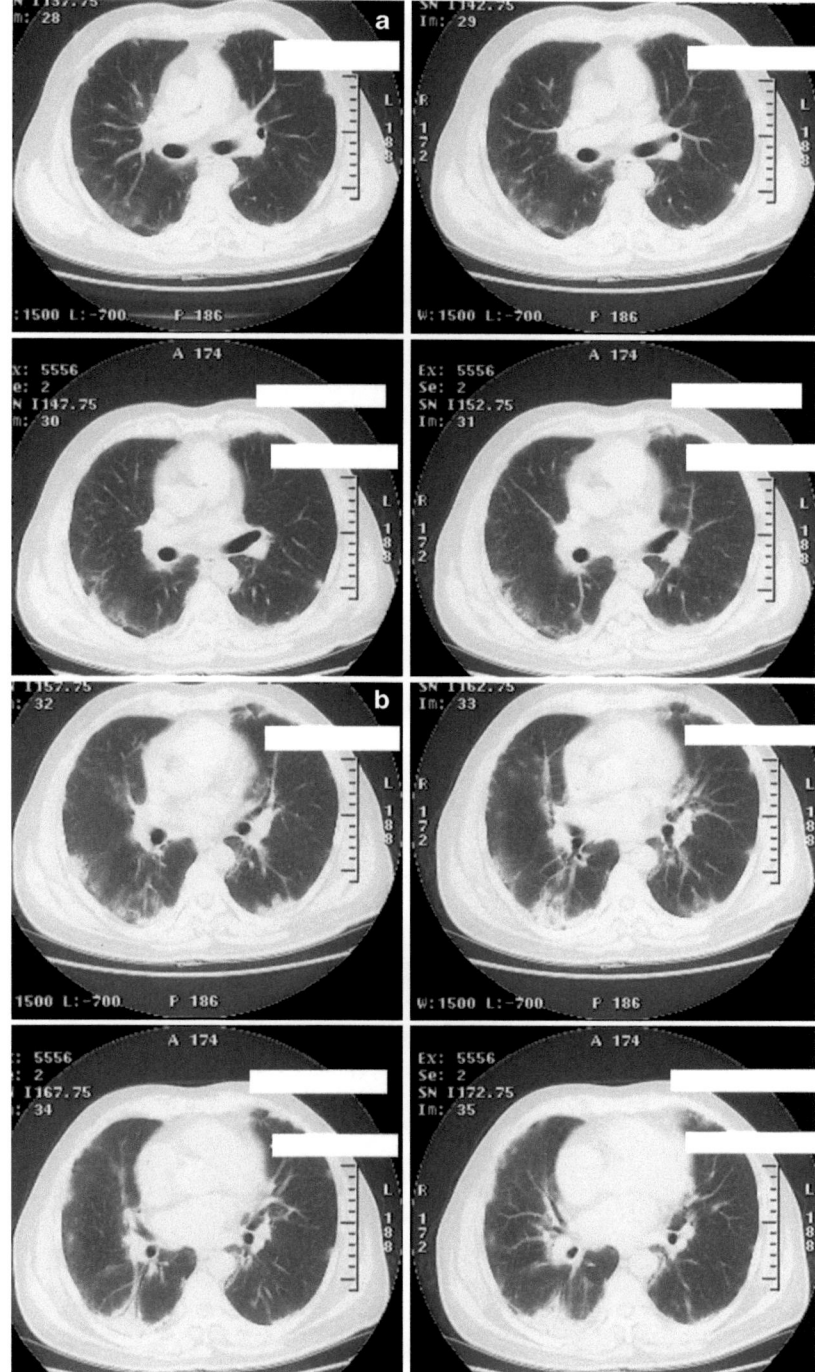

Fig. 8.33 (continued)

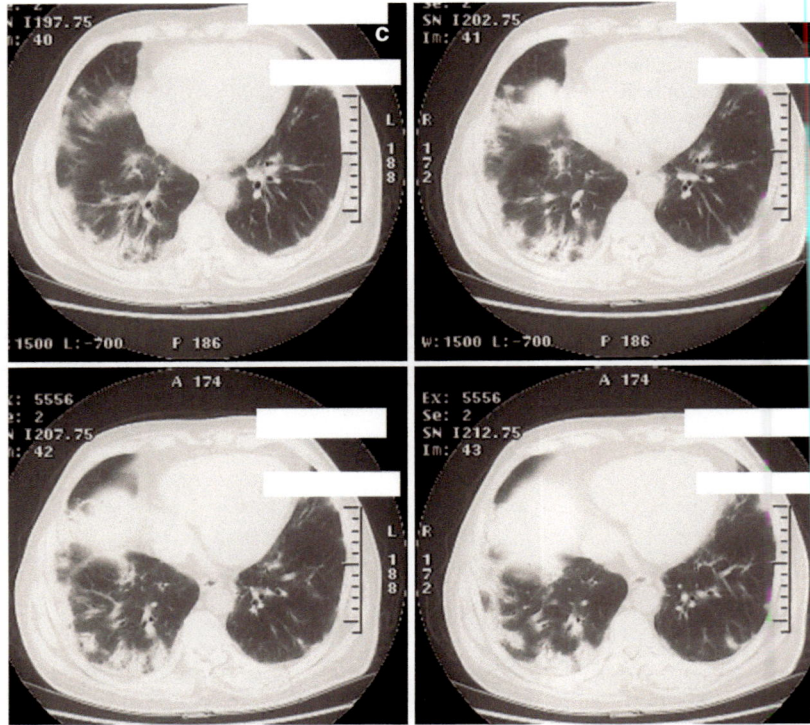

Fig. 8.34 (a–e)
Annotated at the figure
(yellow arrow)

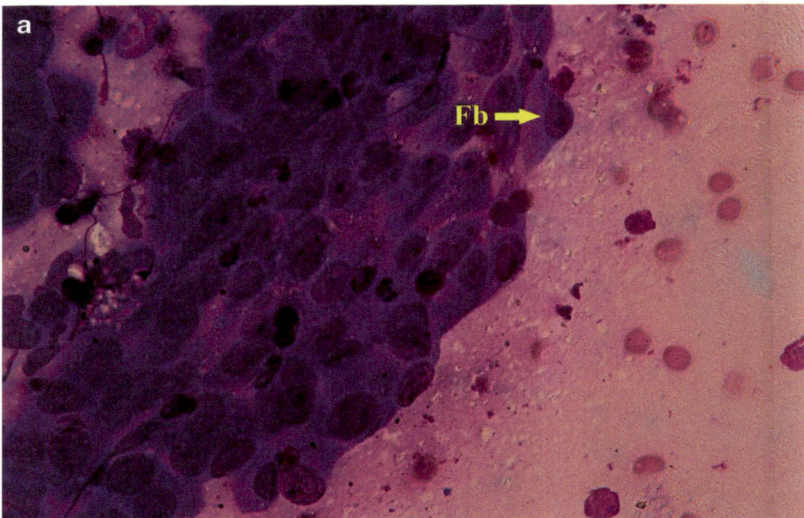

Fig. 8.34 (continued)

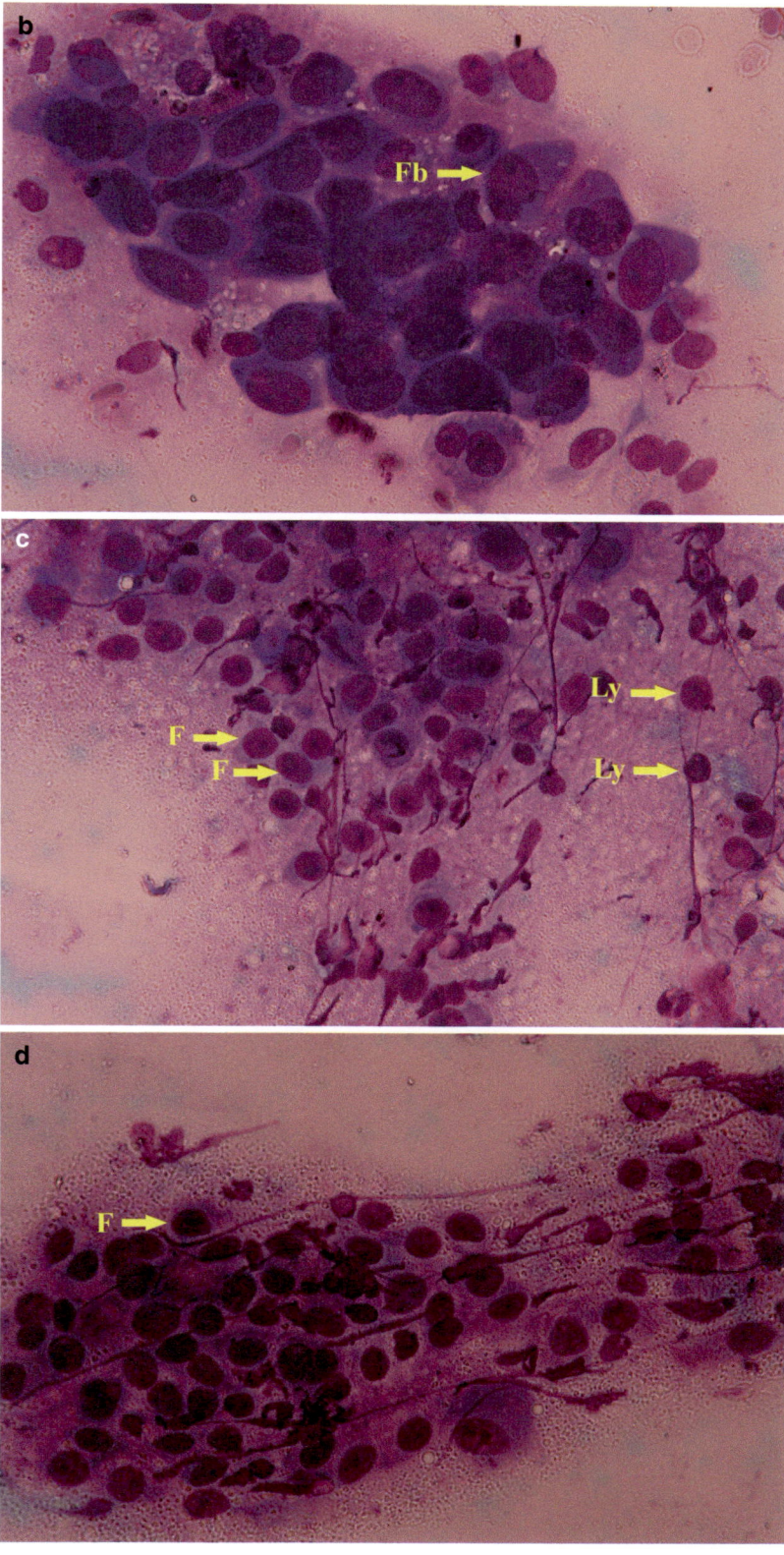

Fig. 8.34 (continued)

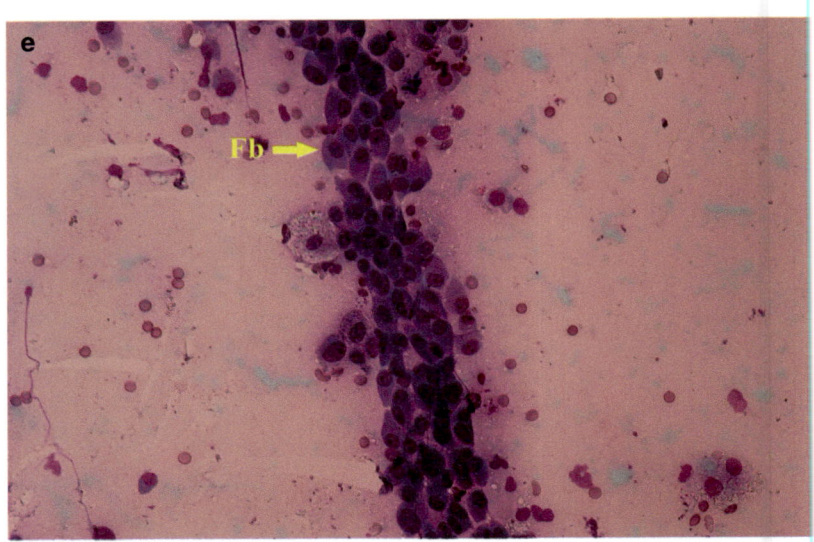

8.7   Pulmonary Involvement from Adult Still Disease

Brief history: Female, 53 years old, persistent coughing with mild shortness of breath, clinically diagnosed as adult Still disease.

Technology to obtain the target lesions: Transbronchial lung biopsy (TBLB).

The preparation of cytological slides for ROSE: Imprinting (rolling).

Clustering (categorizing) analysis in ROSE interpretation:

- "Inflammatory changes".
- Granulomatous inflammation.
- May conform to organization.
- Lymphocyte-based immune inflammatory response.

Fig. 8.35 (a, b)
Extensive ground-glass
opacities and slight
interstitial thickening in
both lungs

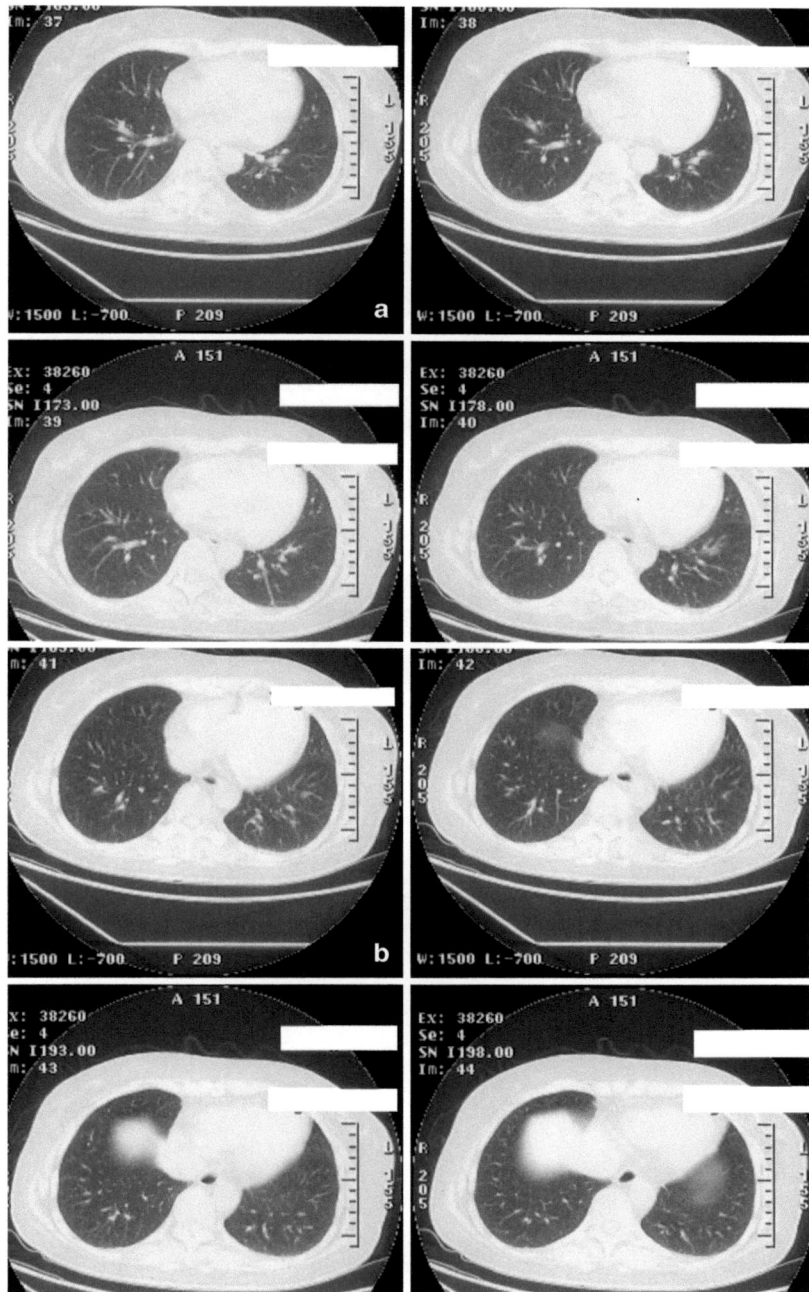

Fig. 8.36 (a–e)
Annotated at the figure
(yellow arrow)

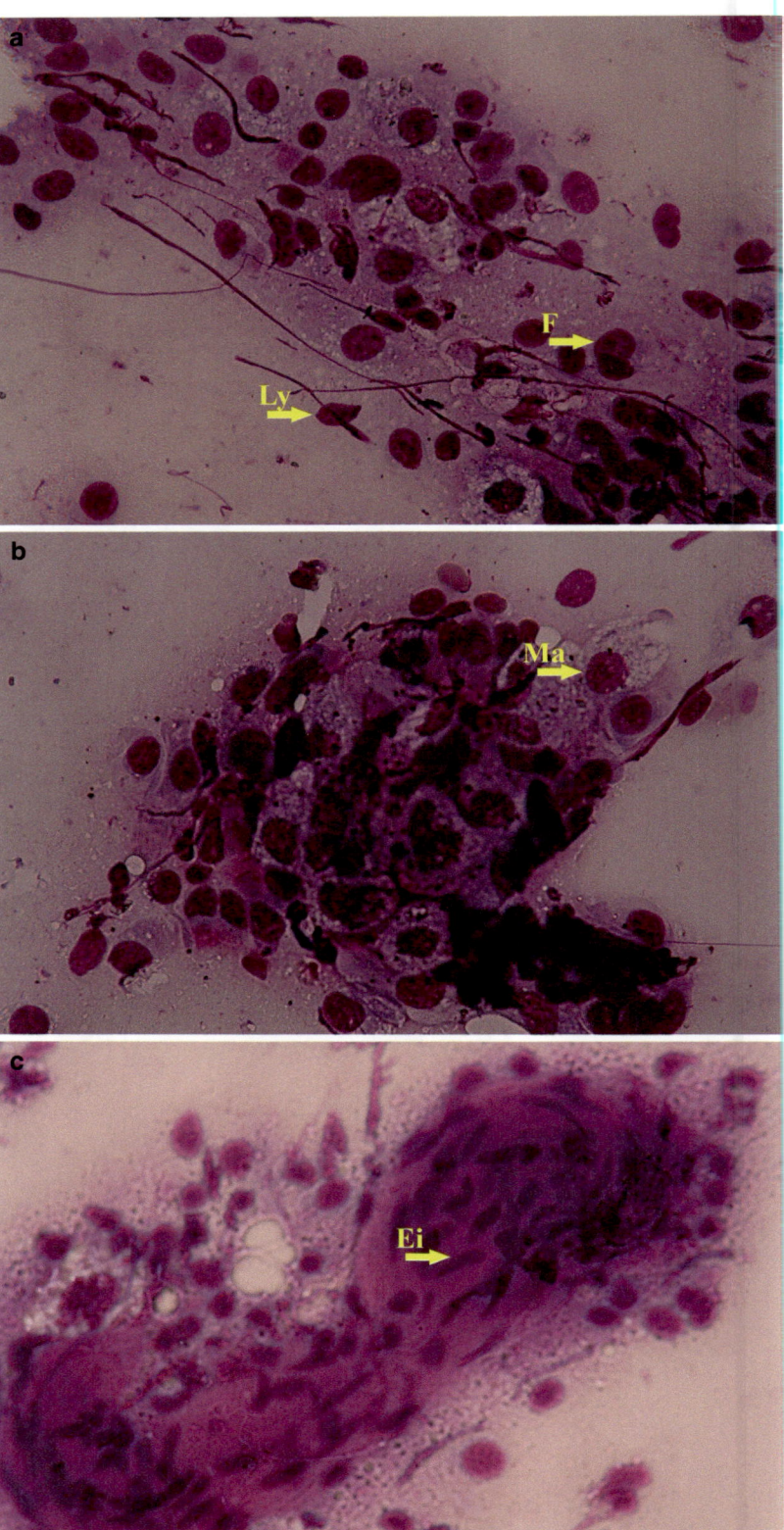

Fig. 8.36   (continued)

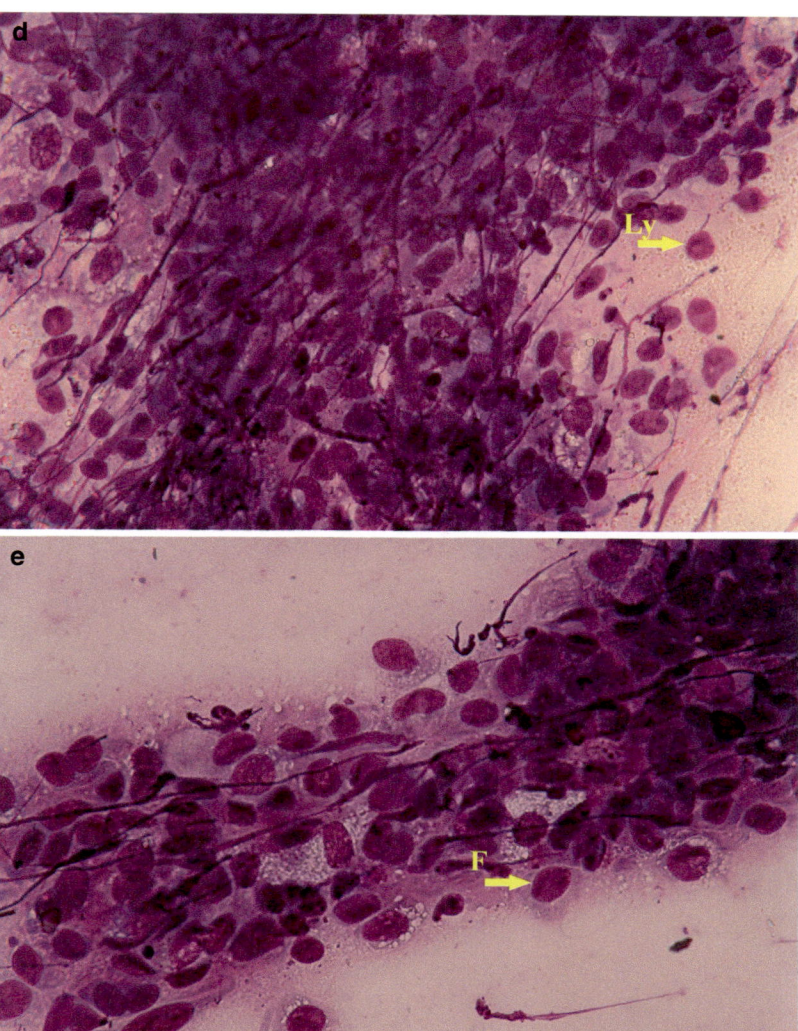

ROSE Cytopathology Cases of Idiopathic Interstitial Lung Diseases

Jing Feng and Dianhua Jiang

9.1 Acute Progression of Pulmonary Interstitial Fibrosis

Brief history: 4 months after peripheral blood stem cell transplantation, the chest CT showed rapid progression of the lesion, the patient developed fever and dyspnea, the arterial oxygen saturation decreased progressively, and type I respiratory failure.

Technology to obtain the target lesions: Transbronchial lung biopsy (TBLB).

The preparation of cytological slides for ROSE: Imprinting (rolling).

Clustering (categorizing) analysis in ROSE interpretation:

- "Inflammatory changes".
- May conform to fibrosis (fibroblast dominant).

J. Feng
Pulmonary and Critical Care Medicine, Tianjin Medical University General Hospital, Tianjin, China
e-mail: zyyhxkfj@126.com

D. Jiang (✉)
Cedars-Sinai Medical Center, Los Angeles, USA
e-mail: Dianhua.Jiang@csmc.edu

© Springer Nature Singapore Pte Ltd. 2020
J. Feng et al. (eds.), *Rapid On-Site Evaluation (ROSE) in Diagnostic Interventional Pulmonology*,
https://doi.org/10.1007/978-981-15-0939-1_9

Fig. 9.1 (a–c) Multiple ground-glass opacities, consolidation and interstitial changes obvious in subpleural areas, and air bronchogram sign

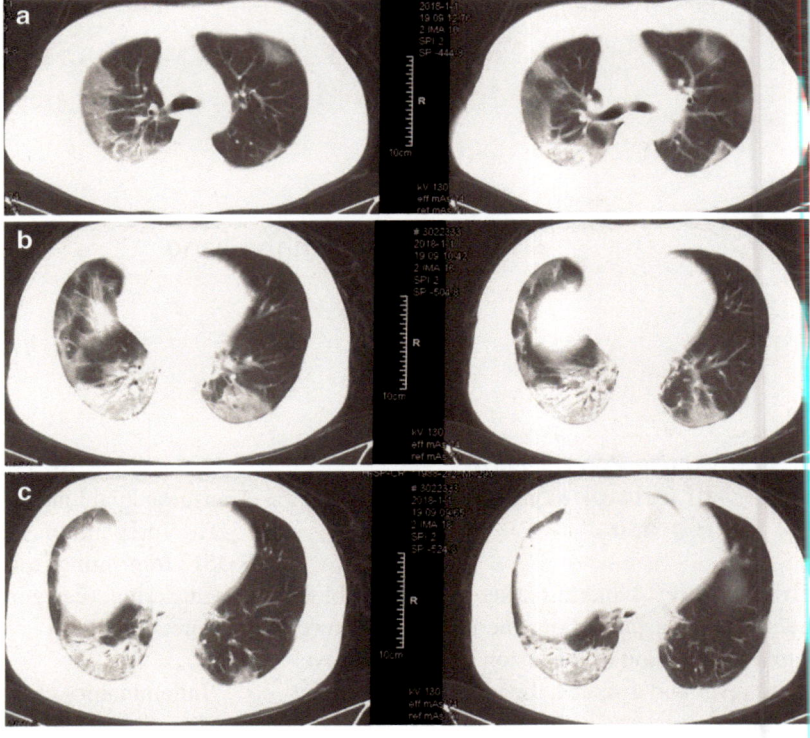

Fig. 9.2 Lots of fibroblasts (yellow arrow) and distal airway short columnar ciliated columnar epithelial cells (red arrow)

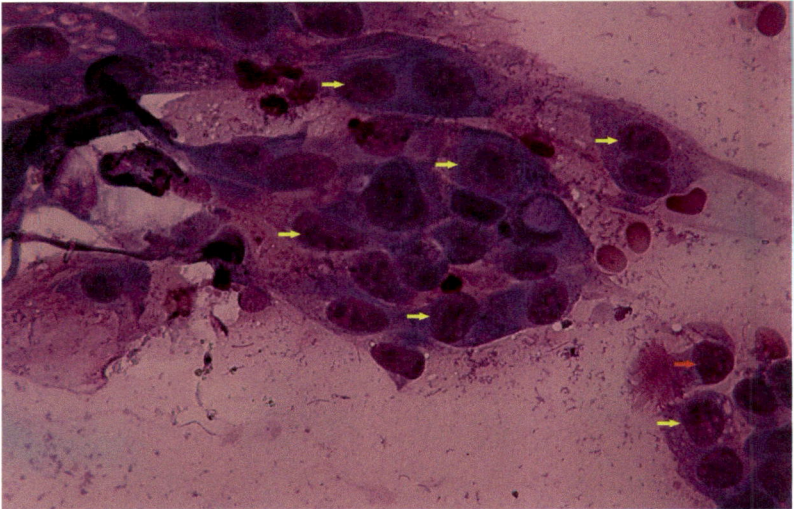

Fig. 9.3 Aggregation of foamy macrophages (yellow arrow)

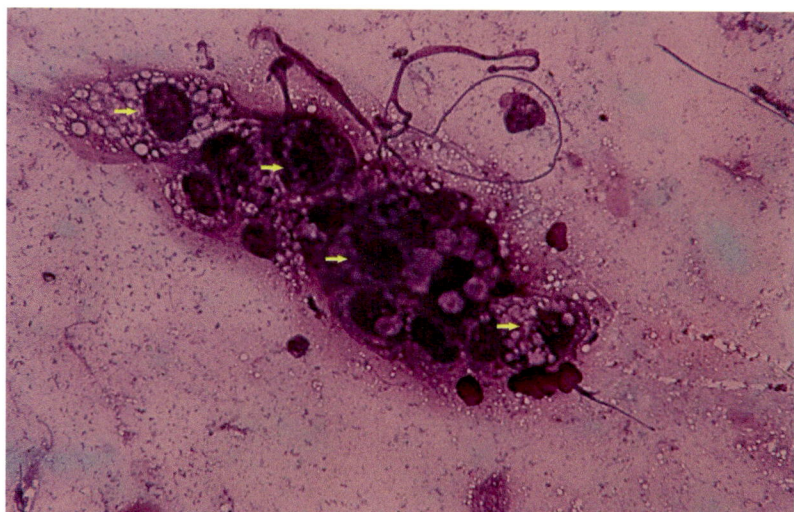

Fig. 9.4 Macrophages, some evolving into histiocytes (yellow arrow) and some developing further into epithelioid cells (red arrow), and type II alveolar epithelial cell hyperplasia (green arrow)

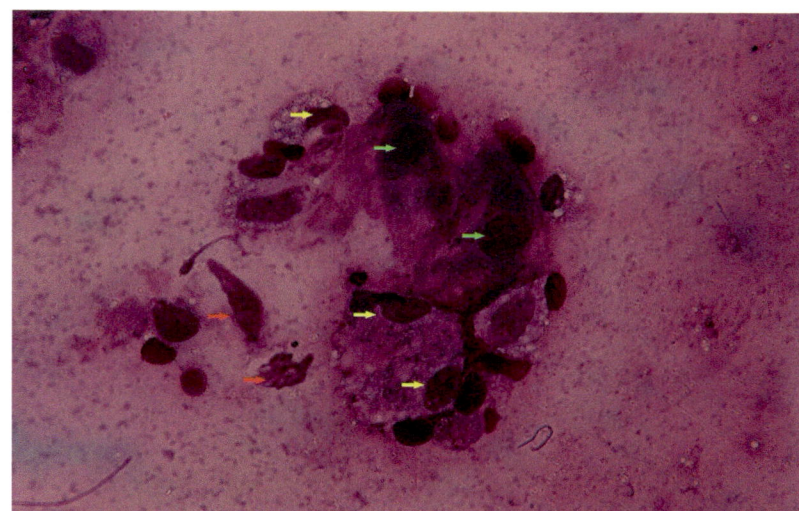

Fig. 9.5 Lots of fibroblasts (yellow arrow)

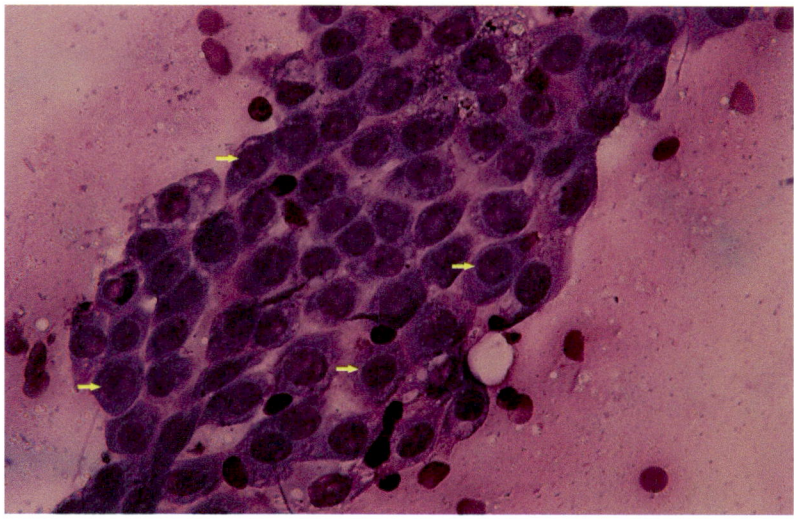

Fig. 9.6 Distal airway
epithelial cell
hyperplasia (yellow
arrow)

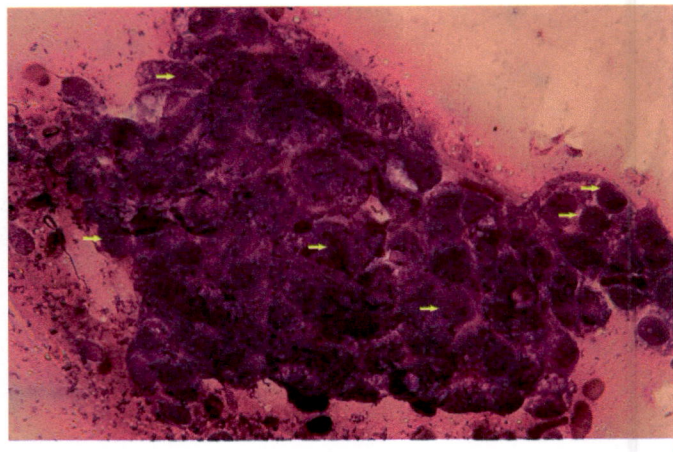

Fig. 9.7 Lots of
fibroblasts (yellow
arrow)

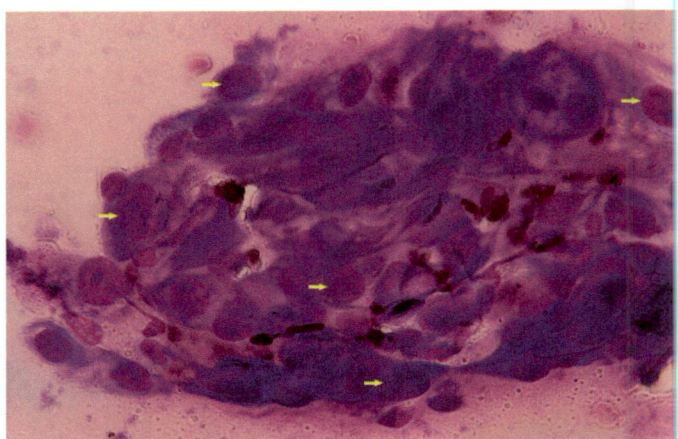

9.2 Bronchiolitis Obliterans Organizing Pneumonia (BOOP)

Brief history: Male, 75 years old, coughing for 2 months with mild shortness of breath, clinically diagnosed as bronchiolitis obliterans organizing pneumonia (BOOP).

Technology to obtain the target lesions: Transbronchial lung biopsy (TBLB).

The preparation of cytological slides for ROSE: Imprinting (rolling).

Clustering (categorizing) analysis in ROSE interpretation:

- May conform to organization.
- May conform to fibrosis (fibroblast dominant or fibrocyte dominant).
- Lymphocyte-based immune inflammatory response.

Fig. 9.8 (a–c) Extensive ground-glass opacities, interlobular septal thickening, and lobular core nodules

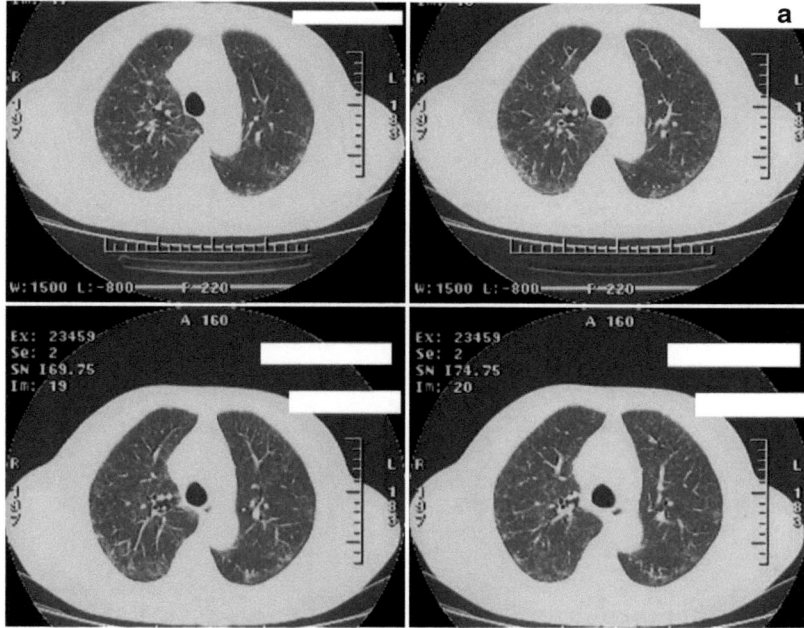

Fig. 9.8 (continued)

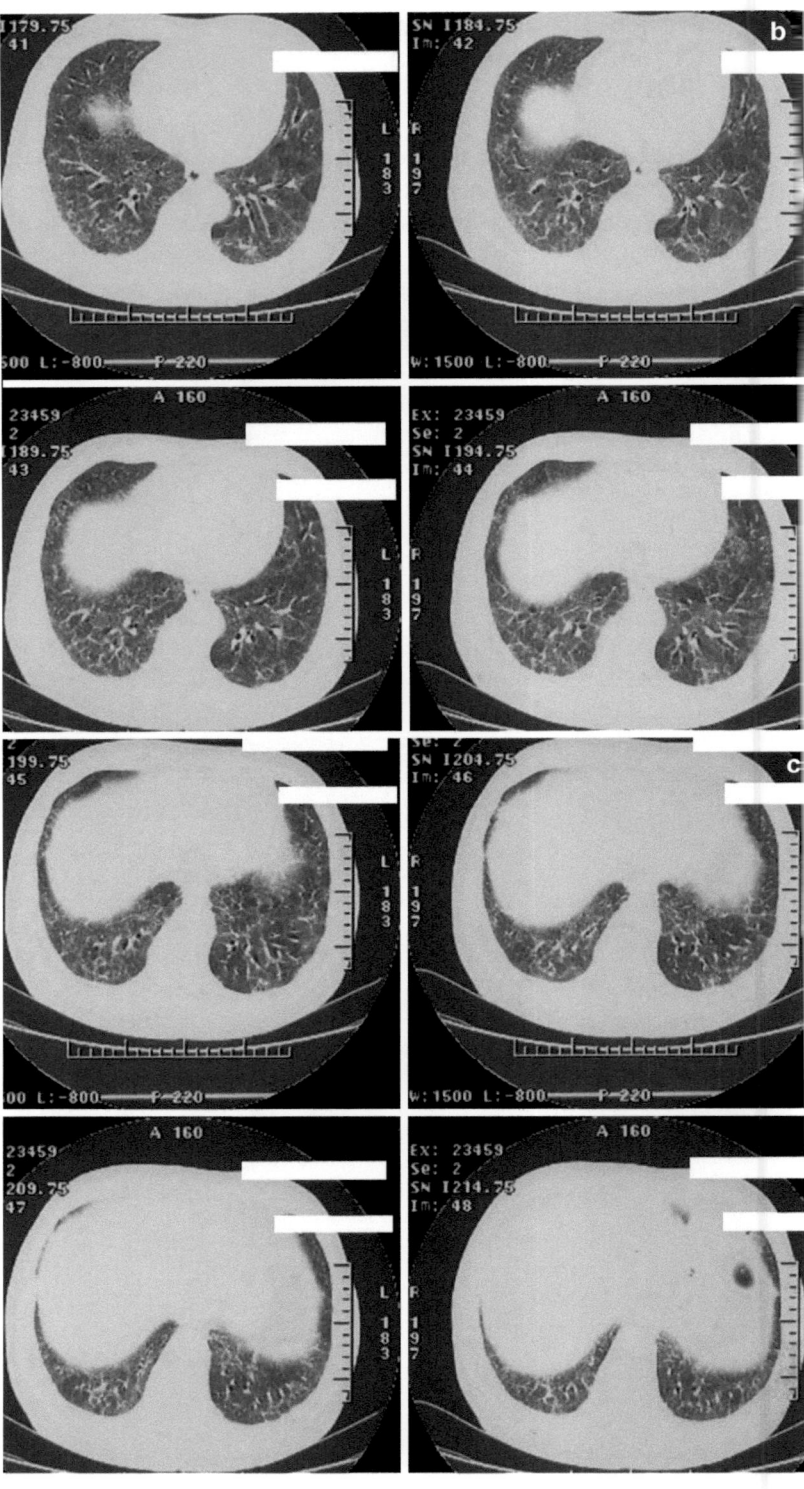

Fig. 9.9 (a–f)
Annotated at the figure
(yellow arrow)

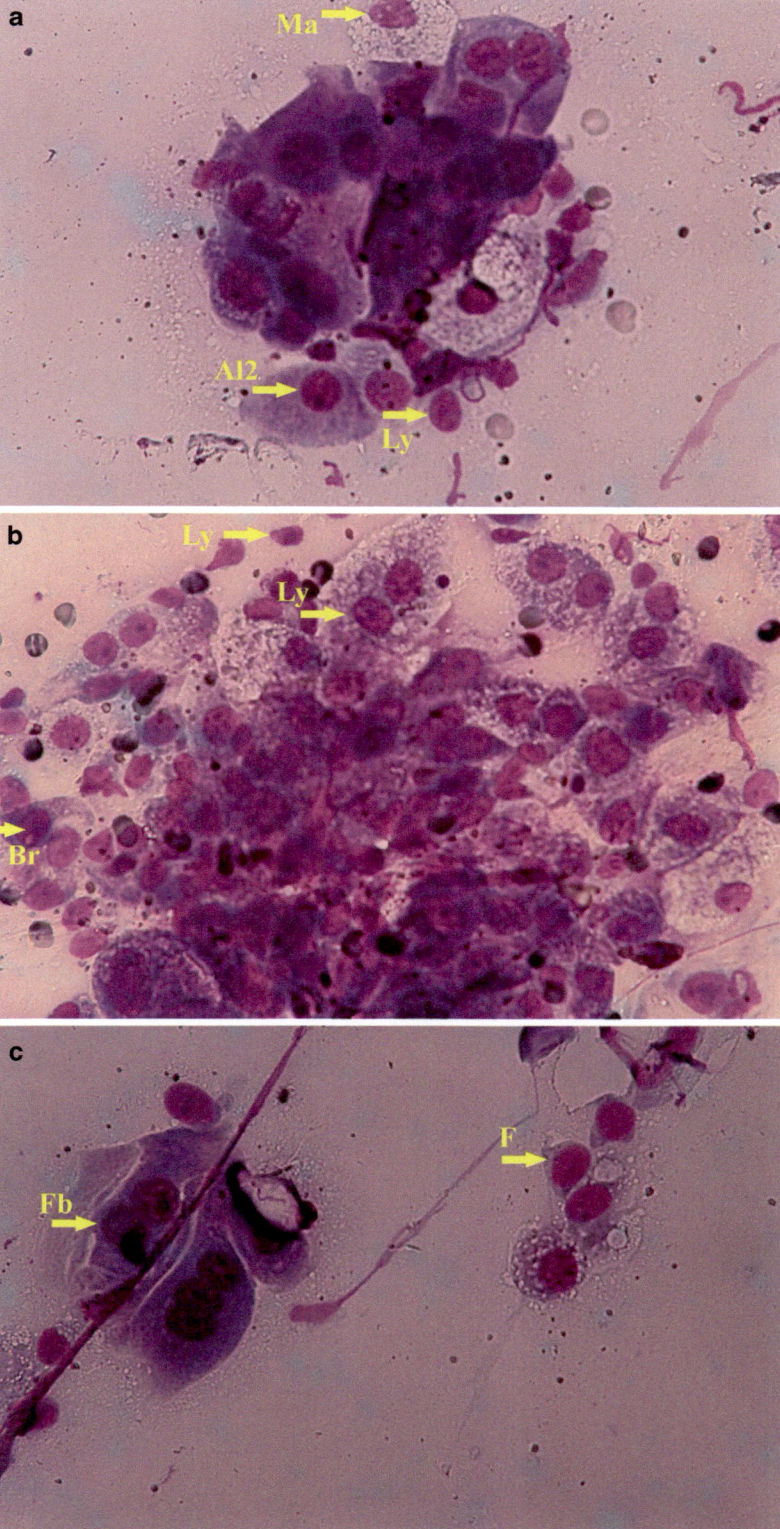

Fig. 9.9 (continued)

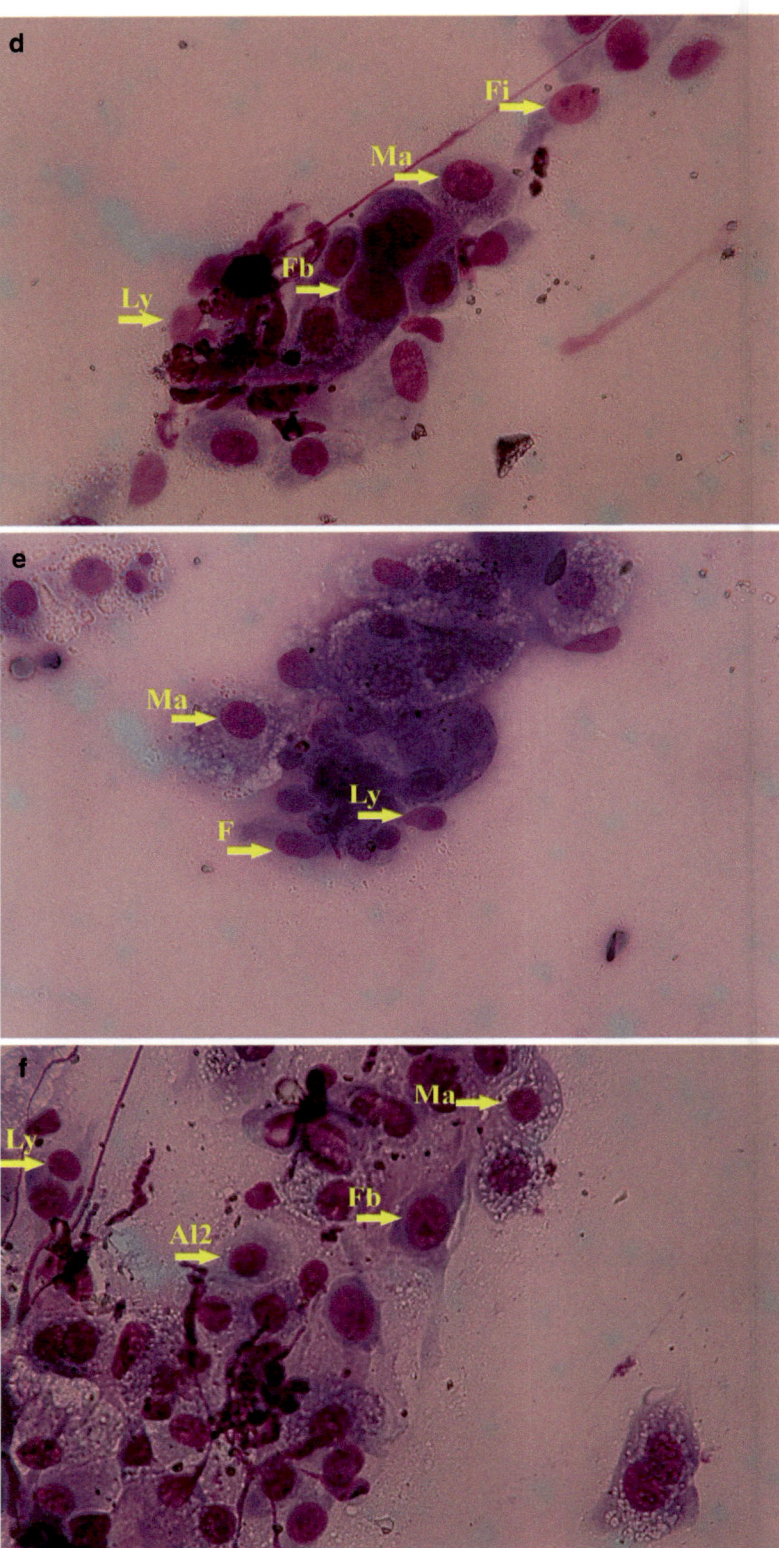

9.3   Lymphocytic Interstitial Pneumonia (LIP)

Brief history: Female, 36 years old, shortness of breath for more than 1 month, mild coughing, clinically diagnosed as lymphocytic interstitial pneumonia.

Technology to obtain the target lesions: Transbronchial lung biopsy (TBLB).

The preparation of cytological slides for ROSE: Imprinting (rolling).

Clustering (categorizing) analysis in ROSE interpretation:

- "Inflammatory changes".
- Lymphocyte-based immune inflammatory response.

Fig. 9.10 (a, b) Extensive ground-glass opacities and interlobular septal thickening

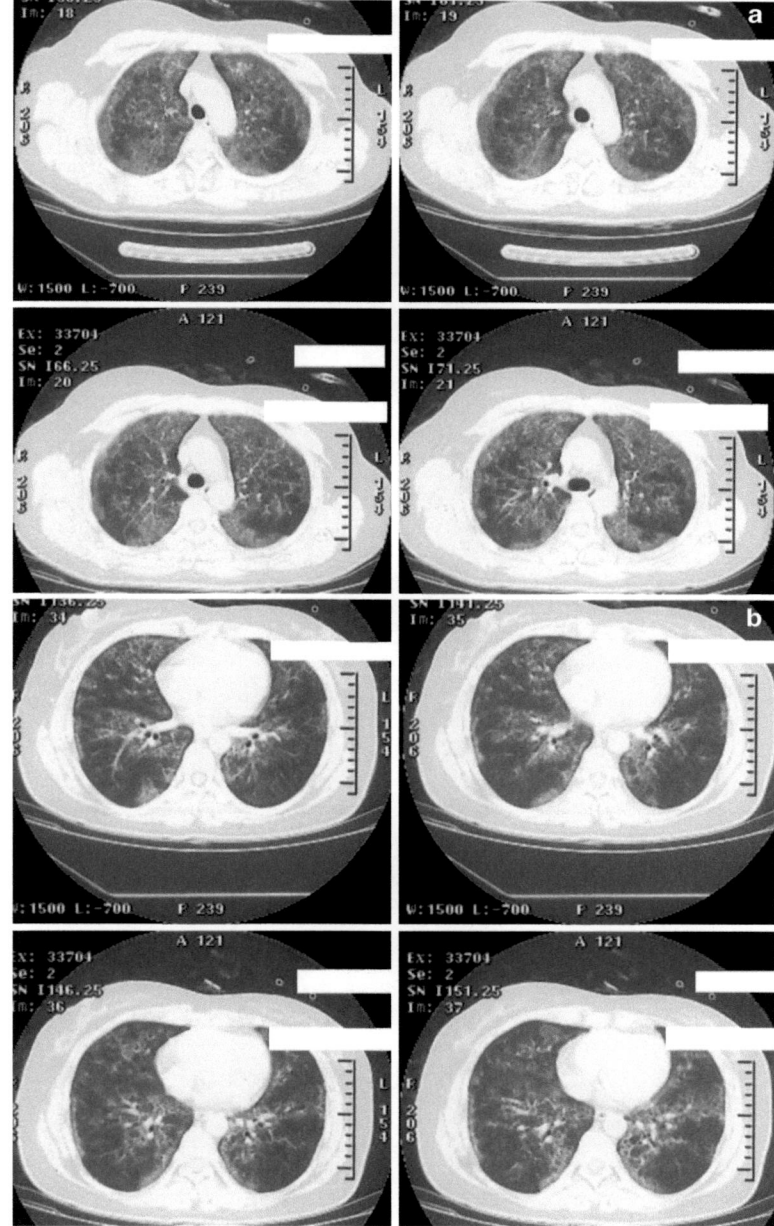

Fig. 9.11 (a–e)
Annotated at the figure
(yellow arrow)

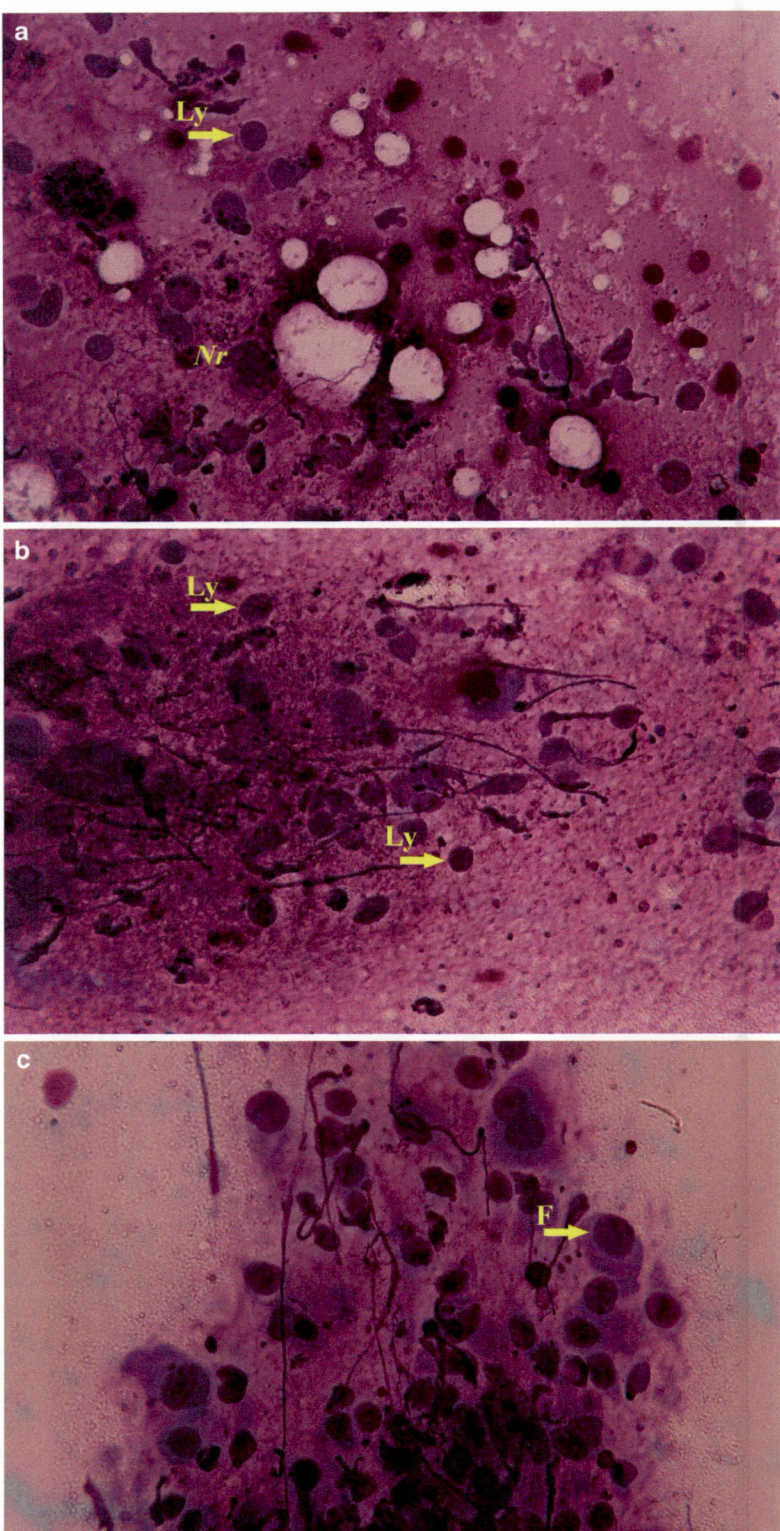

Fig. 9.11 (continued)

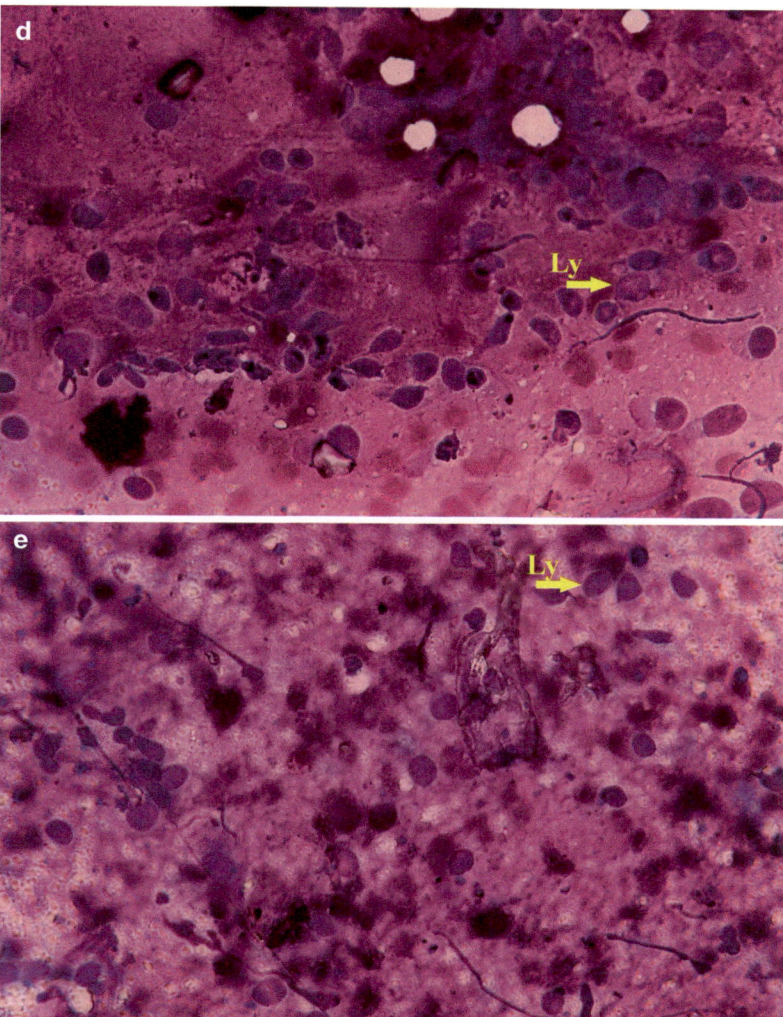

9.4   Idiopathic Interstitial Lung Disease (Undefined Classification)

Brief history: Irritable dry coughing for 3 months, dyspnea for 2 weeks.

Technology to obtain the target lesions: Transbronchial lung biopsy (TBLB).

The preparation of cytological slides for ROSE: Imprinting (rolling).

Clustering (categorizing) analysis in ROSE interpretation:

- Granulomatous inflammation.
- May conform to fibrosis (fibroblast dominant or fibrocyte dominant).
- Lymphocyte-based immune inflammatory response.

Fig. 9.12 Interstitial thickening, interlobular septal thickening, and scattered patches in both upper lungs

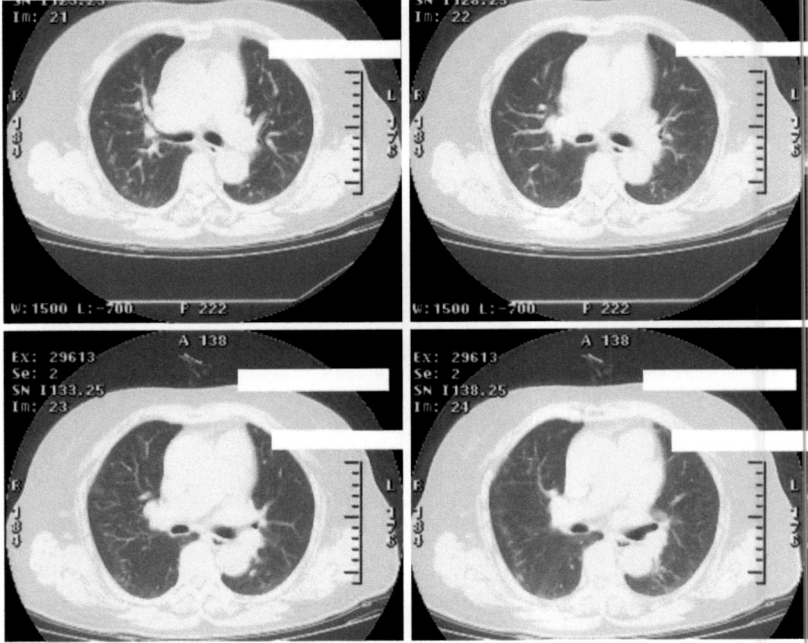

Fig. 9.13 Interstitial thickening, interlobular septal thickening, and scattered patches in both upper lungs, especially both lower lungs

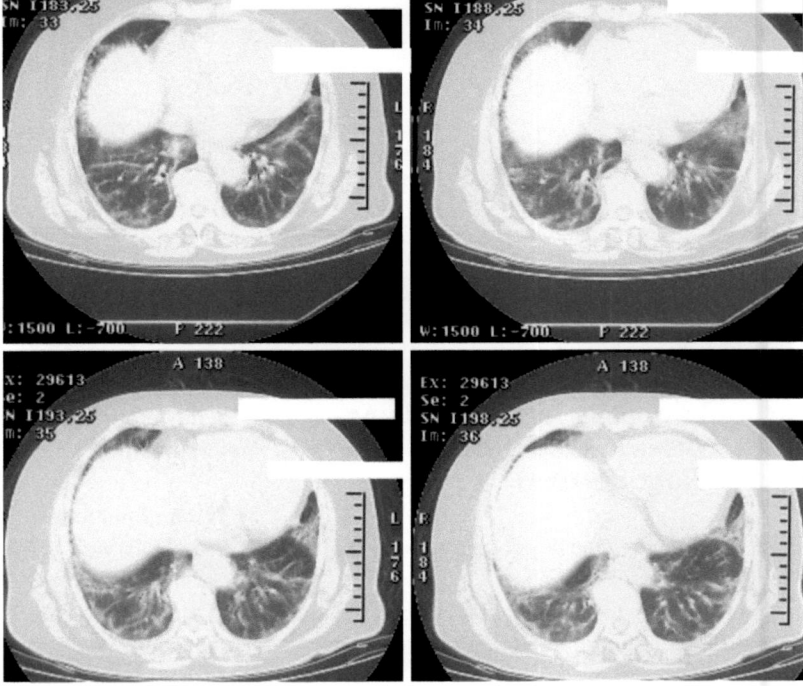

Fig. 9.14 Foamy macrophages, some evolving into histiocytes (yellow arrow)

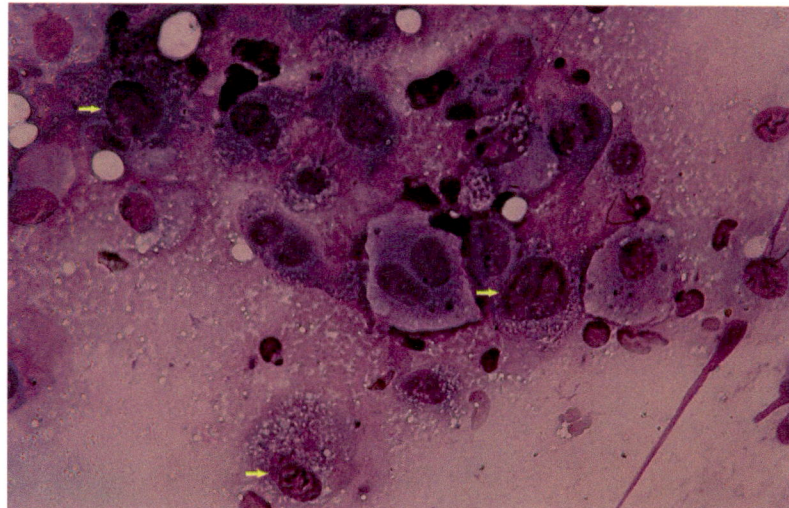

Fig. 9.15 Foamy macrophages, some evolving into histiocytes (yellow arrow), reactive lymphocytes (red arrow), and distal airway epithelial cell proliferation, degeneration, necrosis, and denaturation (green arrow)

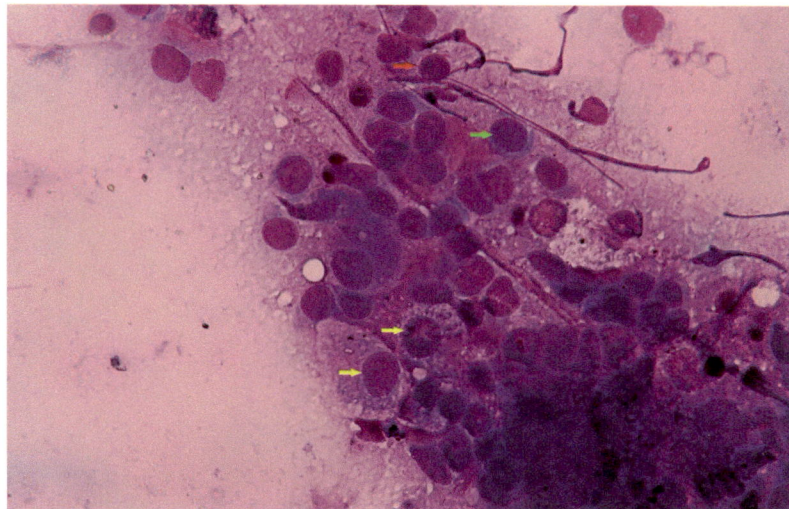

Fig. 9.16 Fibroblasts (yellow arrow)

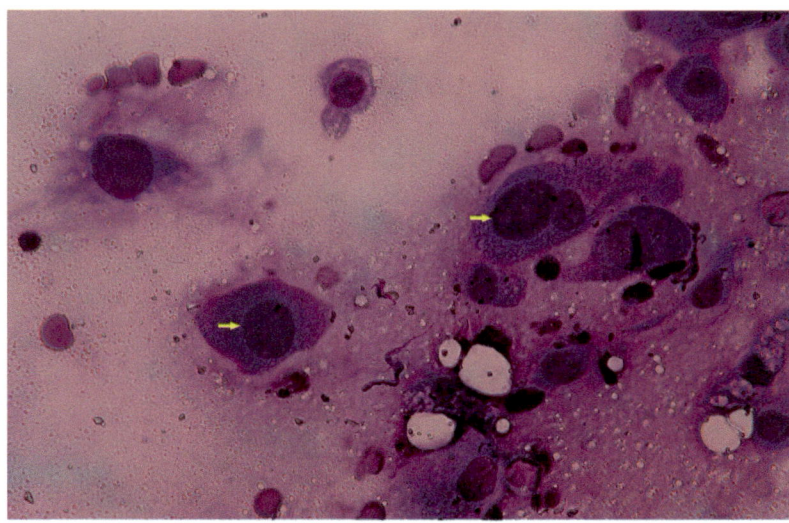

Fig. 9.17 Foamy
macrophages, some
evolving into histiocytes
(yellow arrow), and
distal airway epithelial
cell proliferation,
degeneration, necrosis,
and denaturation (red
arrow)

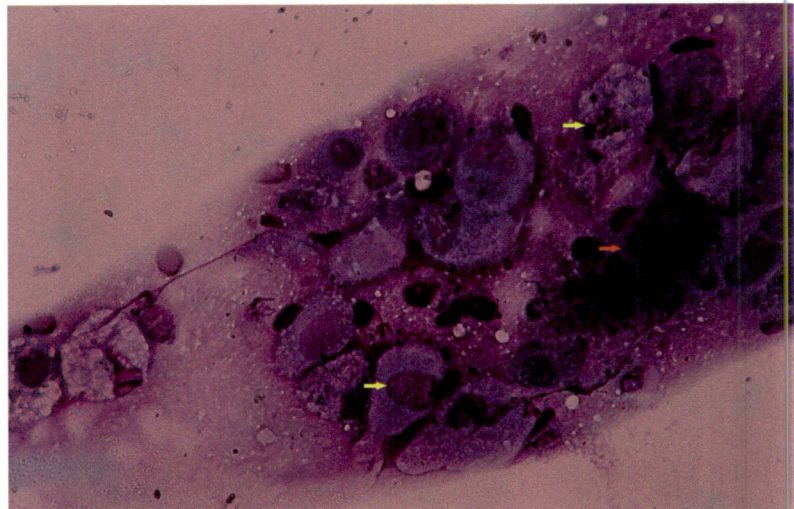

Fig. 9.18 Foamy
macrophages, some
evolving into histiocytes
(yellow arrow)

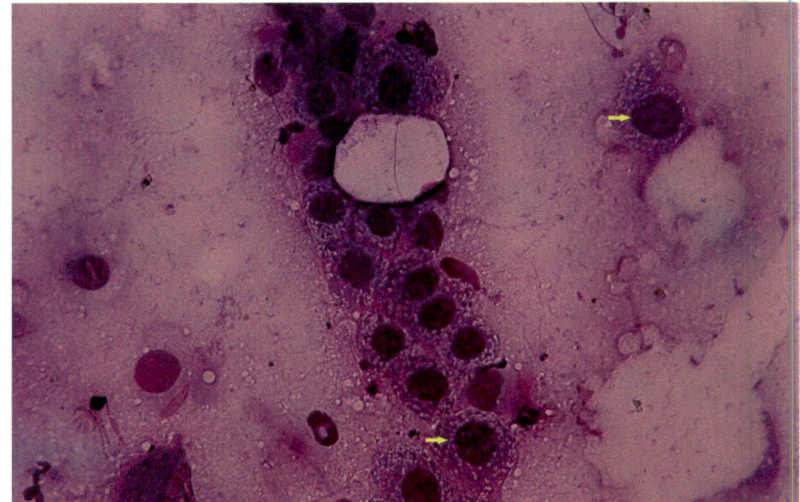

Fig. 9.19 Foamy
macrophages, some
evolving into histiocytes
(yellow arrow), and
distal airway epithelial
cell proliferation,
degeneration, necrosis,
and denaturation
(red arrow)

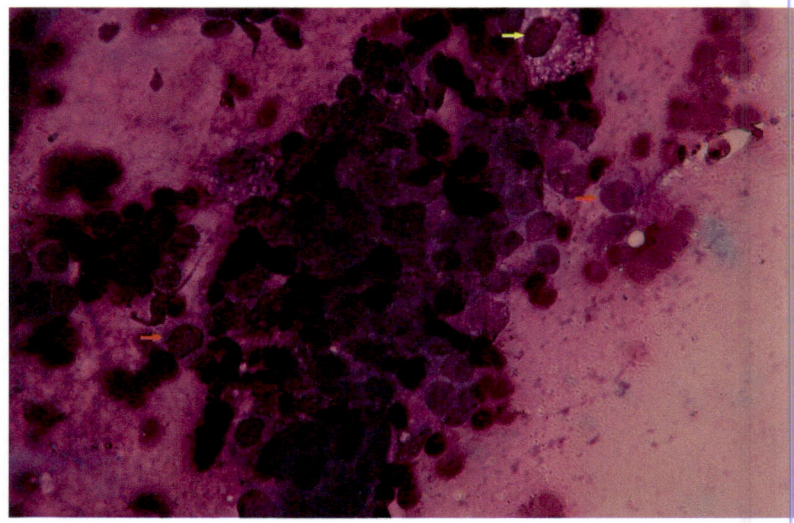

Fig. 9.20 Distal airway epithelial cell proliferation, degeneration, necrosis, and denaturation (yellow arrow)

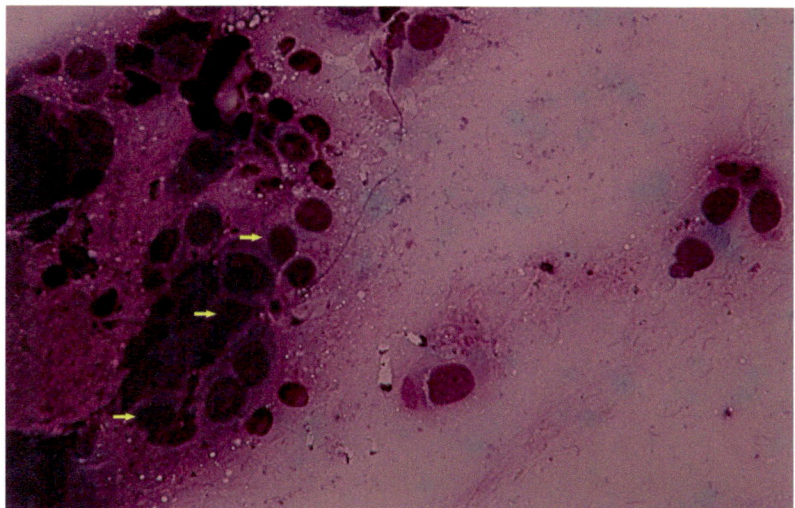

Fig. 9.21 (a–c) Multinuclear giant cells (yellow arrow) and distal airway epithelial cell proliferation, degeneration, necrosis, and denaturation (red arrow)

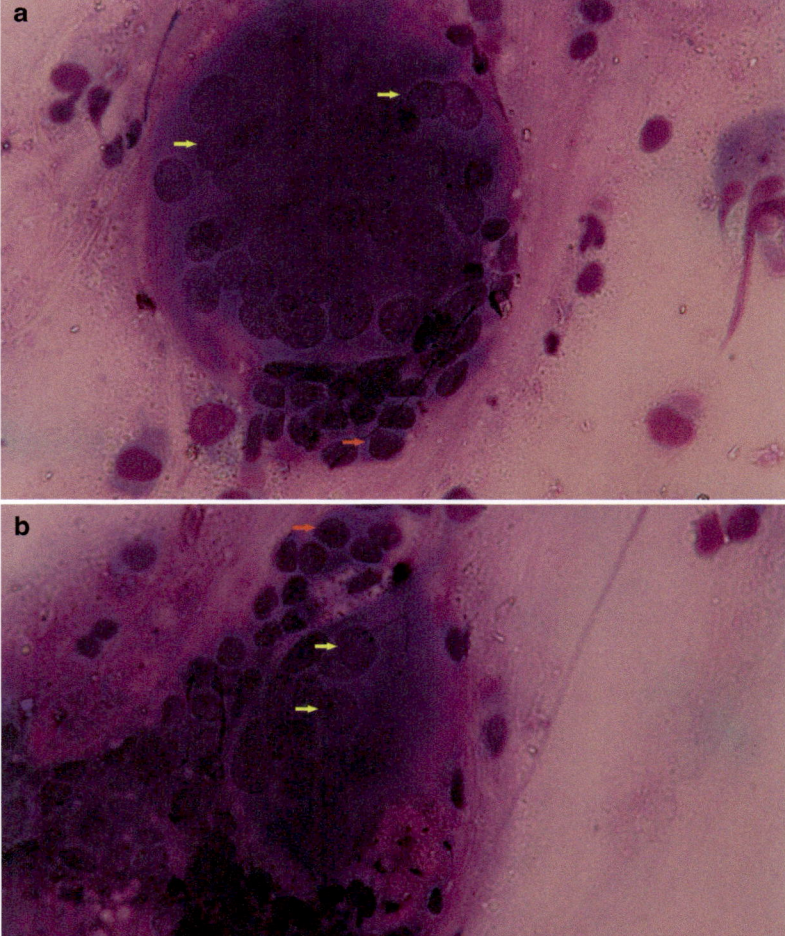

Fig. 9.21 (continued)

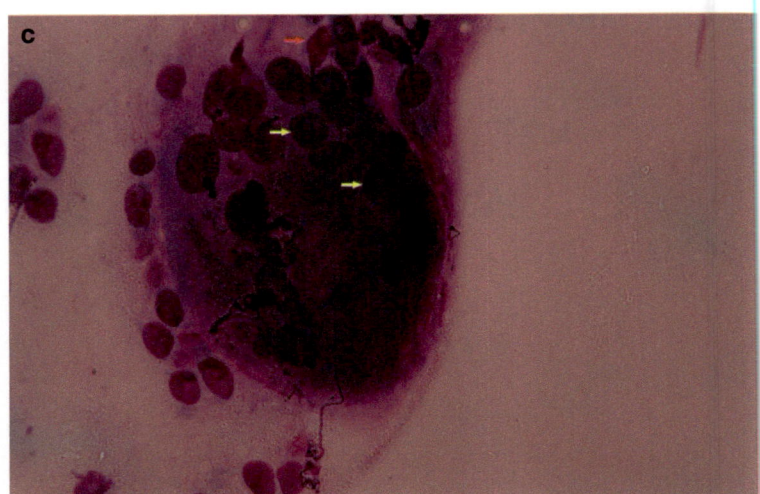

Fig. 9.22 Fibroblasts (yellow arrow); distal airway epithelial cell proliferation, degeneration, necrosis, and denaturation (red arrow); and short columnar distal airway ciliated columnar epithelial cells (green arrow)

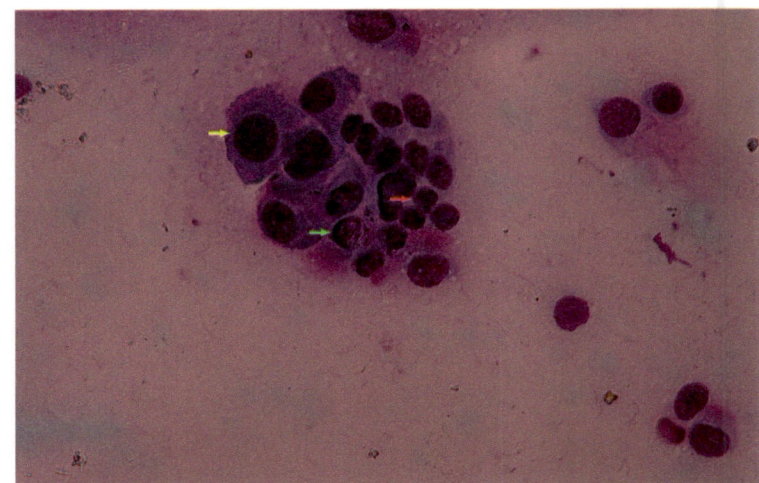

Fig. 9.23 Foamy macrophages, some evolving into histiocytes (yellow arrow), reactive lymphocytes (red arrow), and type II alveolar epithelial cell hyperplasia (green arrow)

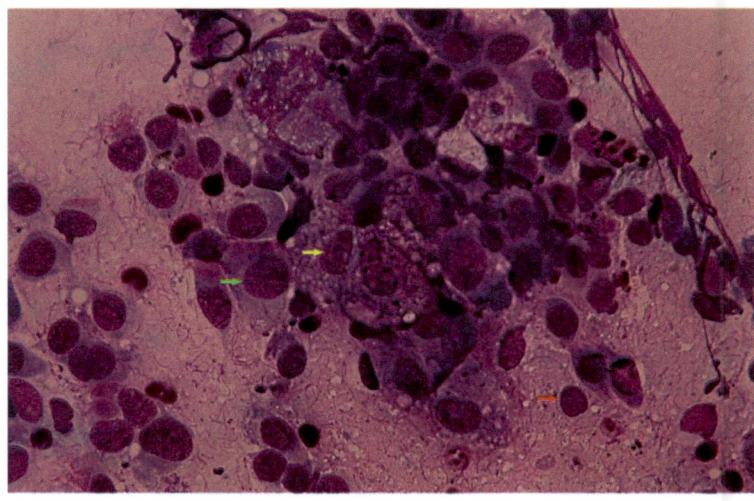

Fig. 9.24 (a, b) Multinuclear giant cells (yellow arrow) and distal airway epithelial cell proliferation, degeneration, necrosis, and denaturation (red arrow)

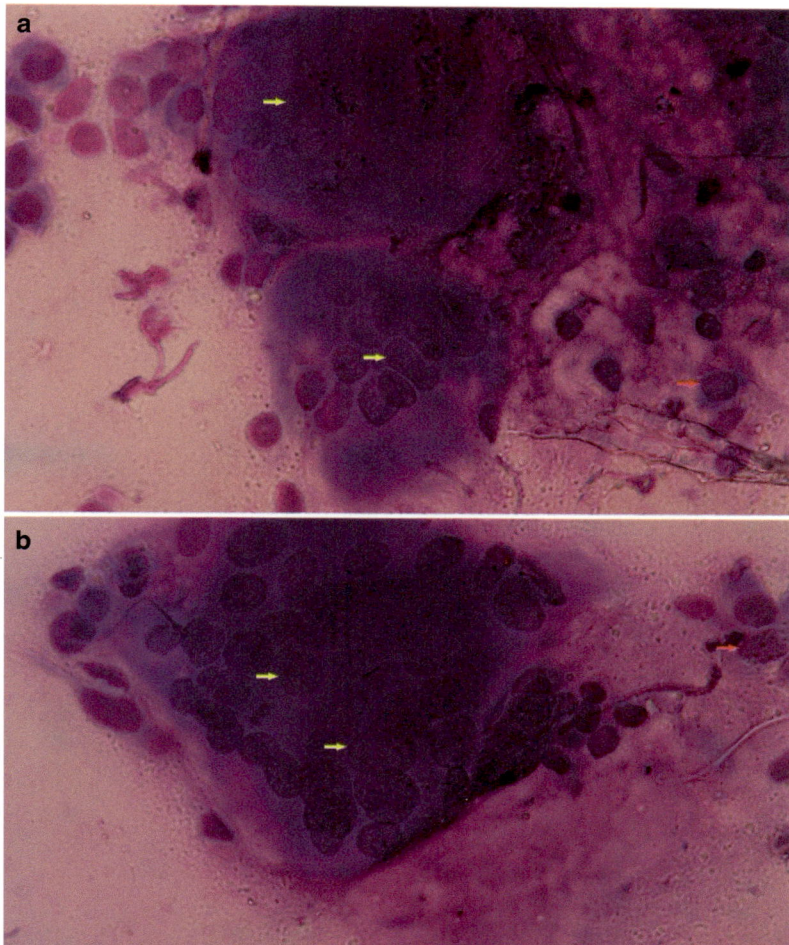

Fig. 9.25 Foamy macrophages, some evolving into histiocytes (yellow arrow), and distal airway epithelial cell proliferation, degeneration, necrosis, and denaturation (red arrow)

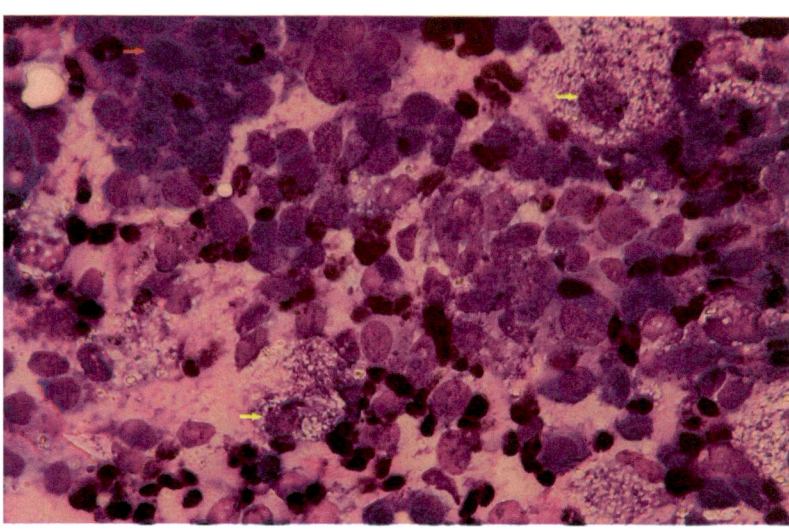

Fig. 9.26 Foamy macrophages, some evolving into histiocytes (yellow arrow), and reactive lymphocytes (red arrow)

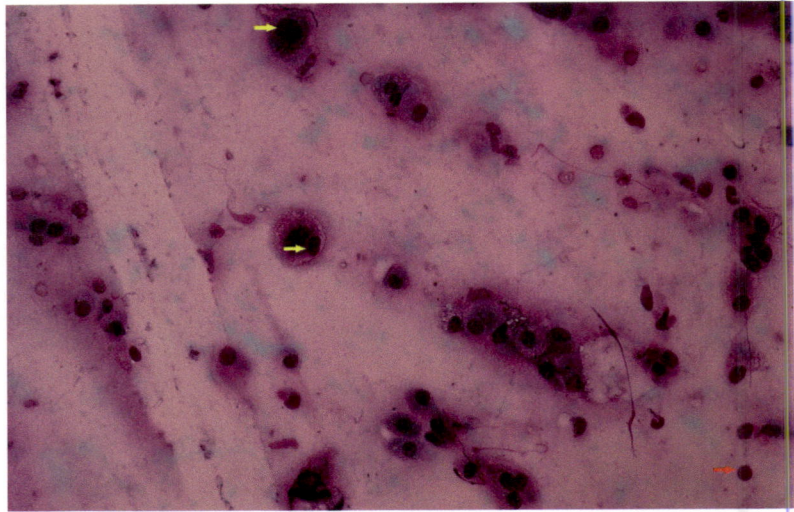

Fig. 9.27 Foamy macrophages, some evolving into histiocytes (yellow arrow), and type II alveolar epithelial cell hyperplasia (red arrow)

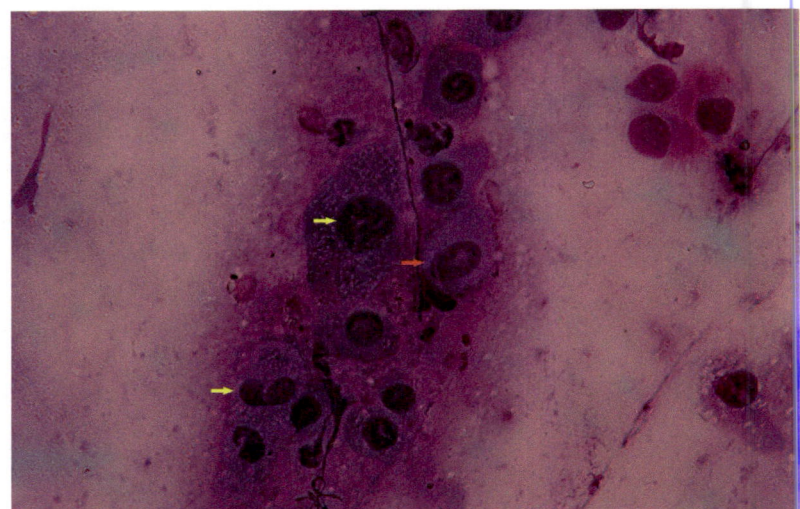

9.5   Idiopathic Interstitial Lung Disease (Undefined Classification)

Brief history: Coughing for more than 3 months with mild dyspnea.

Technology to obtain the target lesions: Transbronchial lung biopsy (TBLB).

The preparation of cytological slides for ROSE: Imprinting (rolling).

Clustering (categorizing) analysis in ROSE interpretation:

- Approximately normal/mild nonspecific inflammatory response.
- May conform to fibrosis (fibrocyte dominant).
- Proliferative/reparative inflammatory response.

Fig. 9.28 (a, b)
Interstitial thickening in
both lungs, especially
subpleural areas, and
extensive ground-glass
opacities

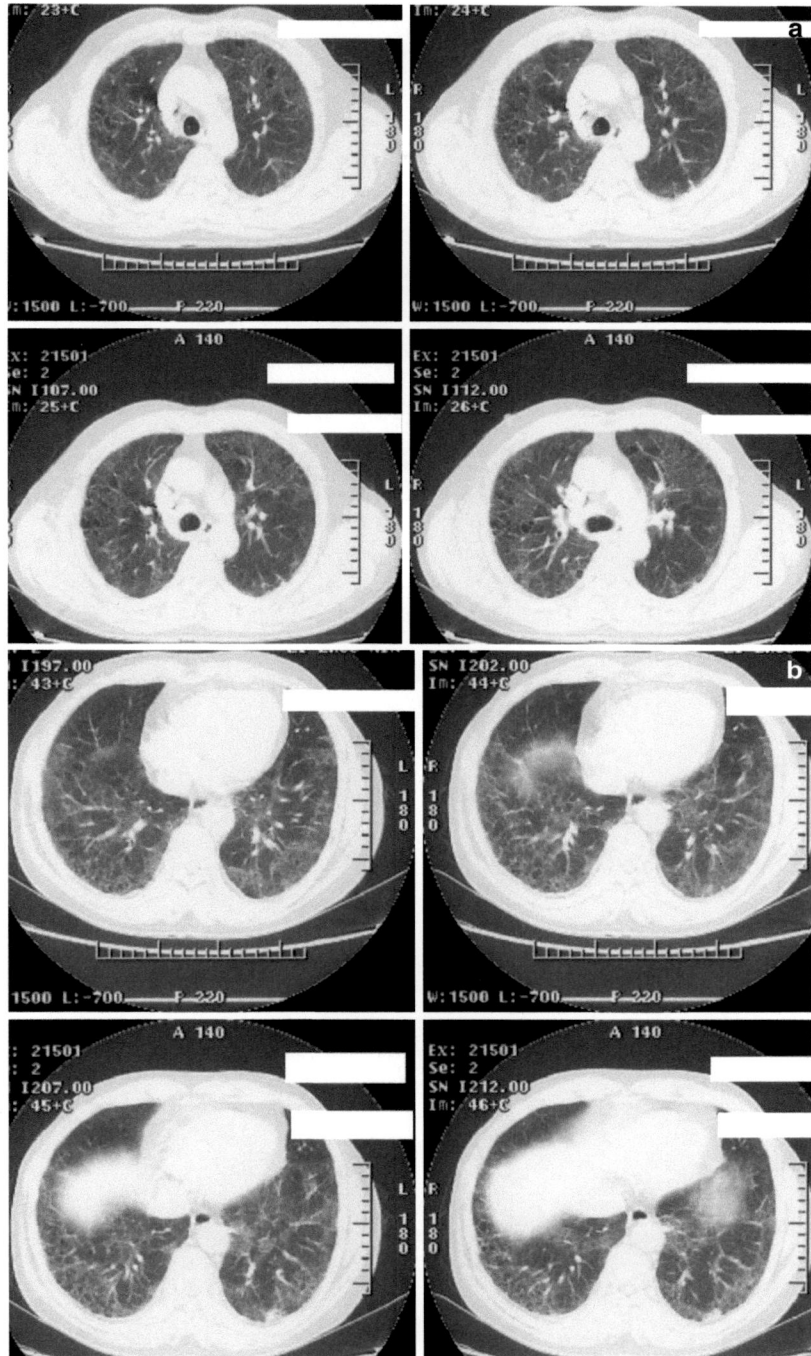

Fig. 9.29 (a–e)
Annotated at the
figure (yellow arrow)

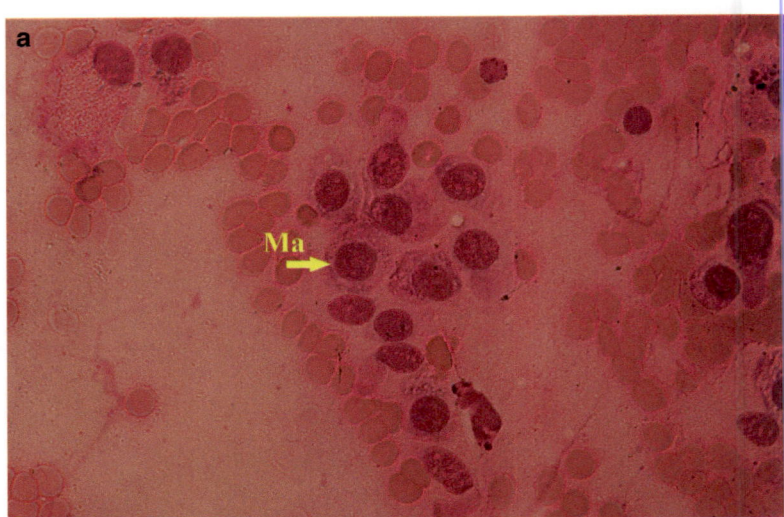

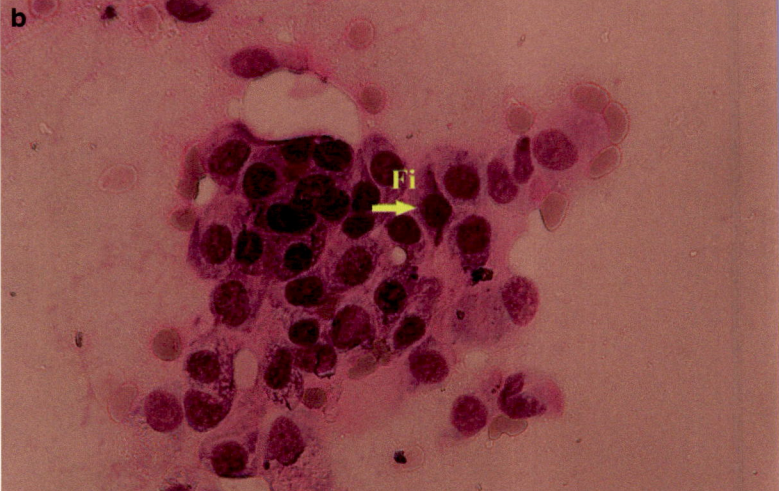

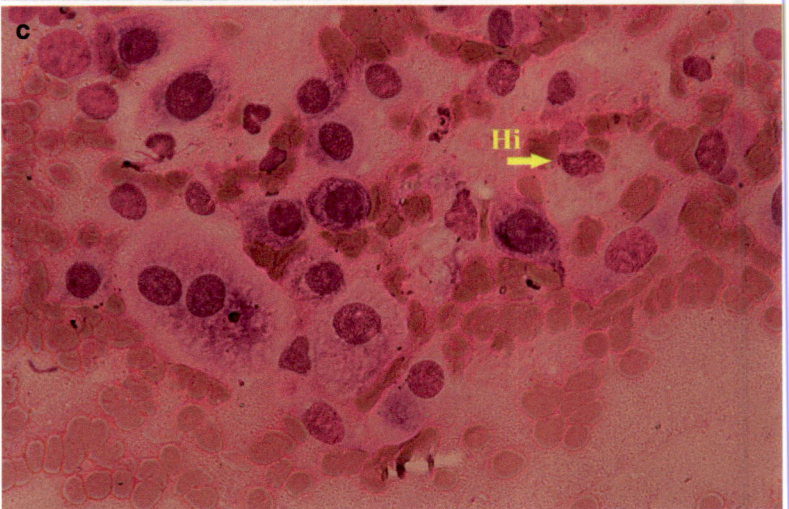

Fig. 9.29 (continued)

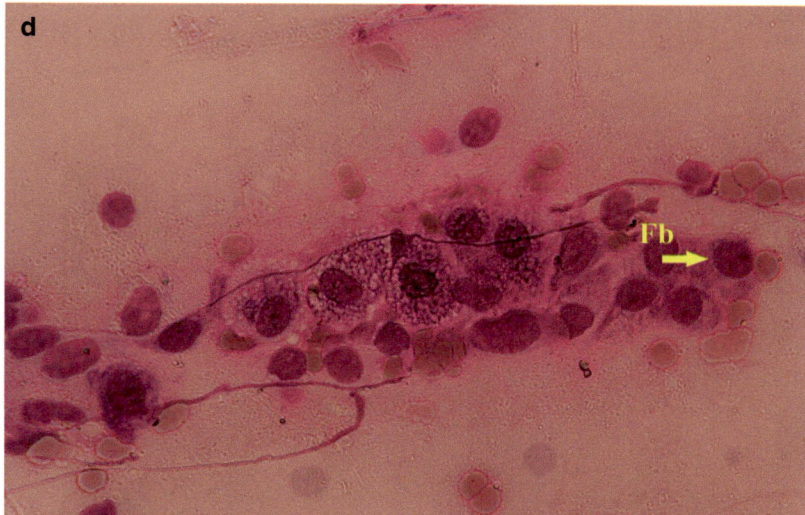

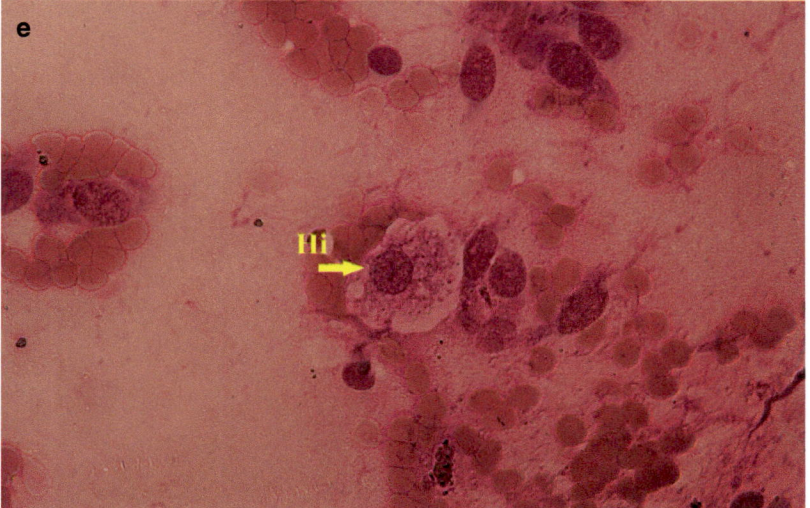

9.6   Idiopathic Interstitial Lung Disease (Undefined Classification), Fibrosing Type

Brief history: Coughing for more than 2 months, dyspnea recently.

Technology to obtain the target lesions: Transbronchial lung biopsy (TBLB).

The preparation of cytological slides for ROSE: Imprinting (rolling).

Clustering (categorizing) analysis in ROSE interpretation:

- May conform to fibrosis (fibroblast dominant).

Fig. 9.30 (**a–c**) Interstitial thickening in both lungs, especially subpleural areas

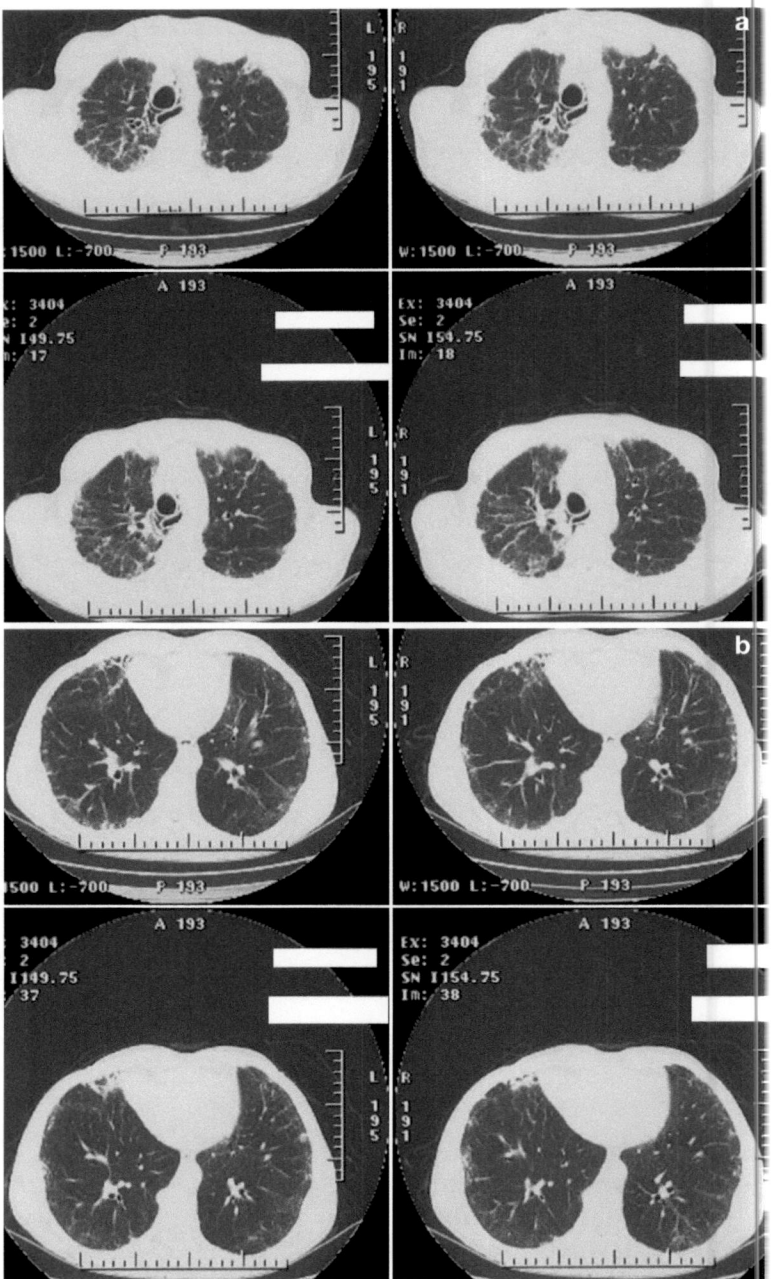

Fig. 9.30 (continued)

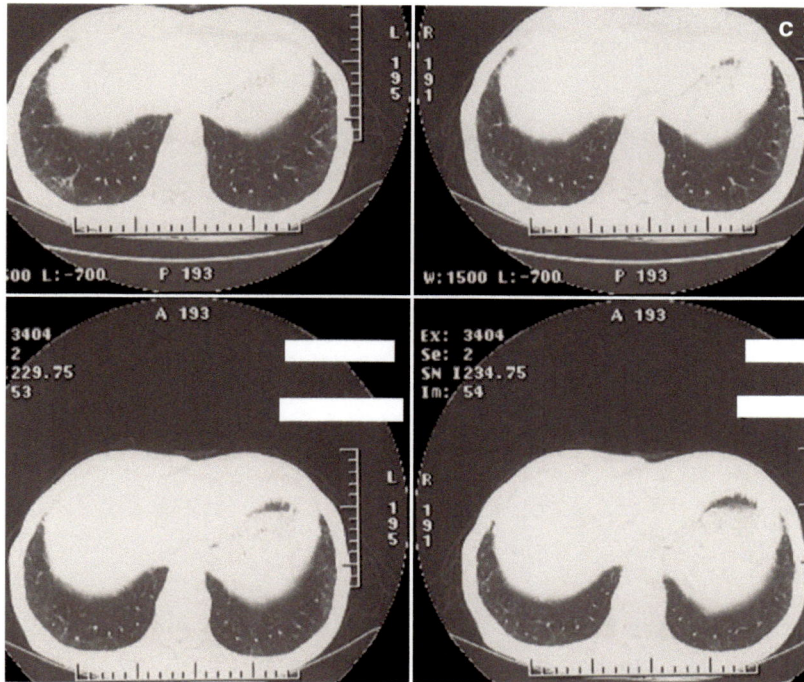

Fig. 9.31 (a–e)
Annotated at the
figure

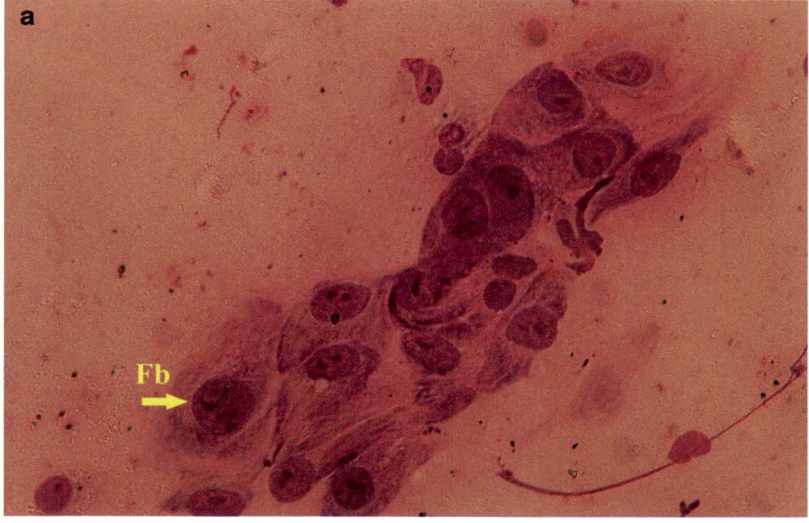

Fig. 9.31 (continued)

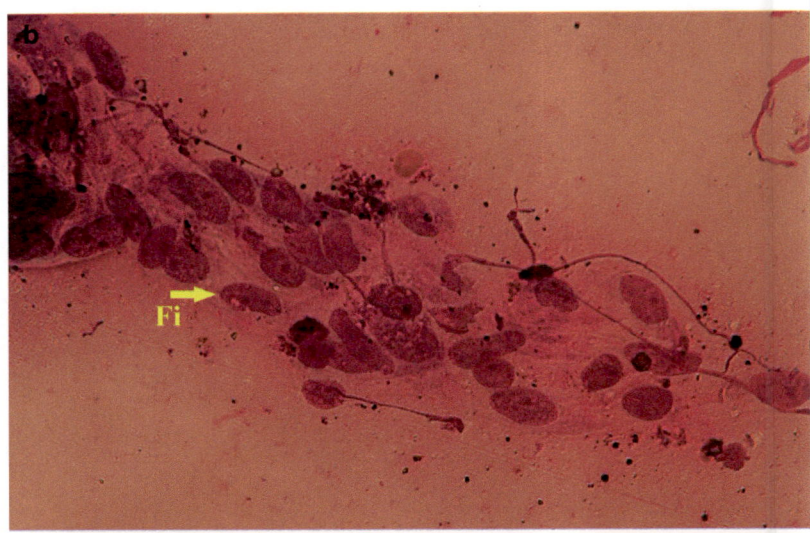

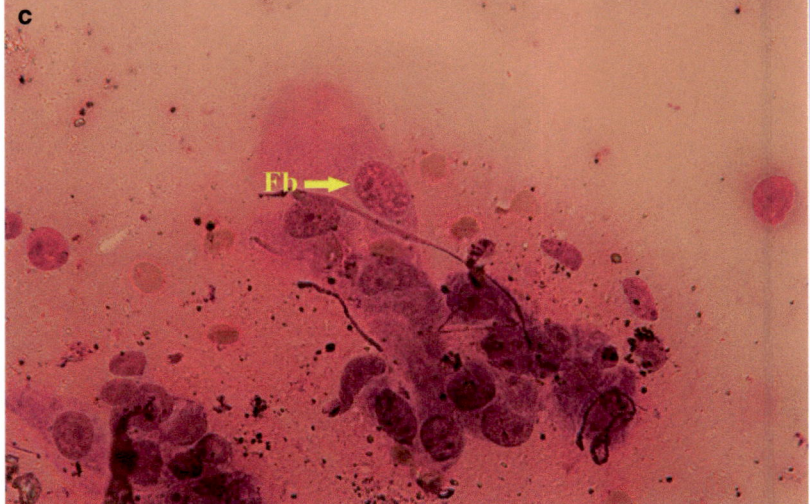

Fig. 9.31 (continued)

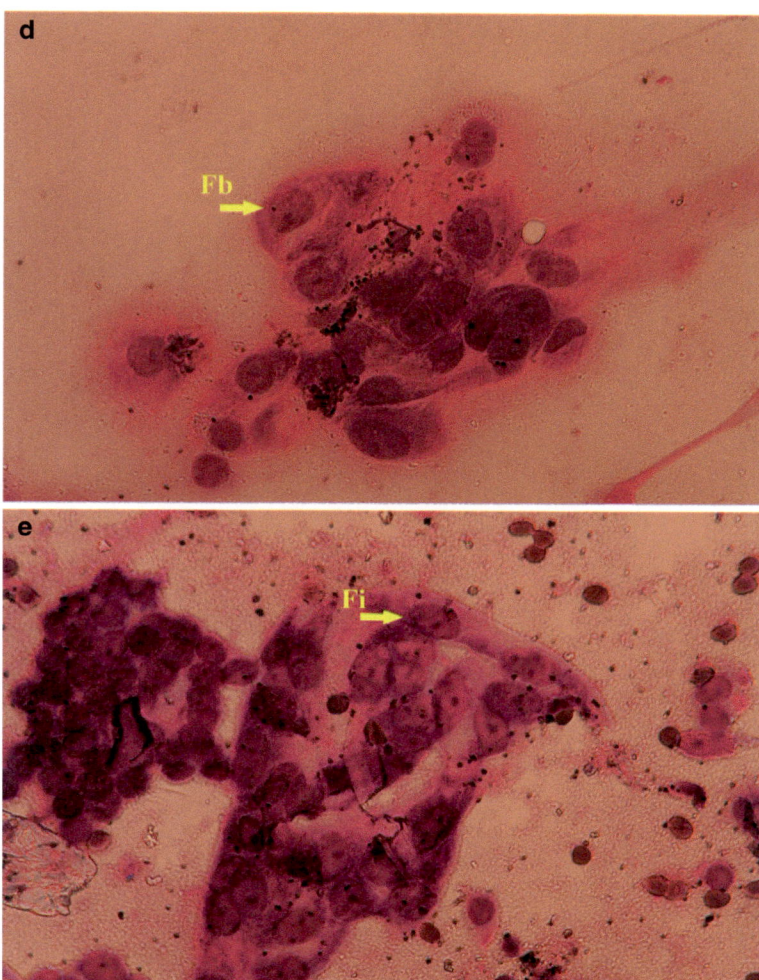

9.7   Pulmonary Alveolar Proteinosis (PAP)

Brief history: Male, 45 years old, coughing with shortness of breath, clinically diagnosed as pulmonary alveolar proteinosis (PAP).

Technology to obtain the target lesions: Transbronchial lung biopsy (TBLB).

The preparation of cytological slides for ROSE: Imprinting (rolling).

Clustering (categorizing) analysis in ROSE interpretation:

- "Inflammatory changes".
- Lymphocyte-based immune inflammatory response.
- There are visible pathogens, characteristic manifestations, or foreign objects.
- Necrotic "inflammatory changes".

Fig. 9.32 (a–c) Diffuse interstitial thickening in both lungs and ground-glass opacities, showing a crazy paving sign

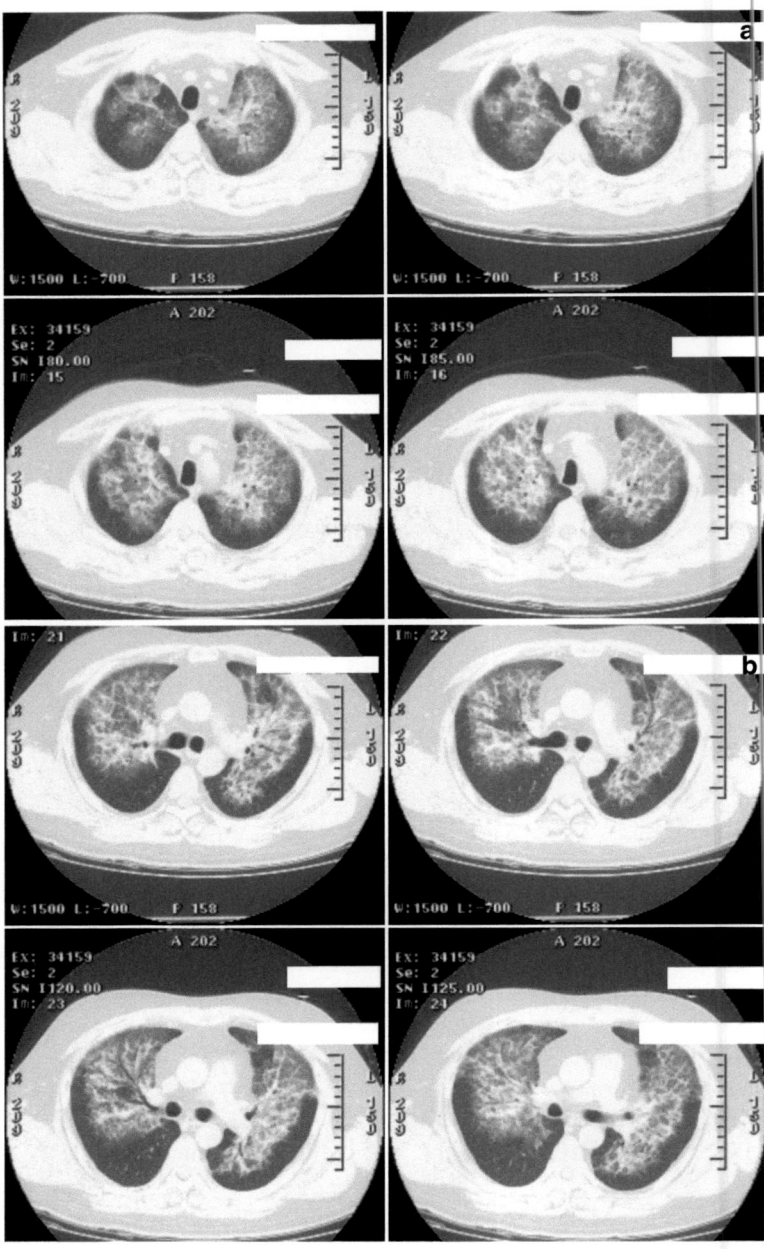

Fig. 9.32 (continued)

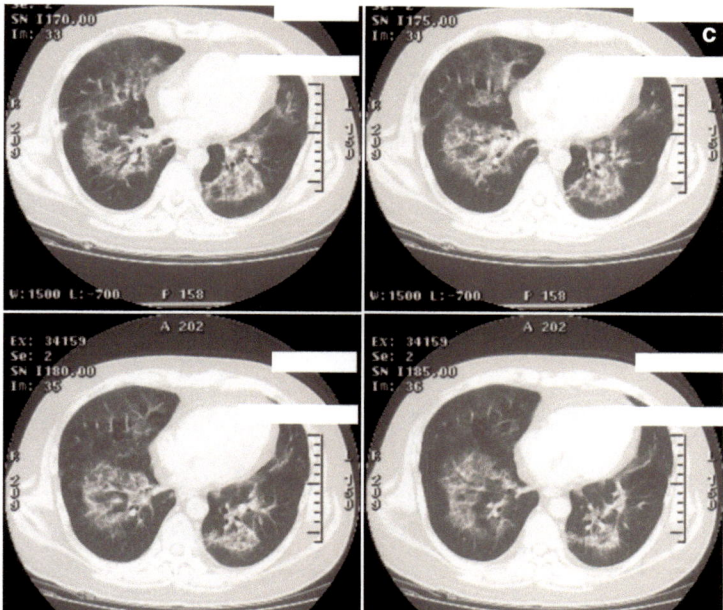

Fig. 9.33 (a–e)
Annotated at the
figure (yellow arrow)
and cyanophilic
amorphous substance
(red arrow)

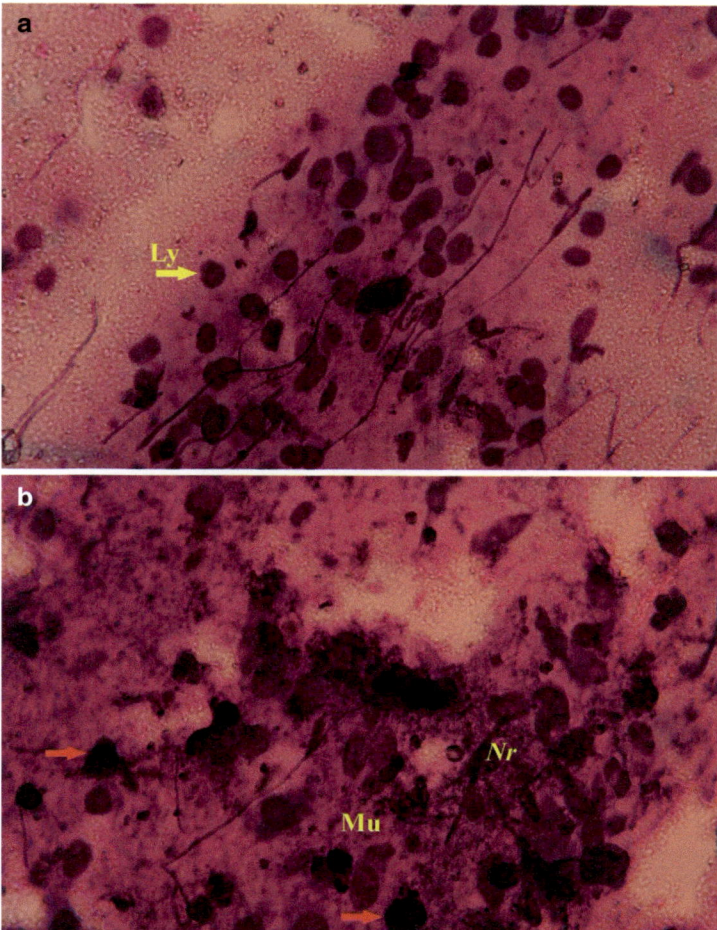

Fig. 9.33 (continued)

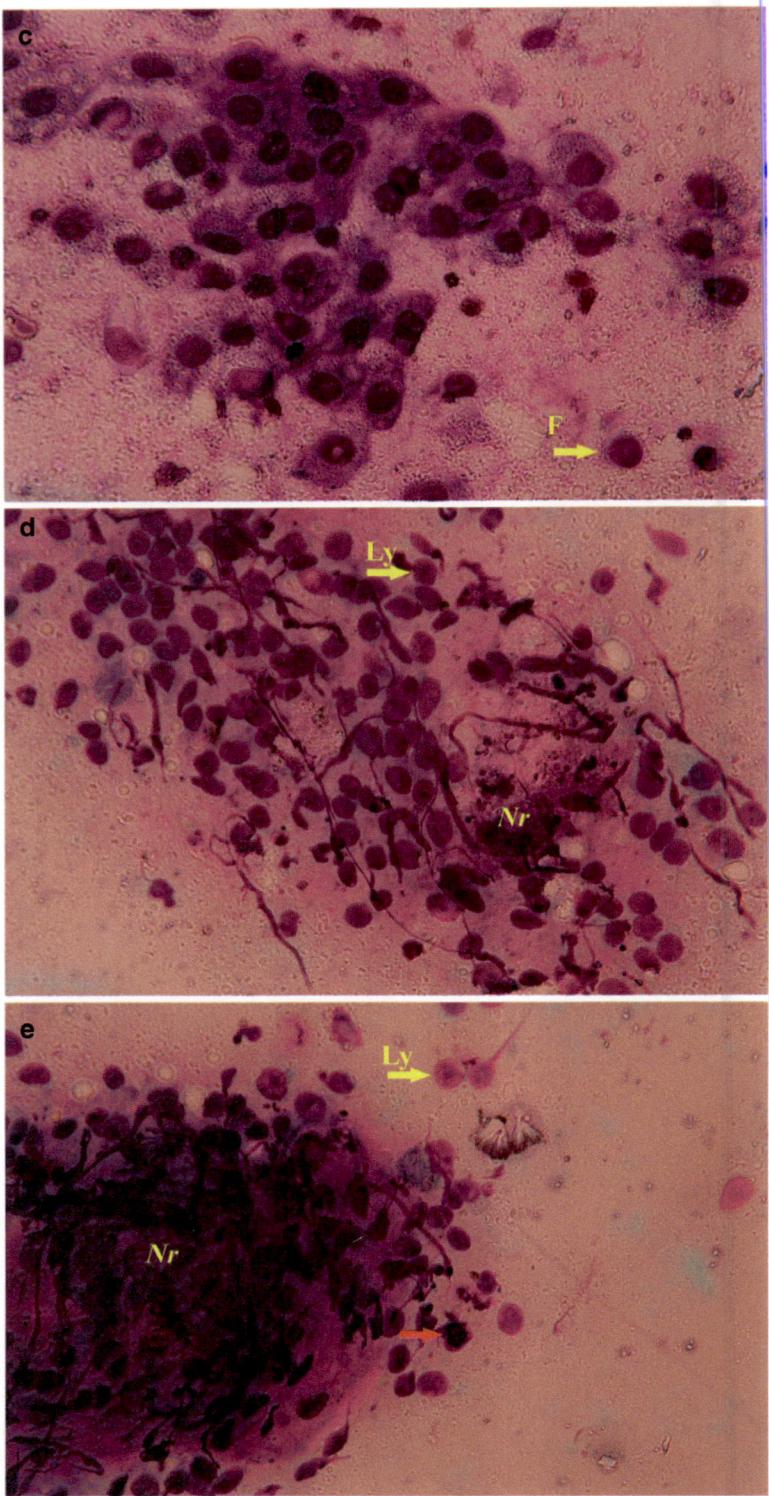

ROSE Cytopathology Cases of Pulmonary Graft-Versus-Host Disease

10

Jing Feng, Dianhua Jiang, and Jingyu Chen

10.1 Pulmonary Graft-Versus-Host Disease

Brief history: Female, 30 years old, 6 months after allogeneic hematopoietic stem cell transplantation due to leukemia, running low fever occasionally, with mild shortness of breath.

Technology to obtain the target lesions: Transbronchial lung biopsy (TBLB).

The preparation of cytological slides for ROSE: Imprinting (rolling).

Clustering (categorizing) analysis in ROSE interpretation:

- "Inflammatory changes".
- May conform to fibrosis (fibroblast dominant or fibrocyte dominant).
- Lymphocyte-based immune inflammatory response.
- Proliferative/reparative inflammatory response.
- Necrotic "inflammatory changes," mild.

J. Feng
Pulmonary and Critical Care Medicine, Tianjin
Medical University General Hospital, Tianjin, China
e-mail: zyyhxkfj@126.com

D. Jiang
Cedars-Sinai Medical Center, Los Angeles, USA
e-mail: Dianhua.Jiang@csmc.edu

J. Chen (✉)
Lung Transplantation Group, Nanjing Medical
University, Wuxi, China
e-mail: chenjy@wuxiph.com

© Springer Nature Singapore Pte Ltd. 2020
J. Feng et al. (eds.), *Rapid On-Site Evaluation (ROSE) in Diagnostic Interventional Pulmonology*,
https://doi.org/10.1007/978-981-15-0939-1_10

Fig. 10.1 (a, b)
Multiple ground-glass
opacities and patches in
both lungs

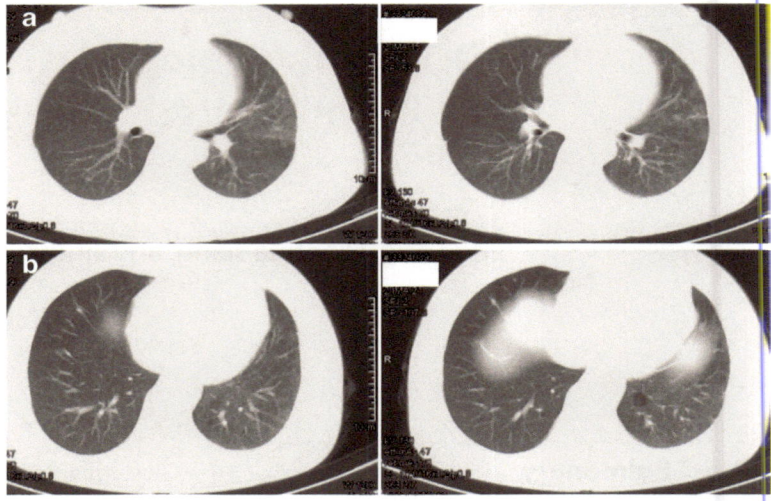

Fig. 10.2 (a–f)
Annotated at the figure
(yellow arrow)

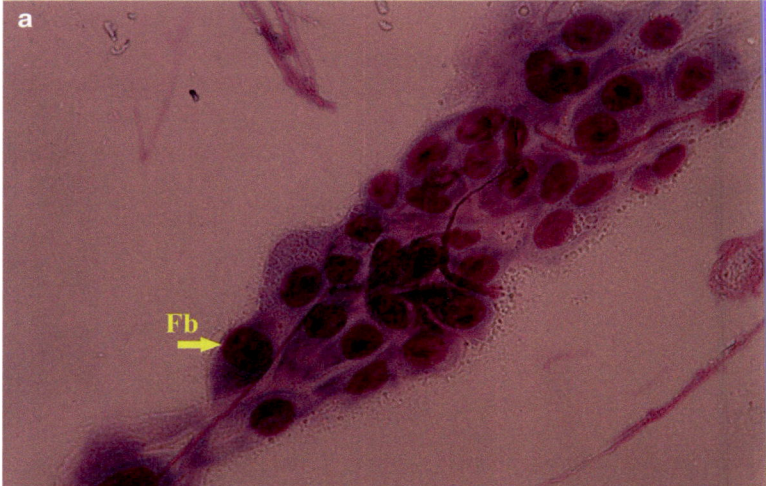

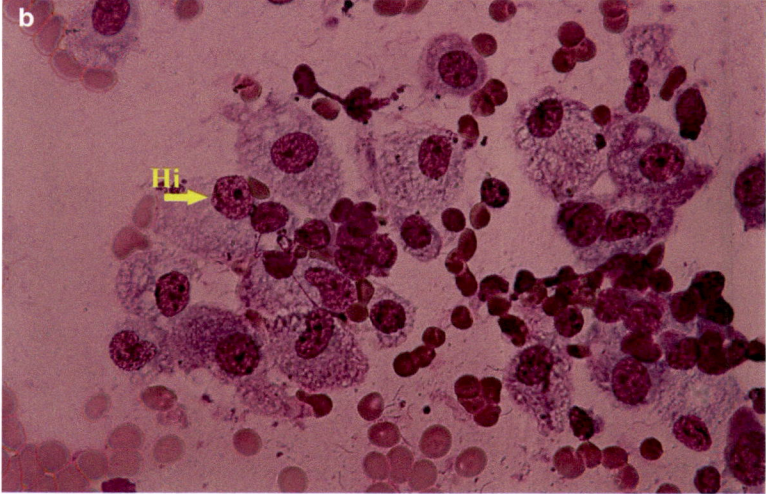

Fig. 10.2 (continued)

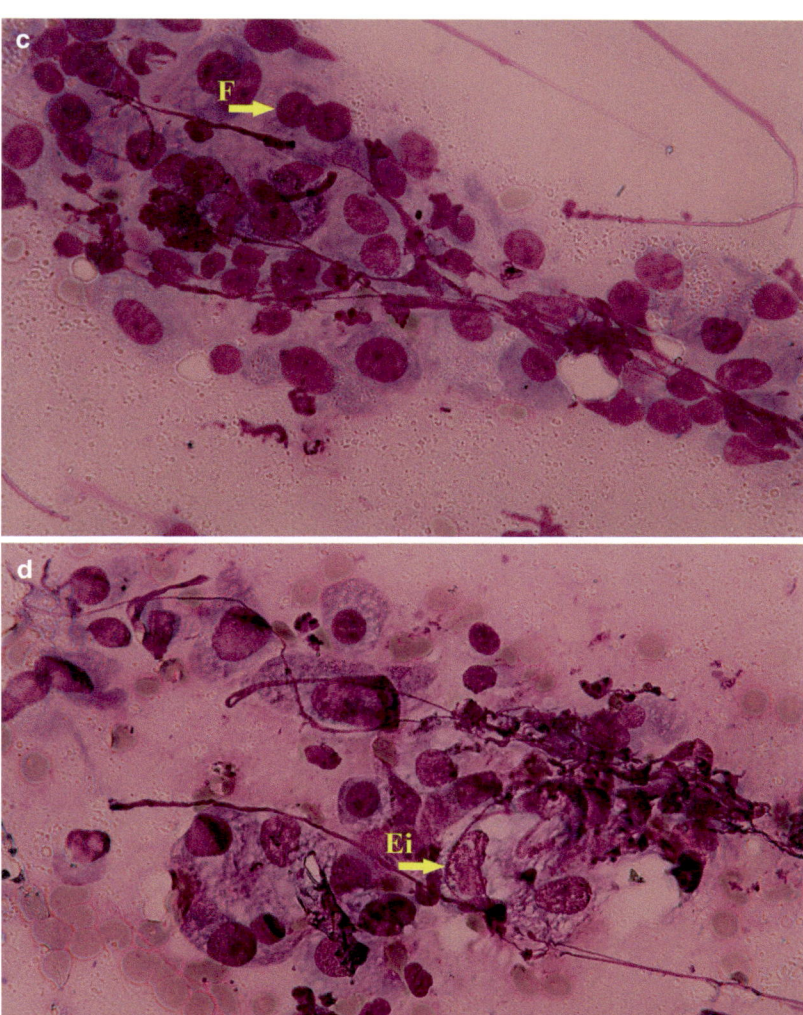

Fig. 10.2 (continued)

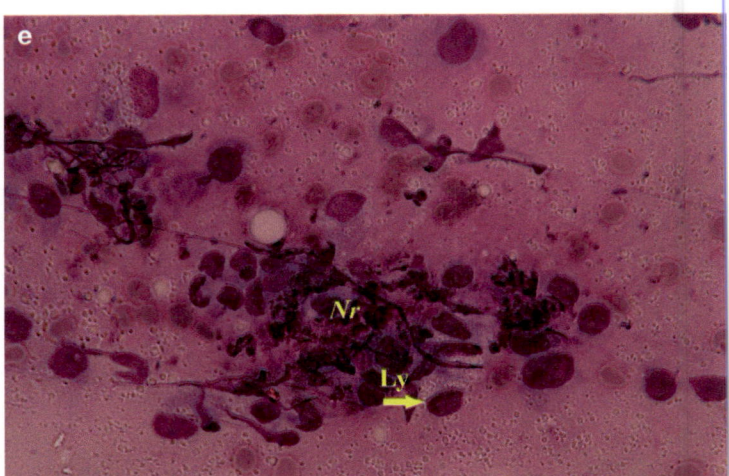

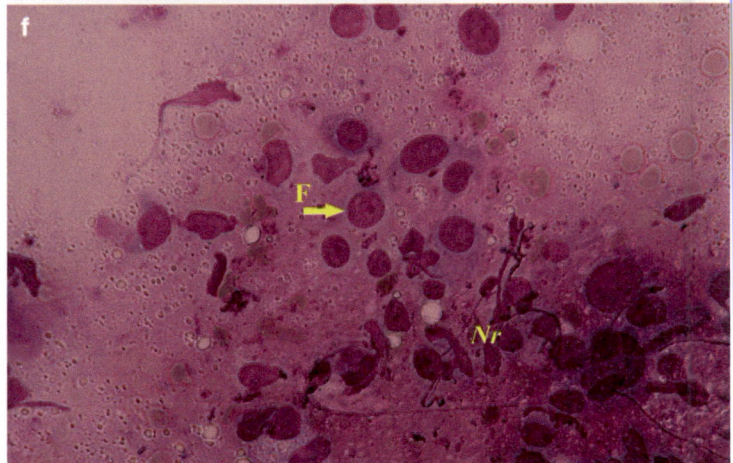

10.2 Pulmonary GVHD After Peripheral Blood Stem Cell Transplantation (Allo-PBSCT)

Brief history: Male, 19 years old, 9 months after peripheral blood stem cell transplantation, clinically diagnosed as systemic GVHD (skin, mucous membrane, digestive system, etc.), dry coughing for 1 week.

Technology to obtain the target lesions: Transbronchial lung biopsy (TBLB).

The preparation of cytological slides for ROSE: Imprinting (rolling).

Clustering (categorizing) analysis in ROSE interpretation:

- Approximately normal/mild nonspecific inflammatory response.
- May conform to fibrosis (fibroblast dominant or fibrocyte dominant).
- Lymphocyte-based immune inflammatory response.
- Proliferative/reparative inflammatory response.

Fig. 10.3 (a, b)
Subpleural
consolidation, interstitial
thickening, and
exudation in the right
lower lobe

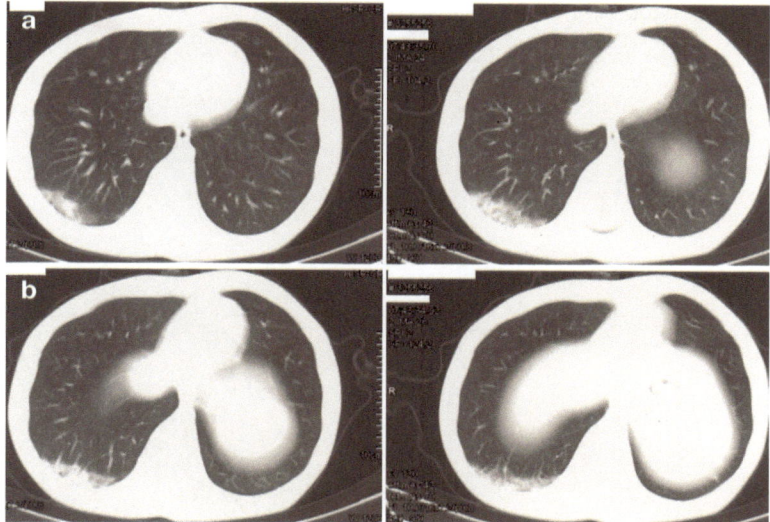

Fig. 10.4 (a–h)
Annotated at the figure
(yellow arrow)

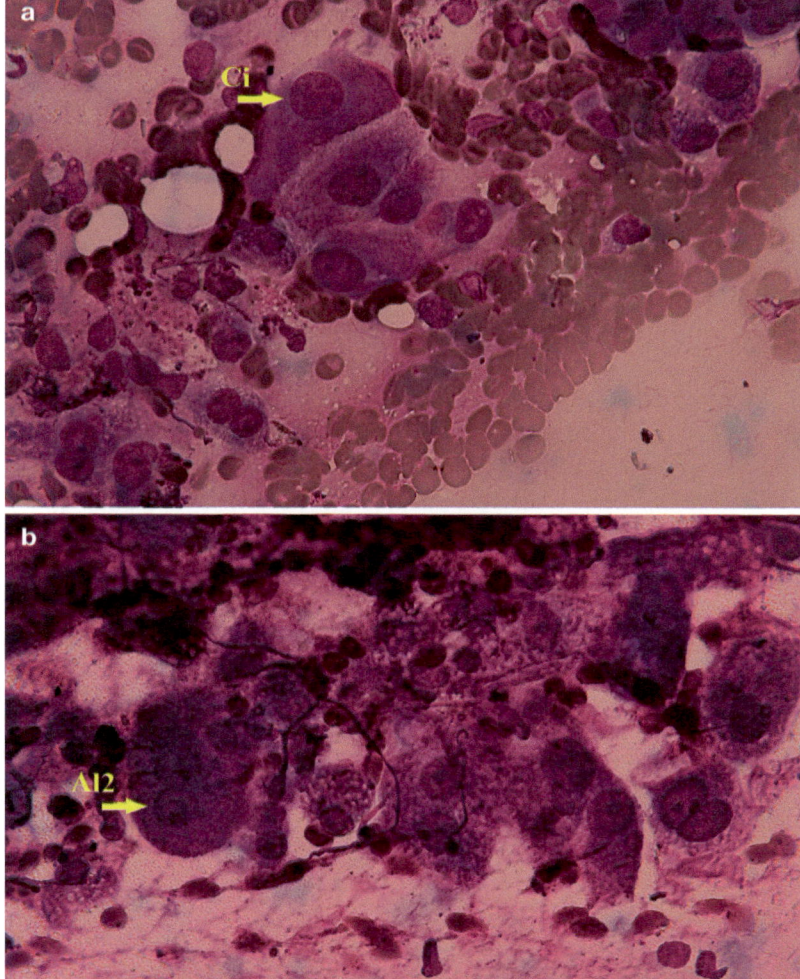

Fig. 10.4 (continued)

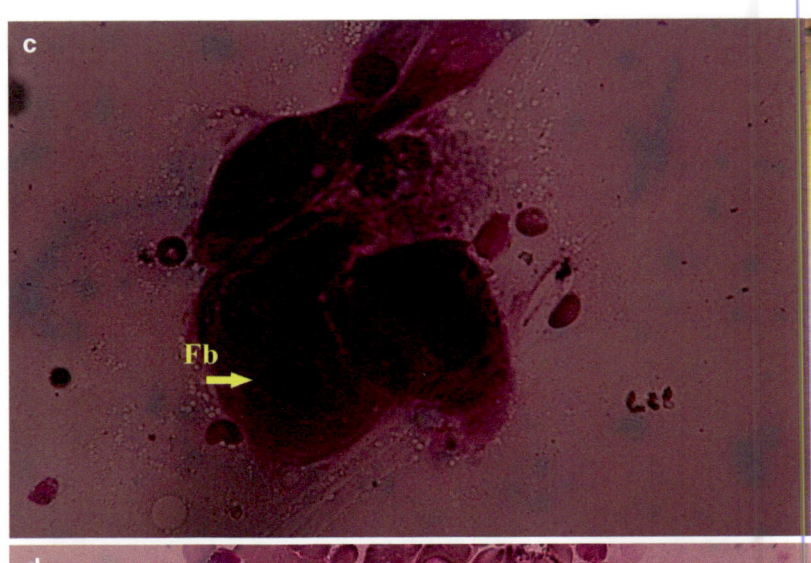

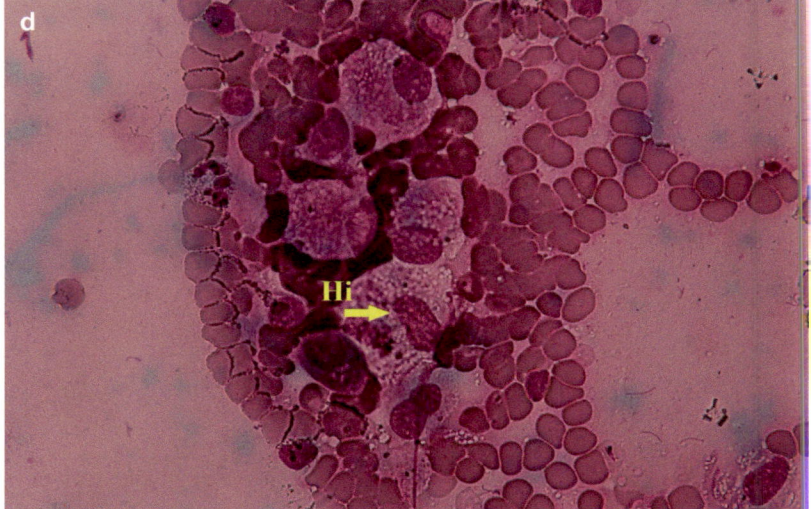

Fig. 10.4   (continued)

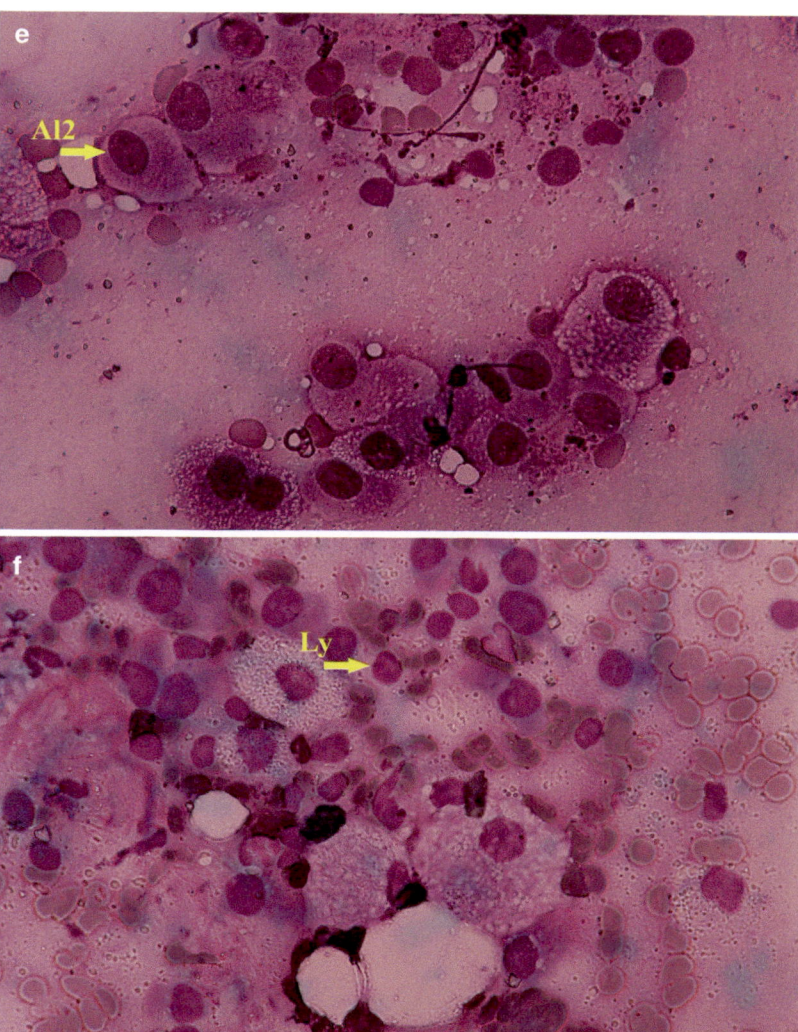

Fig. 10.4 (continued)

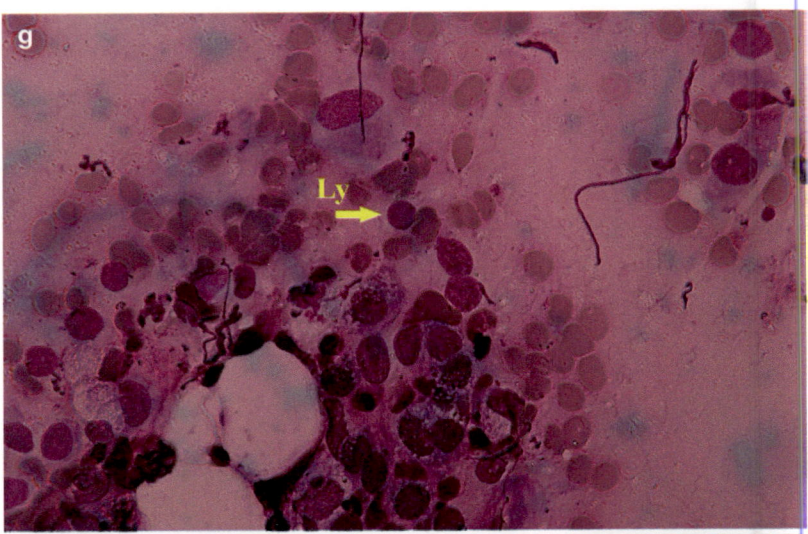

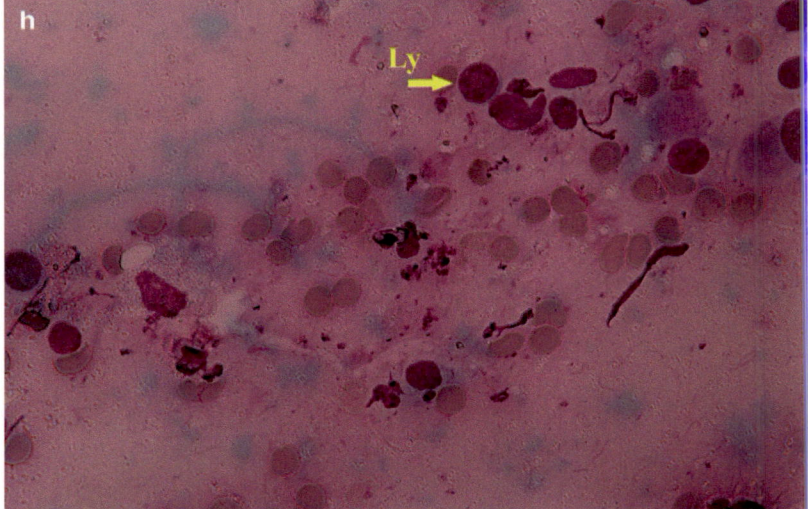

10.3   Pulmonary GVHD After Peripheral Blood Stem Cell Transplantation (Allo-PBSCT)

Brief history: 6 months after allogeneic hematopoietic stem cell transplantation due to acute myeloid leukemia, dyspnea for 10 days, severe mixed ventilatory dysfunction for pulmonary function with a tendency of progressive decline.

Technology to obtain the target lesions: Transbronchial lung biopsy (TBLB).

The preparation of cytological slides for ROSE: Imprinting (rolling).

Clustering (categorizing) analysis in ROSE interpretation:

- Approximately normal/mild nonspecific inflammatory response.
- May conform to fibrosis (fibroblast dominant or fibrocyte dominant).
- Lymphocyte-based immune inflammatory response.
- Proliferative/reparative inflammatory response.

Fig. 10.5 (a–c) Exudation, ground-glass opacities, enhanced visualization of lobular core, and interlobular septal thickening not obvious, especially in both upper lungs

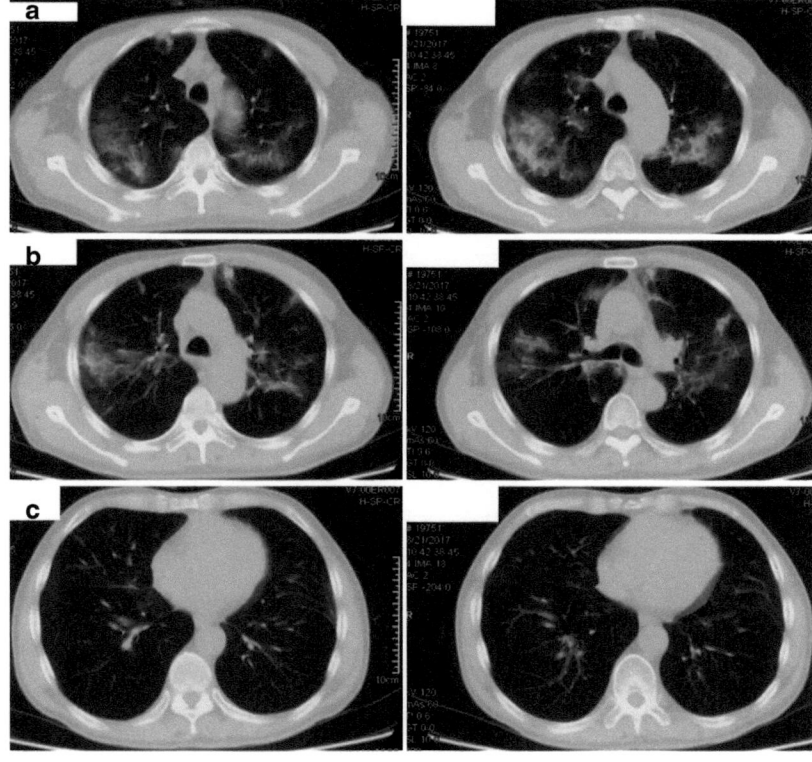

Fig. 10.6 (a–t)
Annotated at the figure
(yellow arrow)

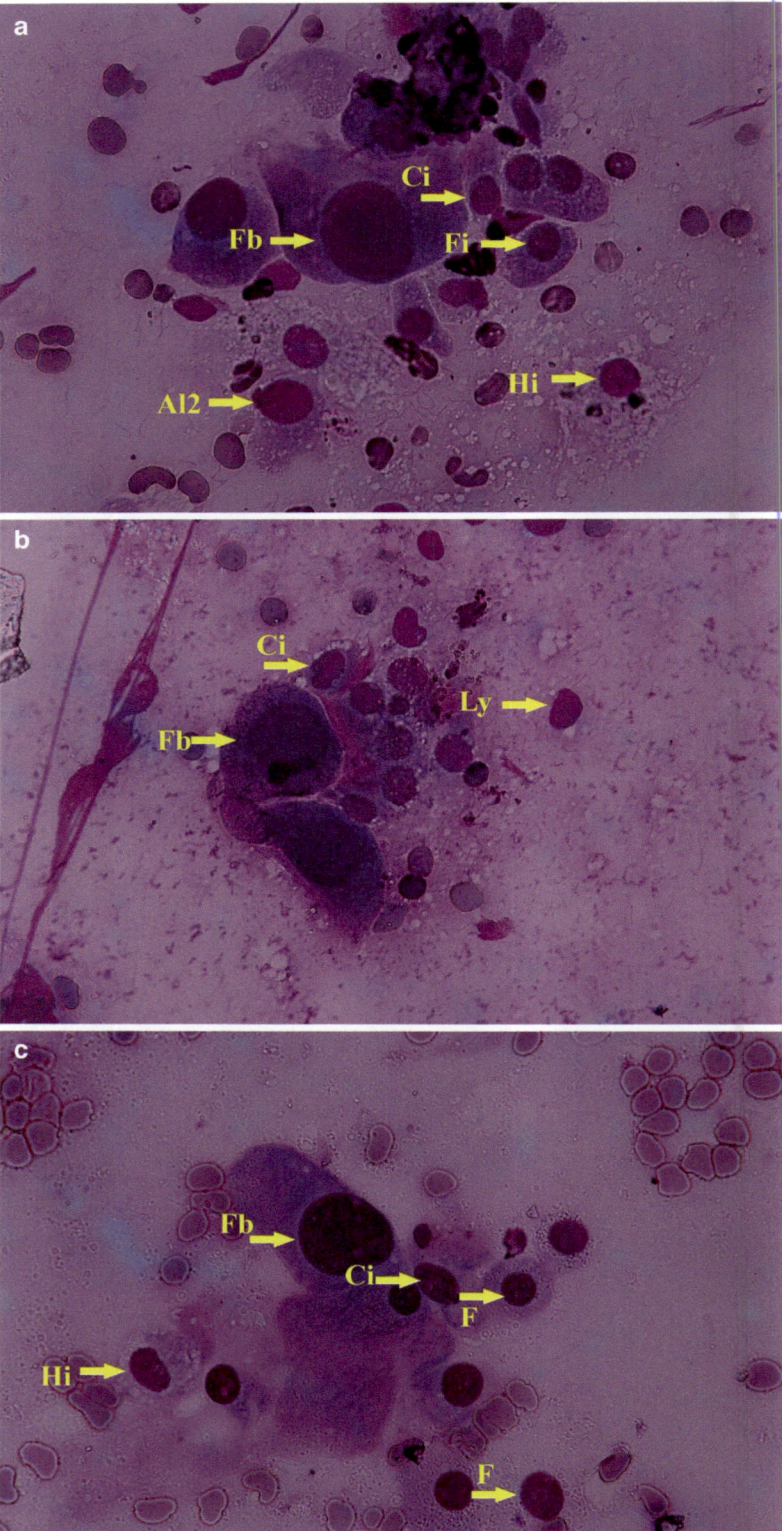

Fig. 10.6 (continued)

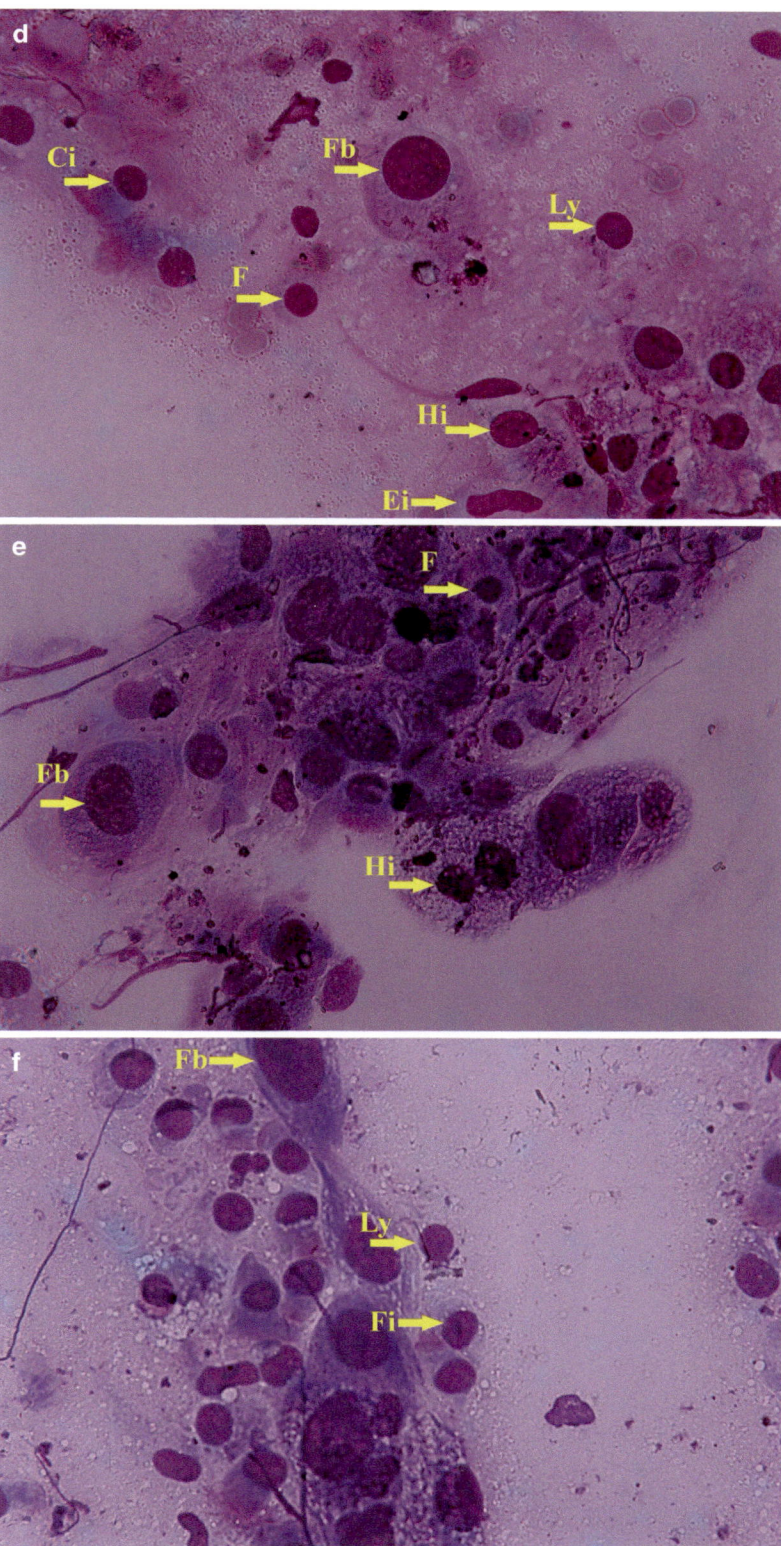

Fig. 10.6 (continued)

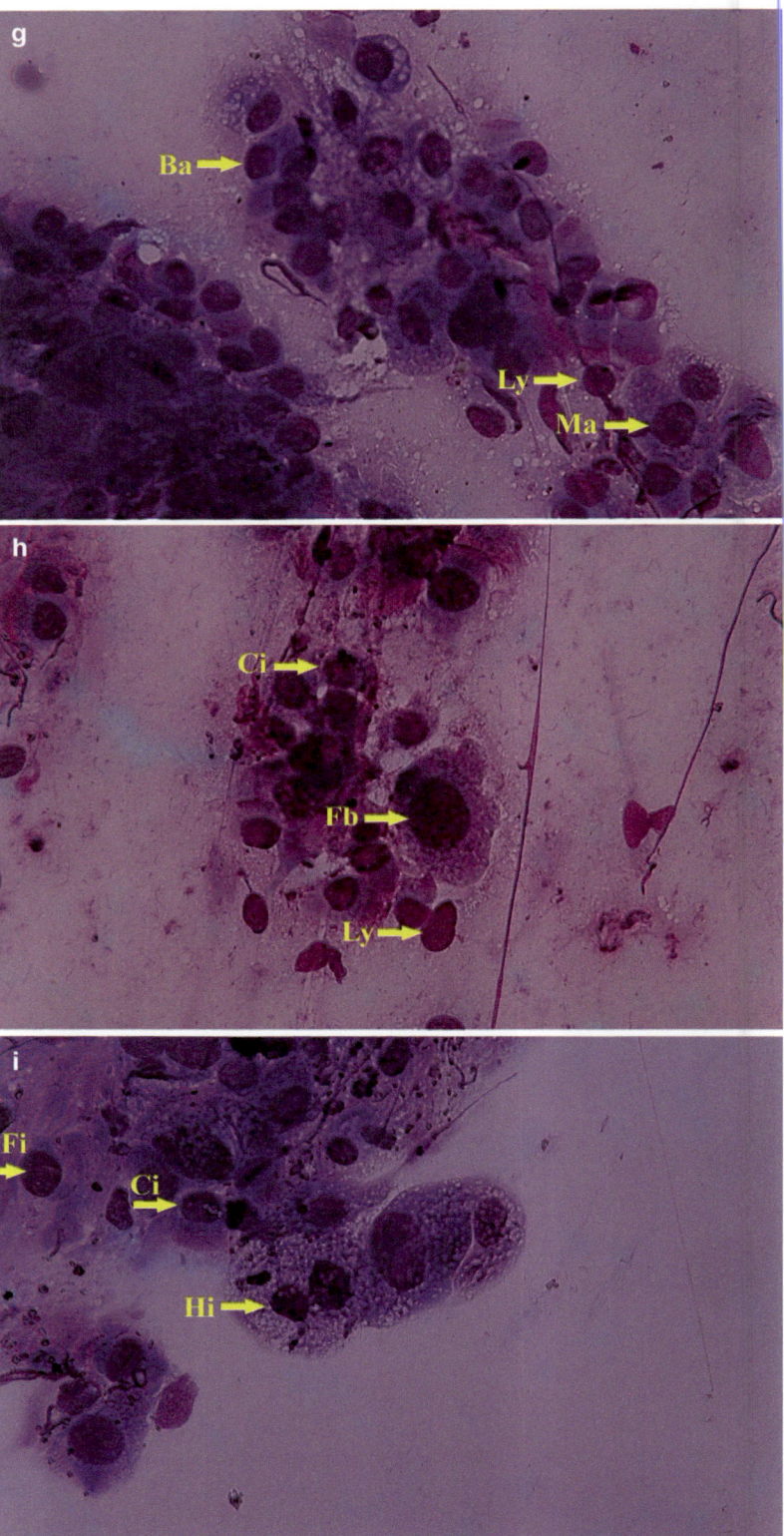

Fig. 10.6 (continued)

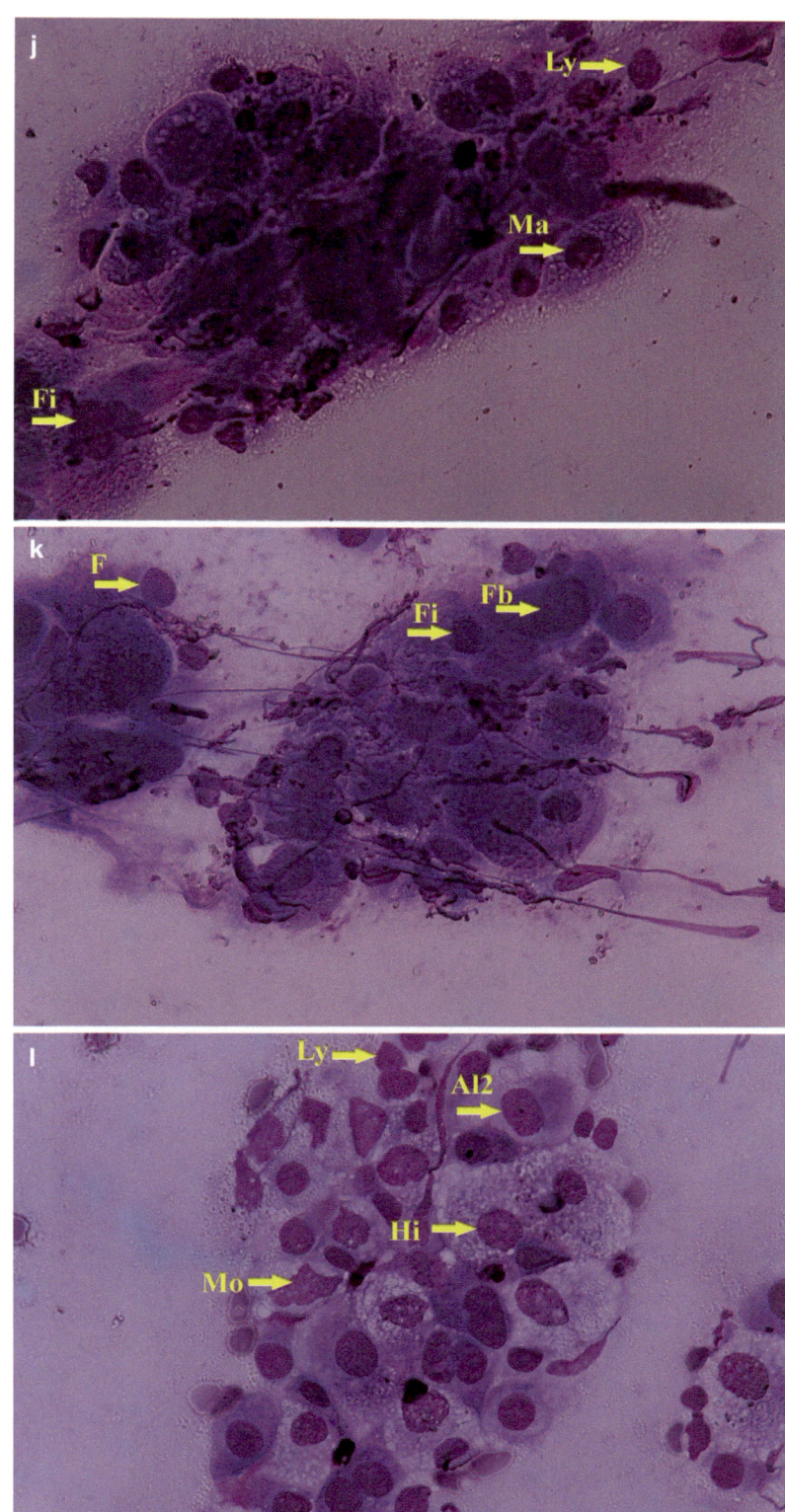

Fig. 10.6 (continued)

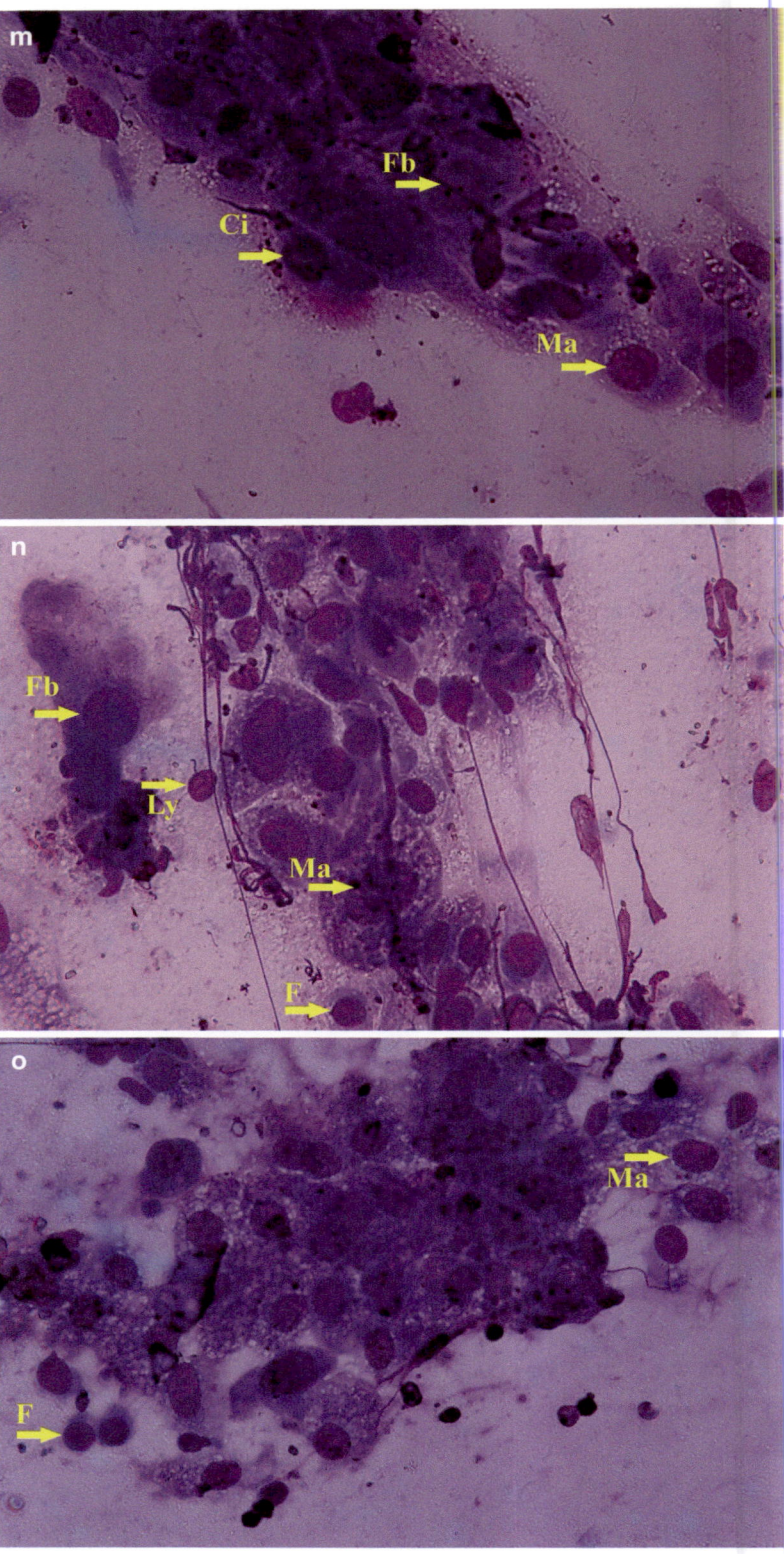

Fig. 10.6 (continued)

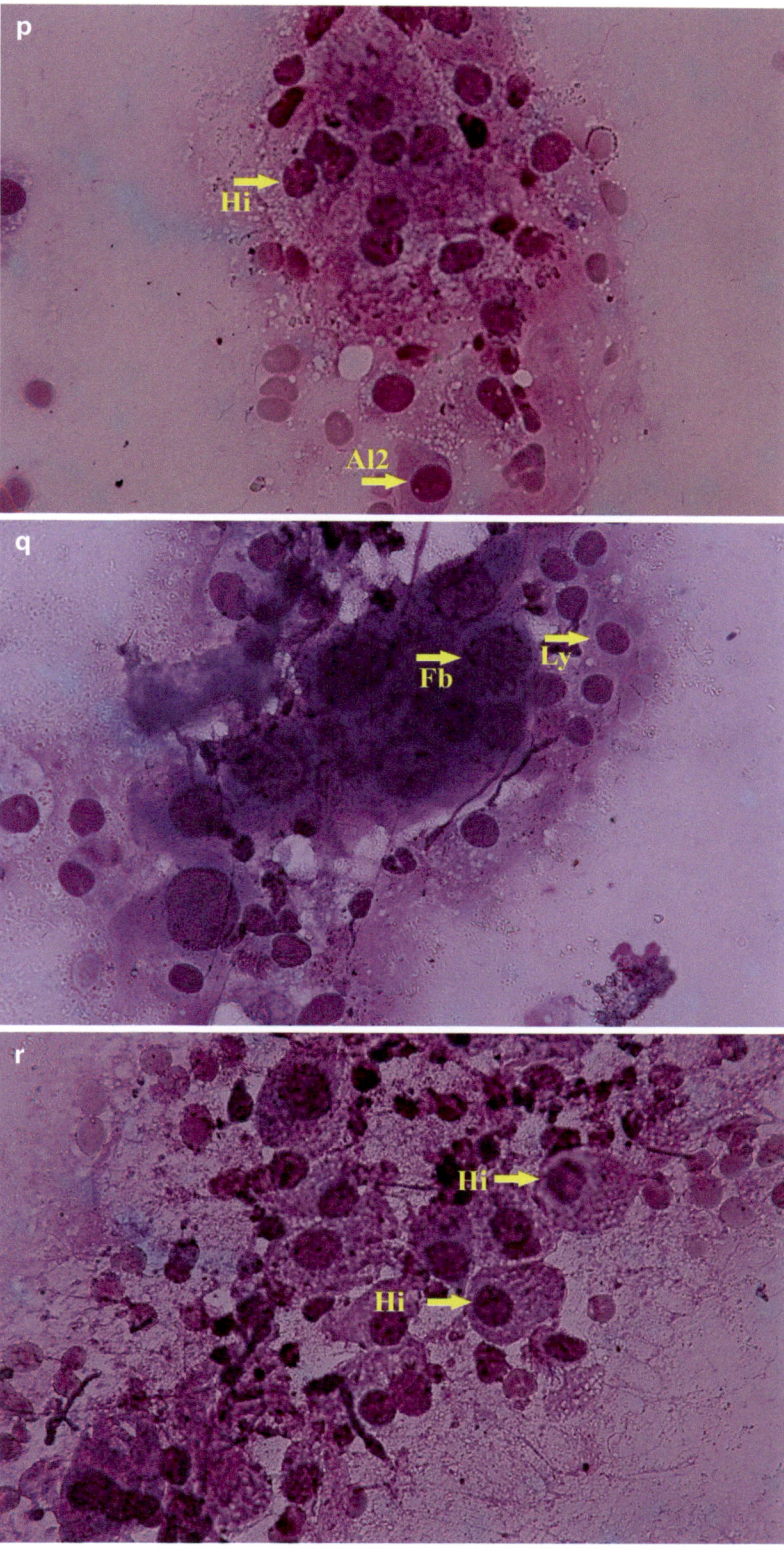

Fig. 10.6 (continued)

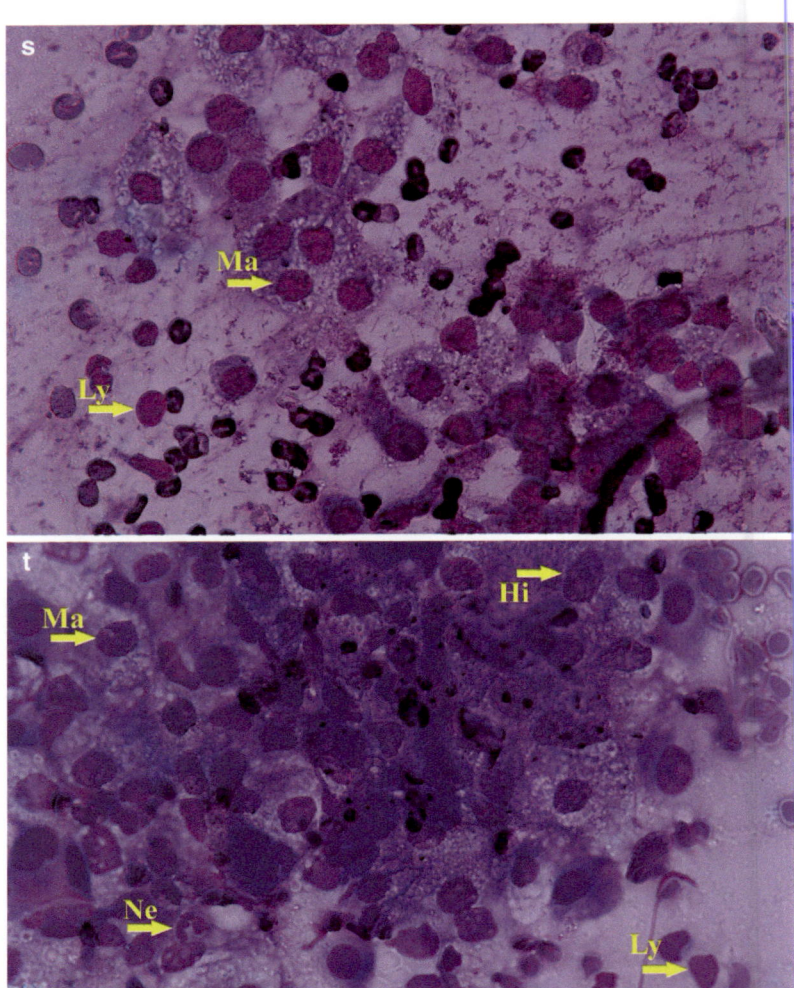

10.4   Pulmonary Graft-Versus-Host Disease (PGVHD)

Brief history: Allogeneic peripheral blood hematopoietic stem cell transplantation for leukemia, 9 months after transplantation, mild dyspnea.

Technology to obtain the target lesions: Transbronchial lung biopsy (TBLB).

The preparation of cytological slides for ROSE: Imprinting (rolling).

Clustering (categorizing) analysis in ROSE interpretation:

- "Inflammatory changes".
- May conform to organization.
- May conform to fibrosis (fibroblast dominant or fibrocyte dominant).
- Proliferative/reparative inflammatory response.

Fig. 10.7 (a–c) Multiple ground-glass opacities in both lungs

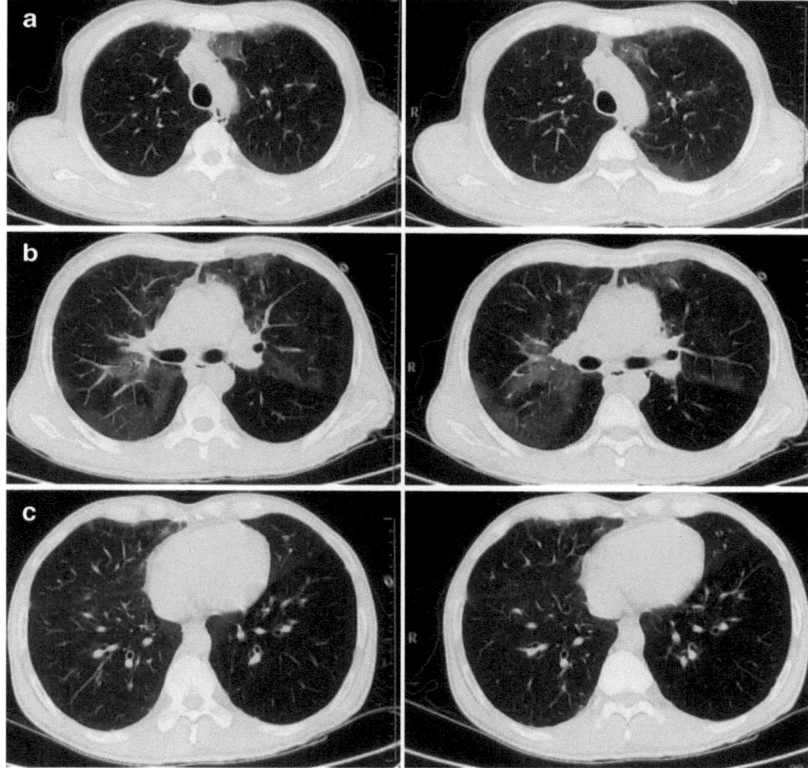

Fig. 10.8 (a–f)
Annotated at the figure
(yellow arrow)

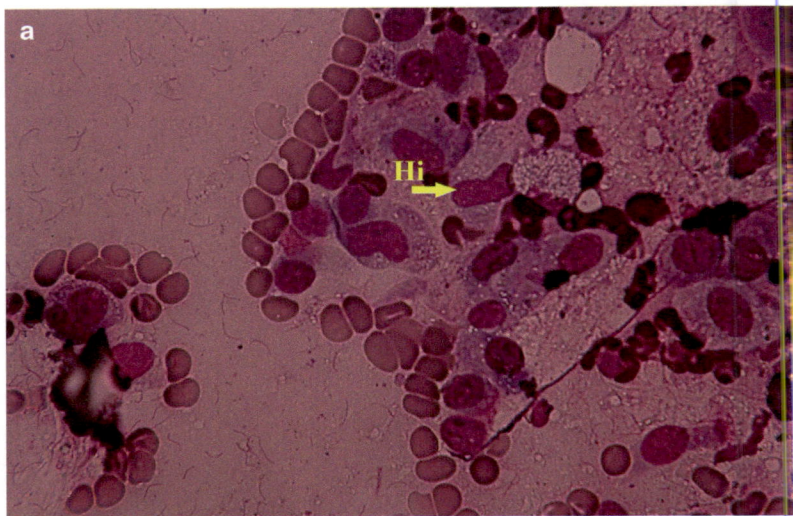

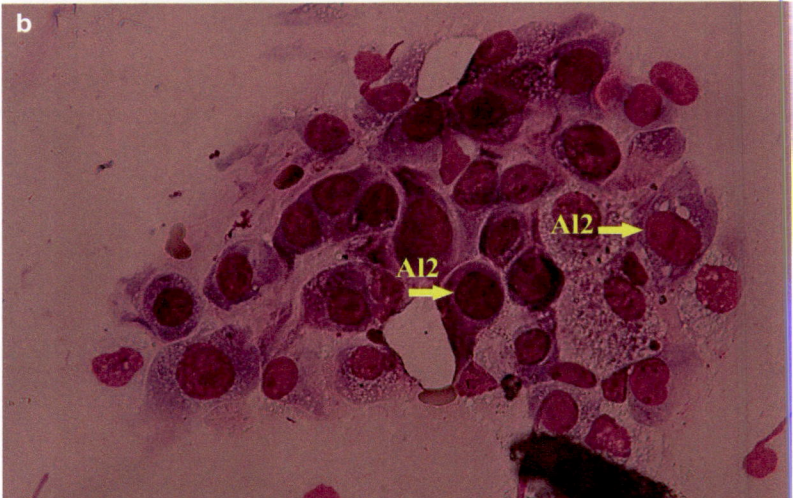

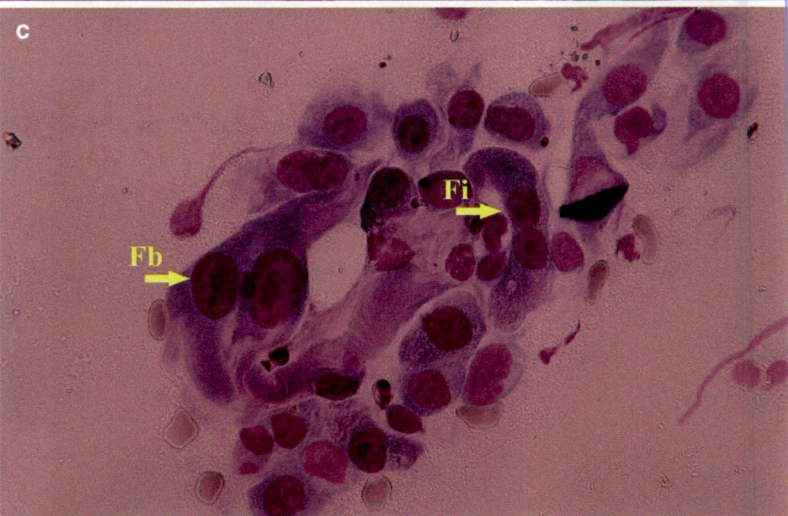

Fig. 10.8   (continued)

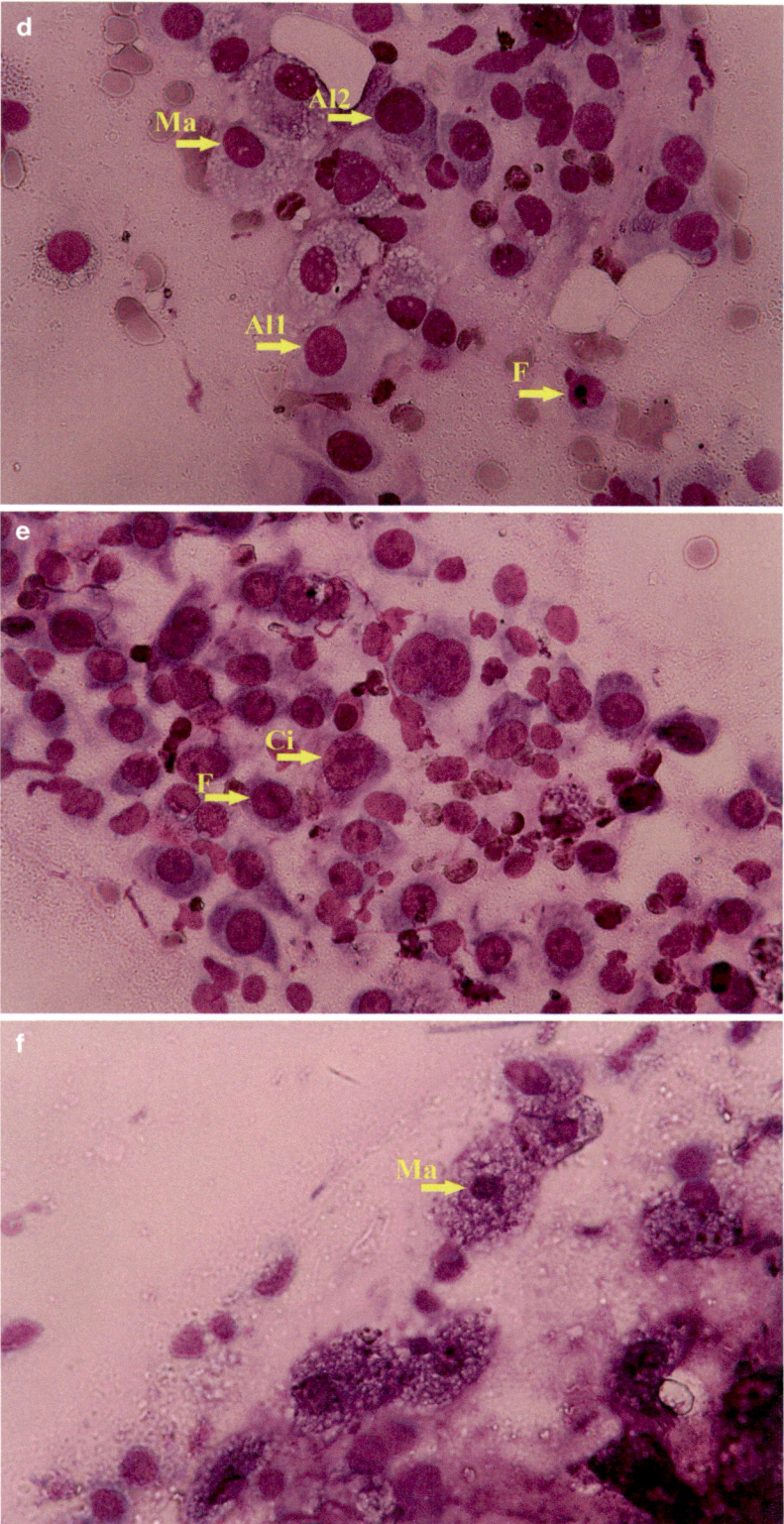

ROSE Cytopathology Cases of Immunogenic Interstitial Changes

11

Jing Feng, Jingyu Chen, and Wen Ning

11.1 Pulmonary Inflammatory Response After Chemotherapy for Myelodysplastic Syndrome (MDS)

Brief history: Male, 24 years old, clinically diagnosed as myelodysplastic syndrome (MDS), running a fever discontinuously with mild shortness of breath.

Technology to obtain the target lesions: Transbronchial lung biopsy (TBLB).

The preparation of cytological slides for ROSE: Imprinting (rolling).

Clustering (categorizing) analysis in ROSE interpretation:

- "Inflammatory changes".
- Lymphocyte-based immune inflammatory response.

J. Feng
Pulmonary and Critical Care Medicine, Tianjin Medical University General Hospital, Tianjin, China
e-mail: zyyhxkfj@126.com

J. Chen
Lung Transplantation Group, Nanjing Medical University, Wuxi, China
e-mail: chenjy@wuxiph.com

W. Ning (✉)
College of Life Sciences, Nankai University, Tianjin, China
e-mail: ningwen108@nankai.edu.cn

© Springer Nature Singapore Pte Ltd. 2020
J. Feng et al. (eds.), *Rapid On-Site Evaluation (ROSE) in Diagnostic Interventional Pulmonology*,
https://doi.org/10.1007/978-981-15-0939-1_11

Fig. 11.1 (a, b) Extensive ground-glass opacities in both lungs, evenly distributed

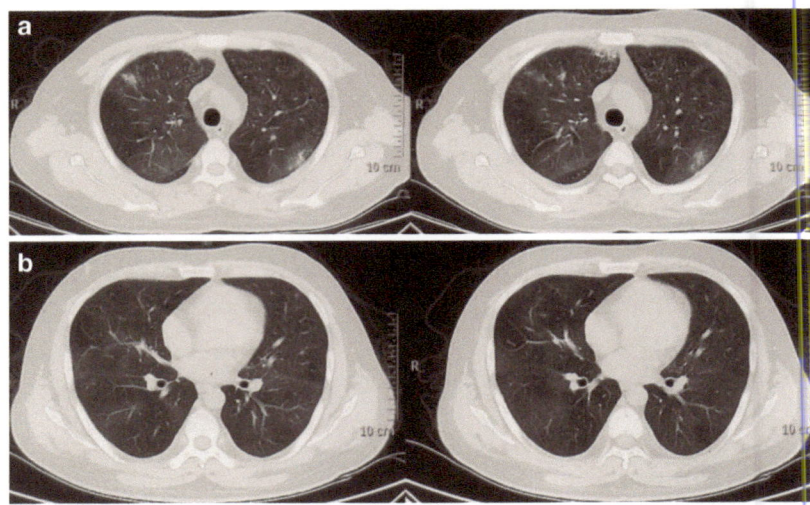

Fig. 11.2 (a–e) Annotated at the figure (yellow arrow)

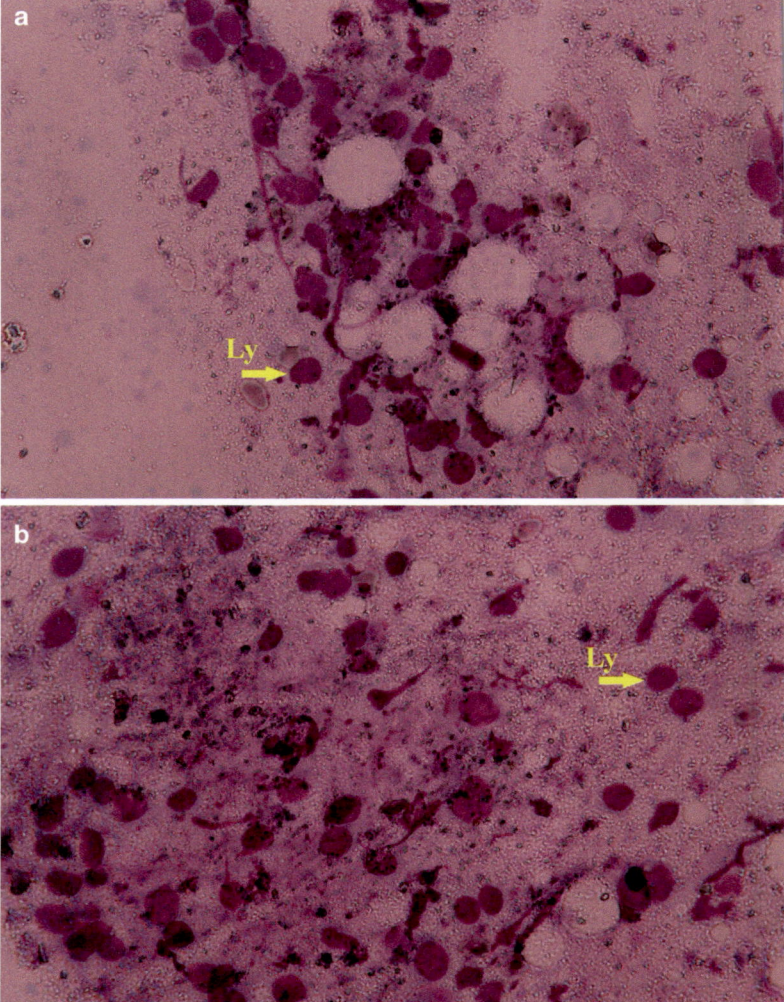

Fig. 11.2   (continued)

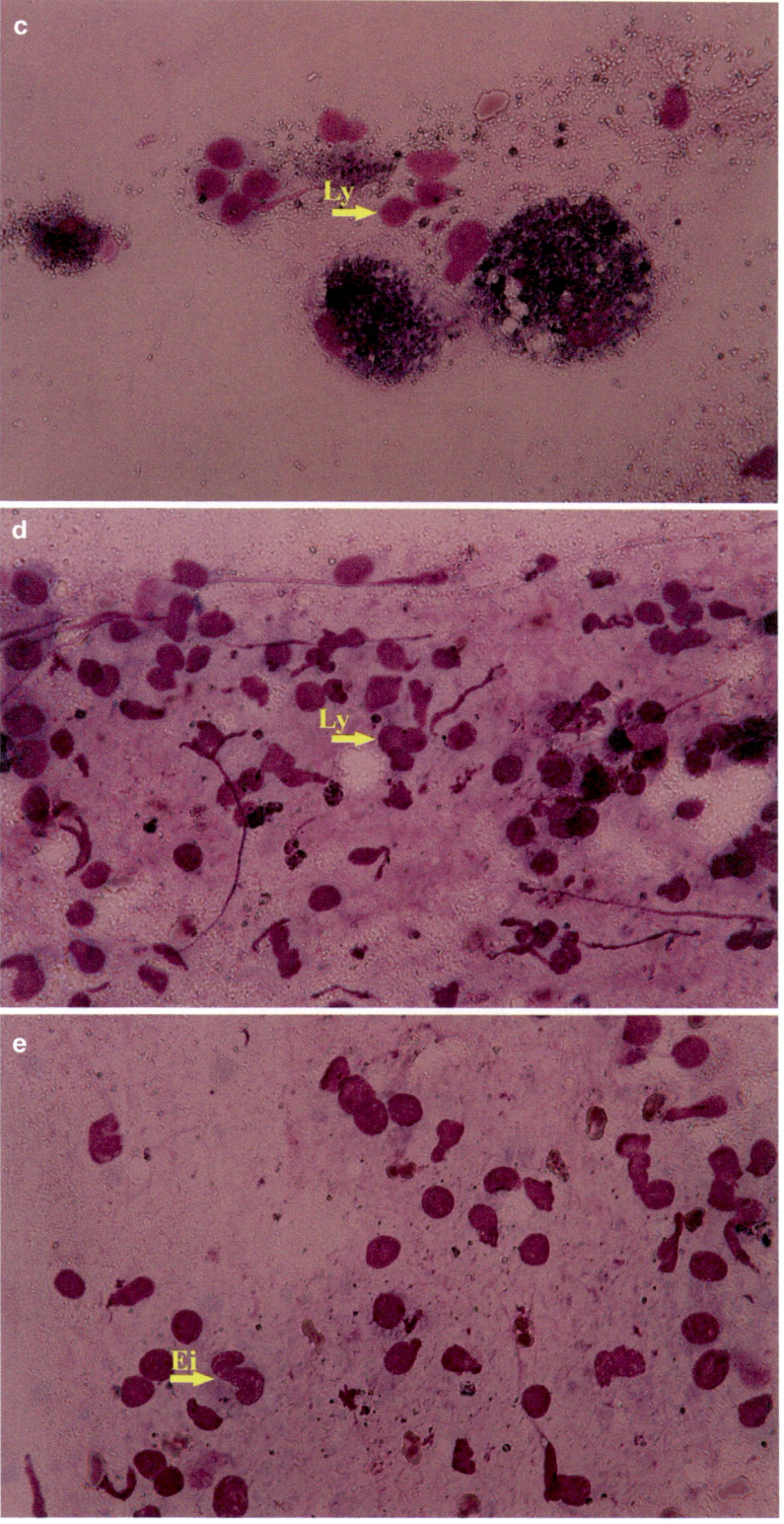

11.2 Pulmonary Involvement Due to Immune Panhematopenia (Pancytopenia)*

Brief history: Clinically diagnosed as immune panhematopenia (pancytopenia), coughing for more than 2 months, with mild shortness of breath.

Technology to obtain the target lesions: Transbronchial lung biopsy (TBLB).

The preparation of cytological slides for ROSE: Imprinting (rolling).

Clustering (categorizing) analysis in ROSE interpretation:

- "Inflammatory changes".
- Granulomatous inflammation.
- May conform to organization.
- Lymphocyte-based immune inflammatory response.

Fig. 11.3 (a–c) Extensive interstitial thickening, scattered exudation and patches, and consolidation in both lower lobes

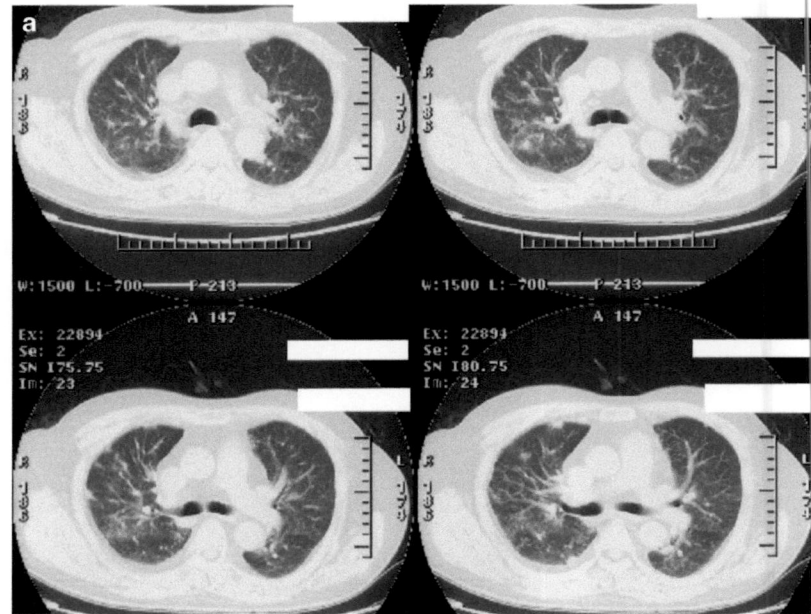

Fig. 11.3 (continued)

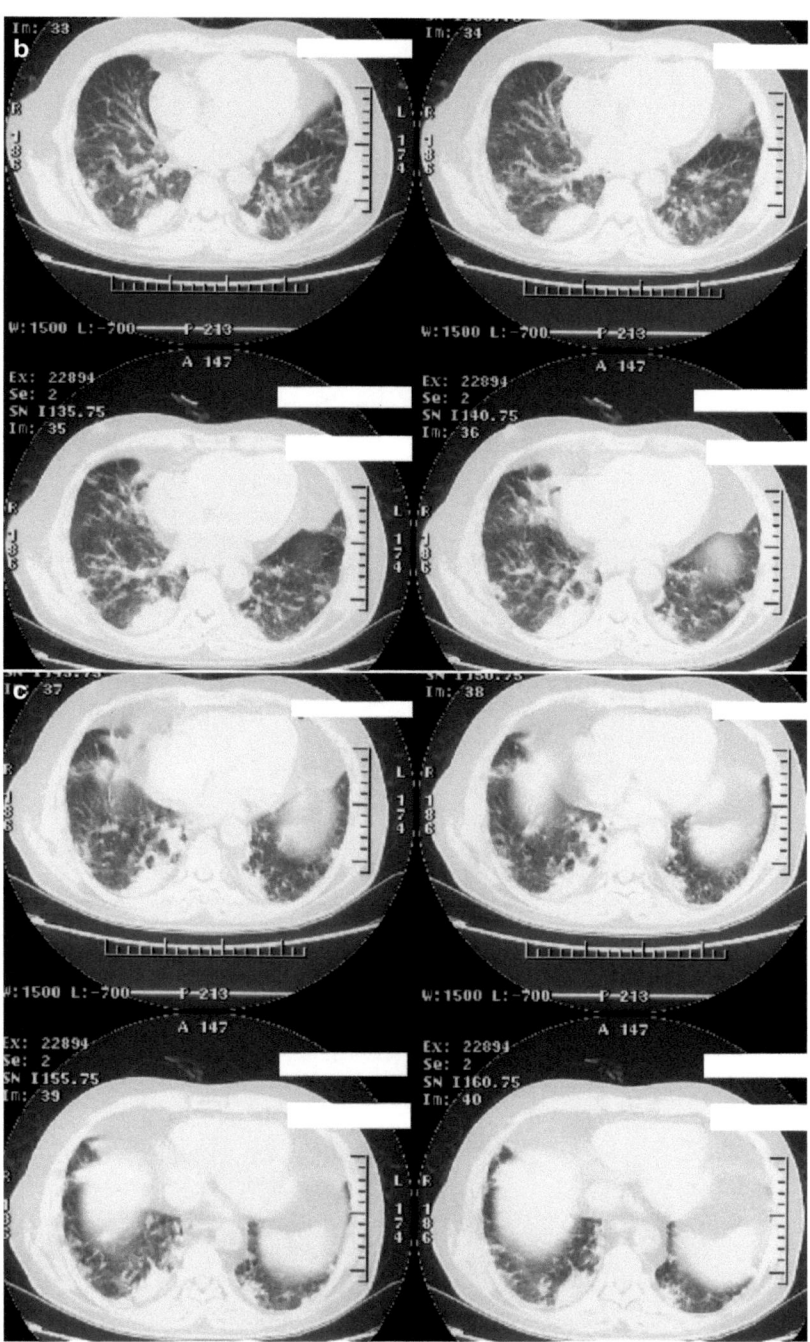

Fig. 11.4 (a–e)
Annotated at the figure
(yellow arrow)

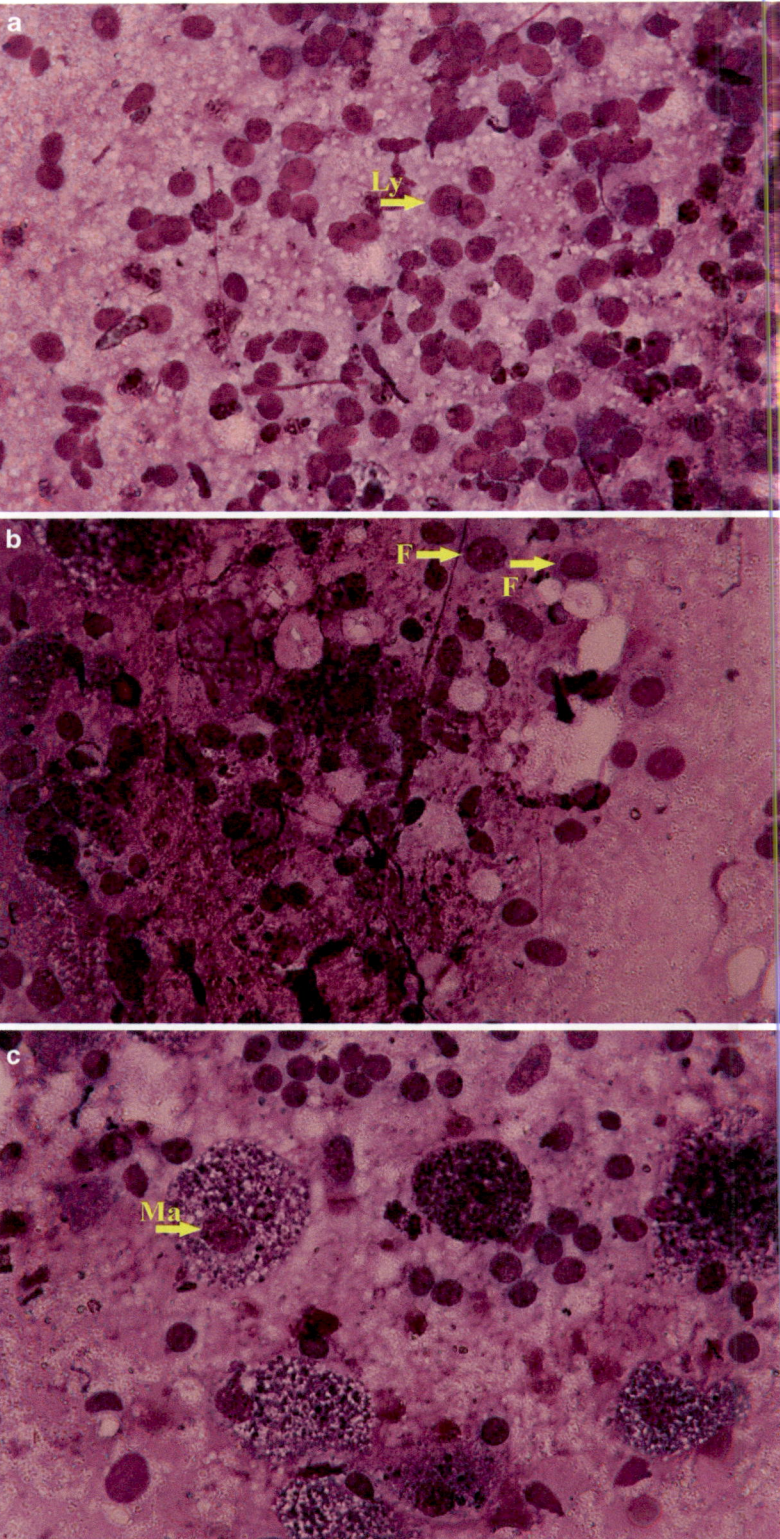

Fig. 11.4   (continued)

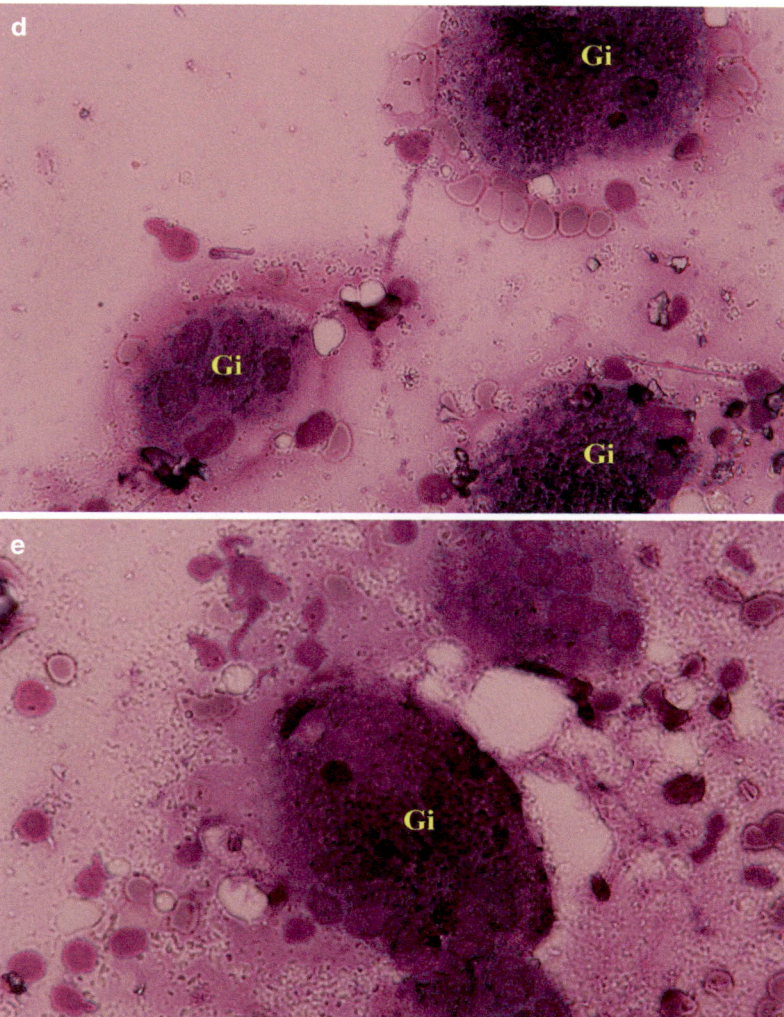

11.3 Chronic Inflammatory Responses After Peripheral Blood Stem Cell Transplantation (PBSCT) for Leukemia

Brief history: Female, 20 years old, 1 year after partially mismatched peripheral blood stem cell transplantation (PBSCT) for leukemia, having ever an acute intestinal graft-versus-host disease, having ever pneumonia 5 months ago, productive coughing for 1 month.

Technology to obtain the target lesions: Transbronchial lung biopsy (TBLB).

The preparation of cytological slides for ROSE: Imprinting (rolling).

Clustering (categorizing) analysis in ROSE interpretation:

- "Inflammatory changes".
- May conform to organization.
- Proliferative/reparative inflammatory response.

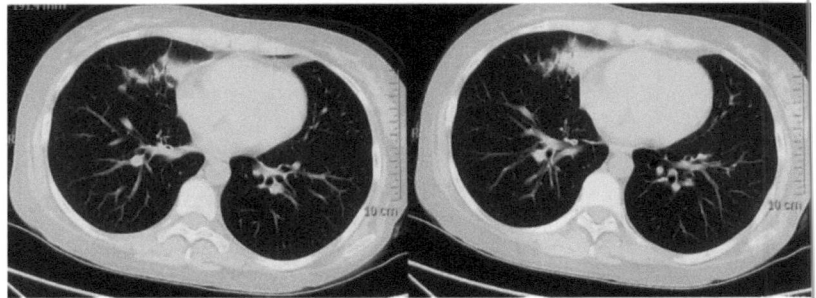

Fig. 11.5 Area of consolidation and exudation in the right middle lobe

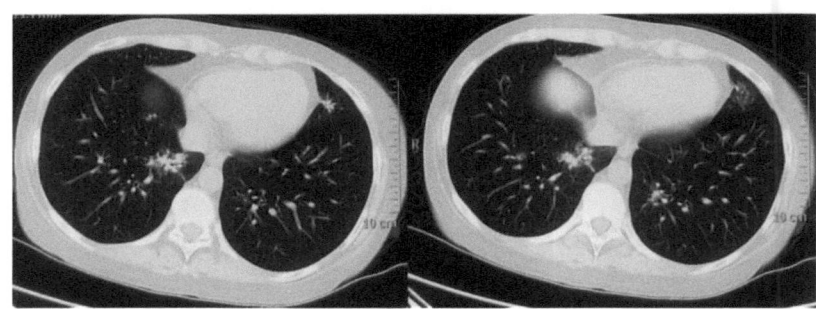

Fig. 11.6 Exudation in the inner basal segment of the right lower lobe

Fig. 11.7 (a–e)
Annotated at the figure
(yellow arrow)

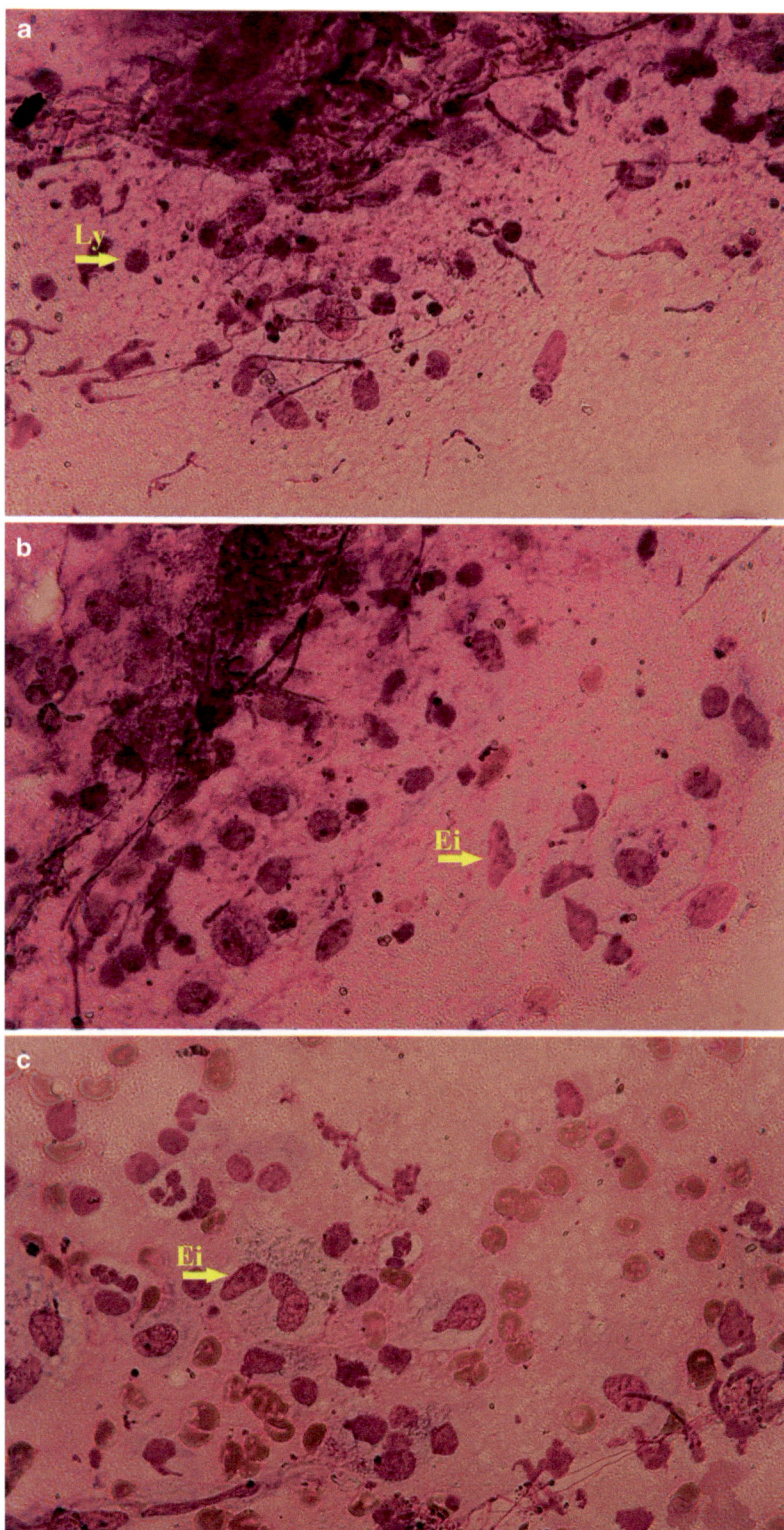

Fig. 11.7 (continued)

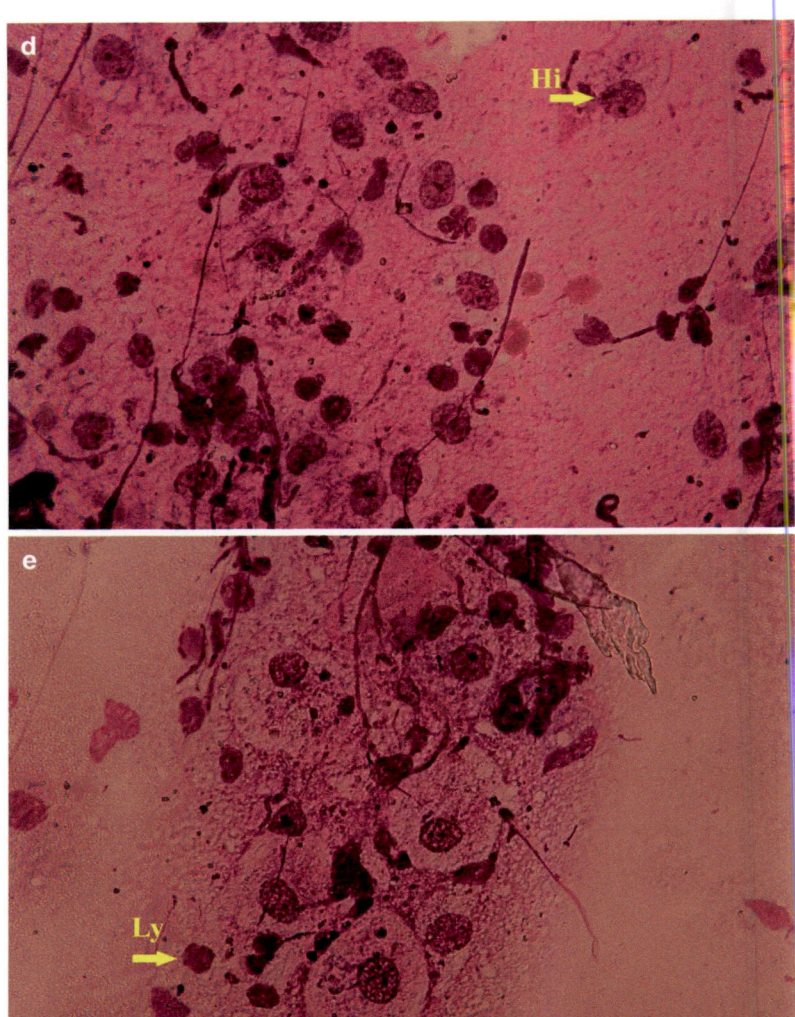

Other Non-neoplastic Non-infectious Lung Diseases

12

Jing Feng, Dianhua Jiang, and Jingyu Chen

12.1 Pulmonary Lymphangioleiomyomatosis (PLAM)

Brief history: Female, 48 years old, shortness of breath after activities, pulmonary imaging and final histopathological findings suggesting pulmonary lymphangioleiomyomatosis (PLAM).

Technology to obtain the target lesions: Transbronchial lung biopsy (TBLB).

The preparation of cytological slides for ROSE: Imprinting (rolling).

Clustering (categorizing) analysis in ROSE interpretation:

- Granulomatous inflammation.
- Lymphocyte-based immune inflammatory response.
- Necrotic "inflammatory changes" (mild).

J. Feng
Pulmonary and Critical Care Medicine, Tianjin
Medical University General Hospital, Tianjin, China
e-mail: zyyhxkfj@126.com

D. Jiang (✉)
Cedars-Sinai Medical Center, Los Angeles, USA
e-mail: Dianhua.Jiang@csmc.edu

J. Chen
Lung Transplantation Group, Nanjing Medical
University, Wuxi, China
e-mail: chenjy@wuxiph.com

© Springer Nature Singapore Pte Ltd. 2020
J. Feng et al. (eds.), *Rapid On-Site Evaluation (ROSE) in Diagnostic Interventional Pulmonology*,
https://doi.org/10.1007/978-981-15-0939-1_12

Fig. 12.1 Non-foamy macrophages (yellow arrow), some evolving into histiocytes (red arrow) and further evolving into epithelioid cells (green arrow), and reactive lymphocytes (blue arrow), a tendency to form atypical granuloma

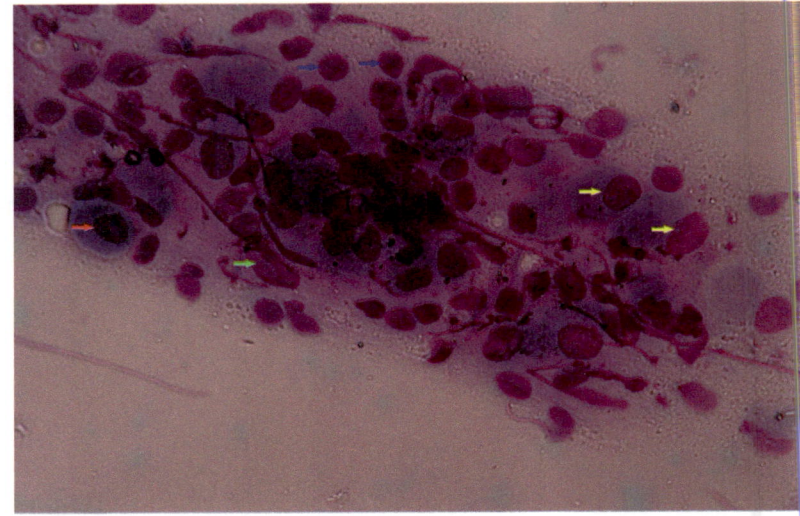

Fig. 12.2 Histiocytes (yellow arrow), epithelioid cells and granuloma-forming (red arrow), and reactive lymphocytes (green arrow)

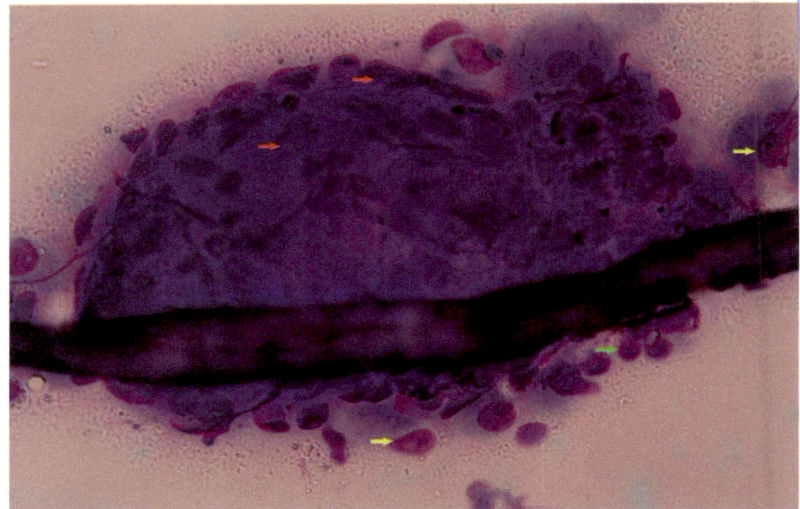

Fig. 12.3 Non-foamy macrophages (yellow arrow), some evolving into histiocytes (red arrow) and further evolving into epithelioid cells (green arrow), and reactive lymphocytes (blue arrow), a tendency to form atypical granuloma

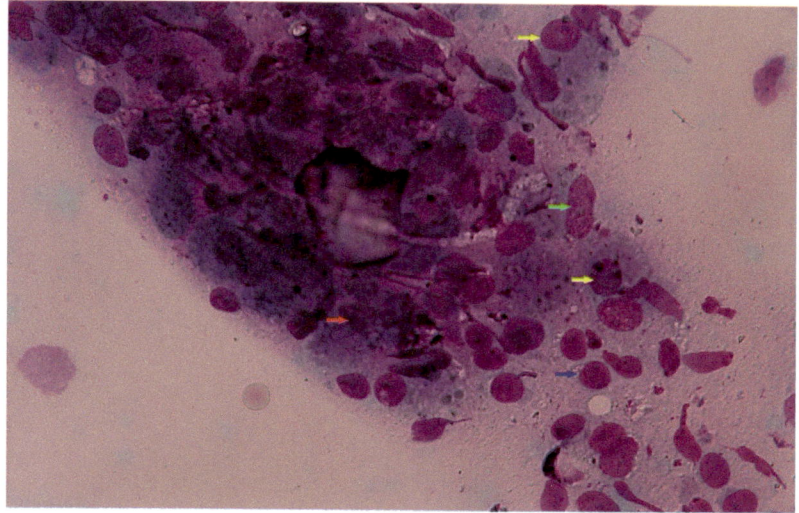

Fig. 12.4 Non-foamy macrophages (yellow arrow), some evolving into histiocytes (red arrow) and further evolving into epithelioid cells (green arrow); reactive lymphocytes (blue arrow), a tendency to form atypical granuloma; and distal airway epithelial cells (pink arrow)

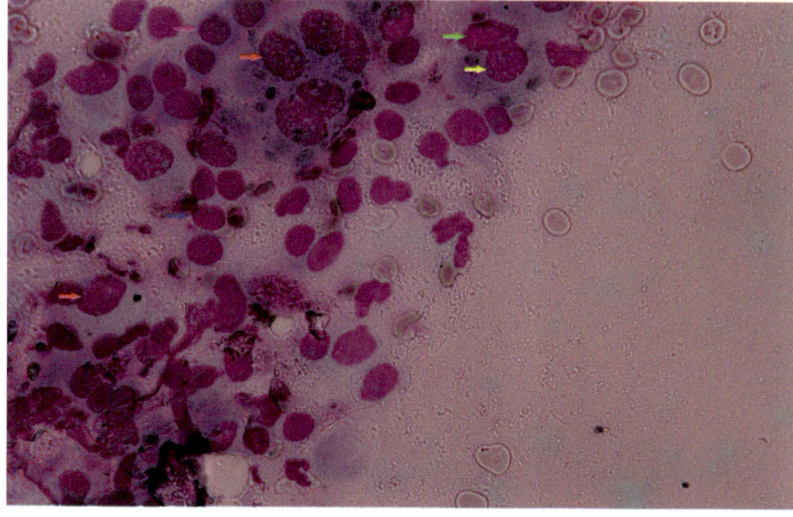

Fig. 12.5 Non-foamy macrophages (yellow arrow), some evolving into histiocytes (red arrow) and further evolving into epithelioid cells (green arrow), reactive lymphocytes (blue arrow), and nuclear filaments from necrotic cells (pink arrow)

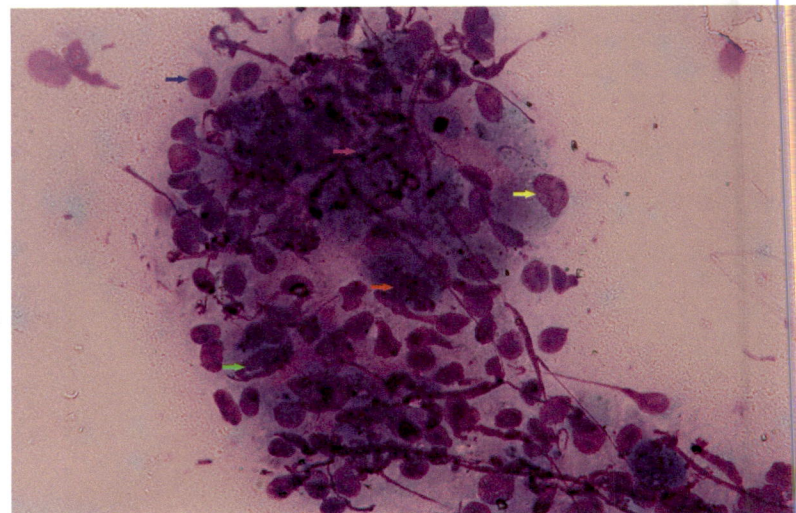

Fig. 12.6 Non-foamy macrophages (yellow arrow), some evolving into histiocytes (red arrow), reactive lymphocytes (green arrow), and nuclear filaments from necrotic cells (blue arrow)

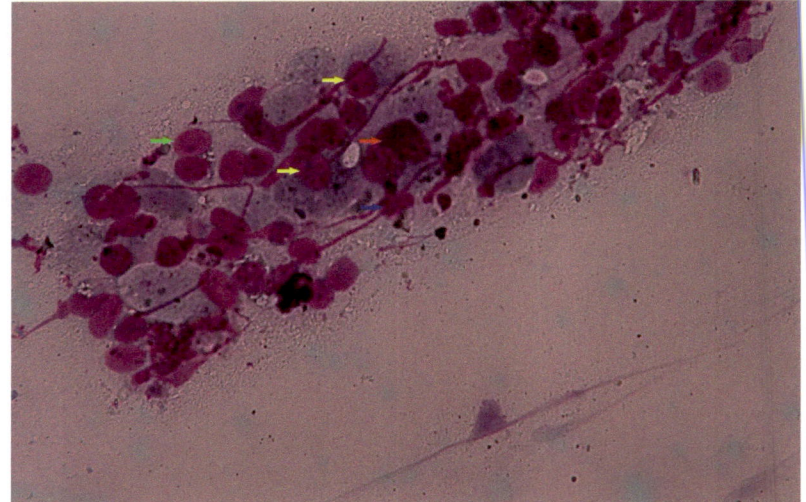

12.2 Pulmonary Lymphangioleiomyomatosis (PLAM)

Brief history: Clinically diagnosed as pulmonary lymphangioleiomyomatosis (PLAM).

Technology to obtain the target lesions: Transbronchial lung biopsy (TBLB).

The preparation of cytological slides for ROSE: Imprinting (rolling).

Clustering (categorizing) analysis in ROSE interpretation:

- "Inflammatory changes".
- Lymphocyte-based immune inflammatory response.
- Proliferative/reparative inflammatory response.

Fig. 12.7 (a, b)
Thin-walled cysts of
varying sizes, evenly
distributed in both lungs

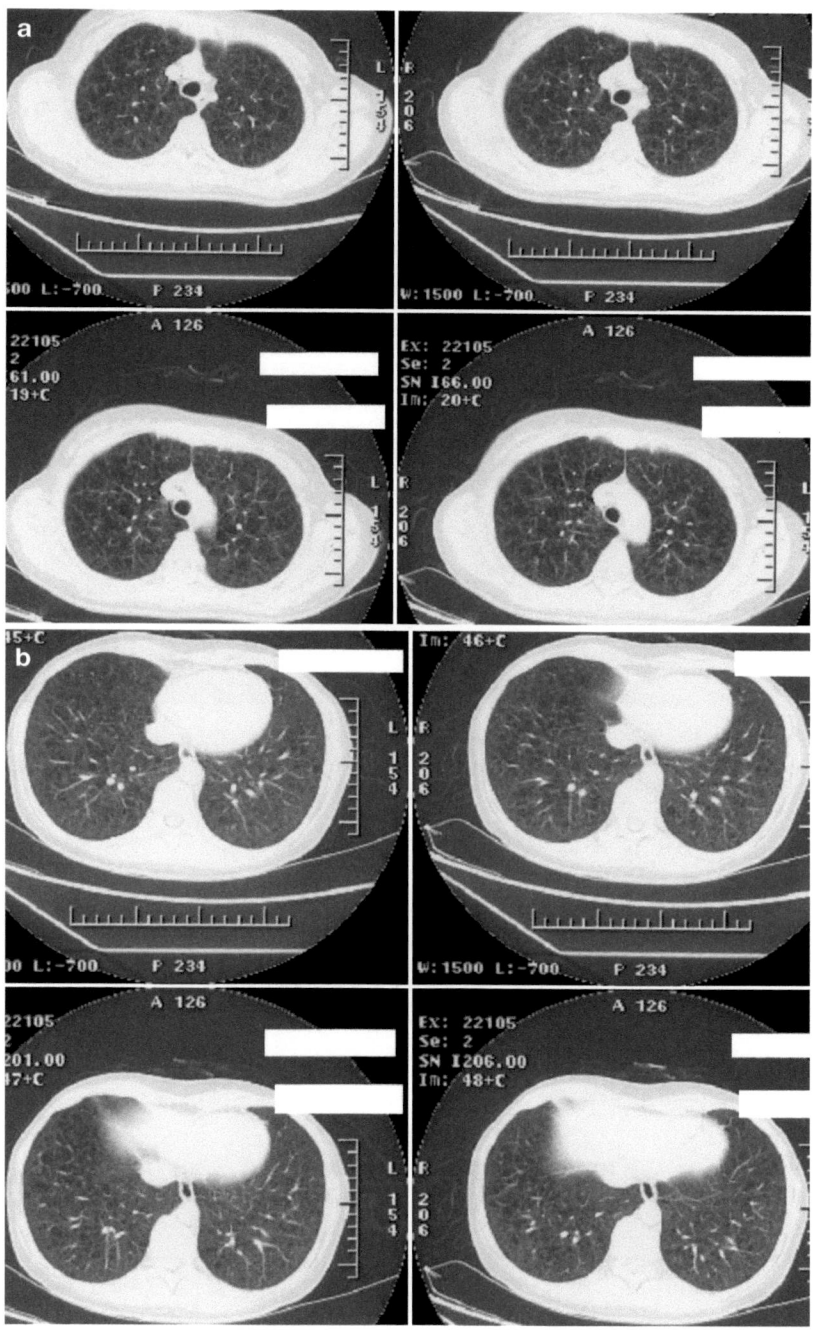

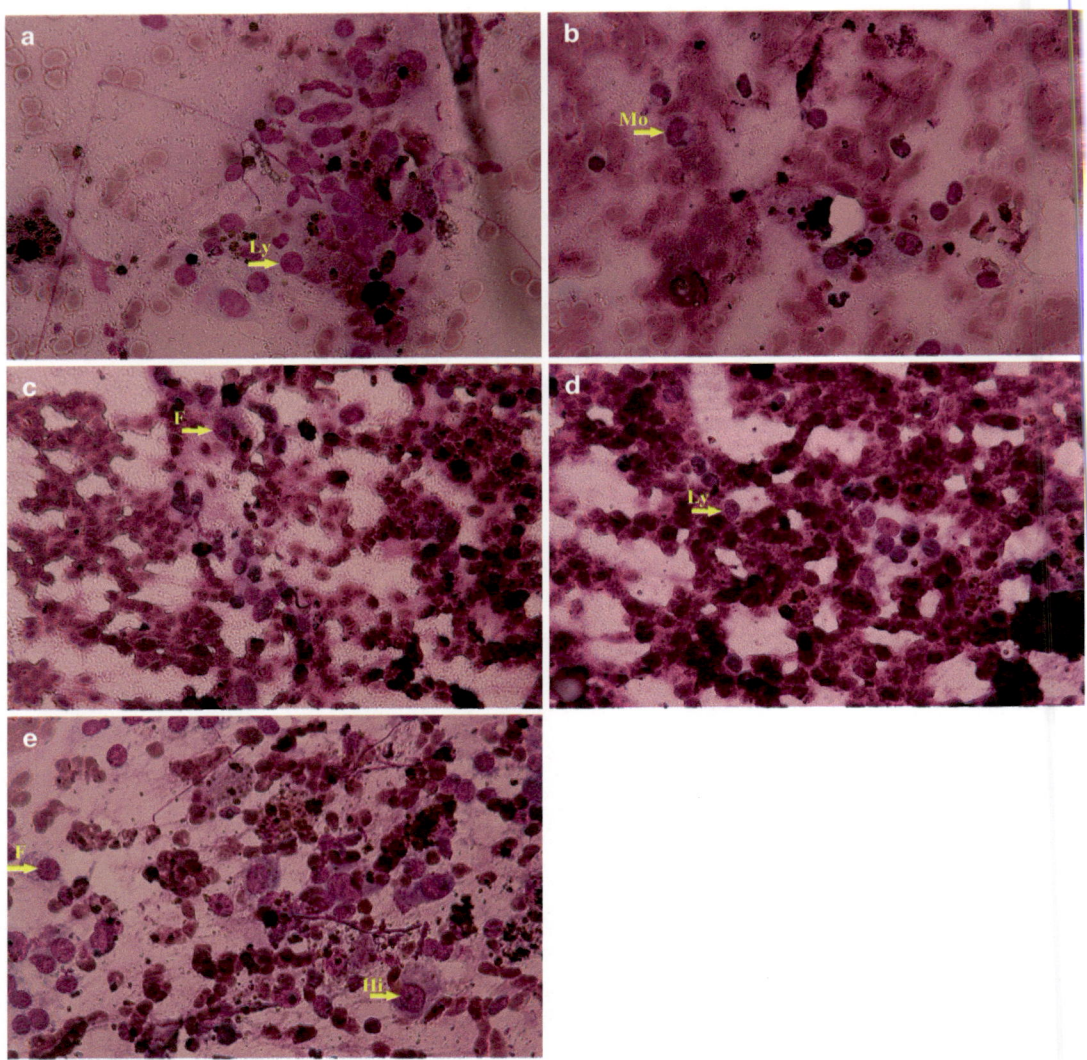

Fig. 12.8 (a–e) Annotated at the figure (yellow arrow)

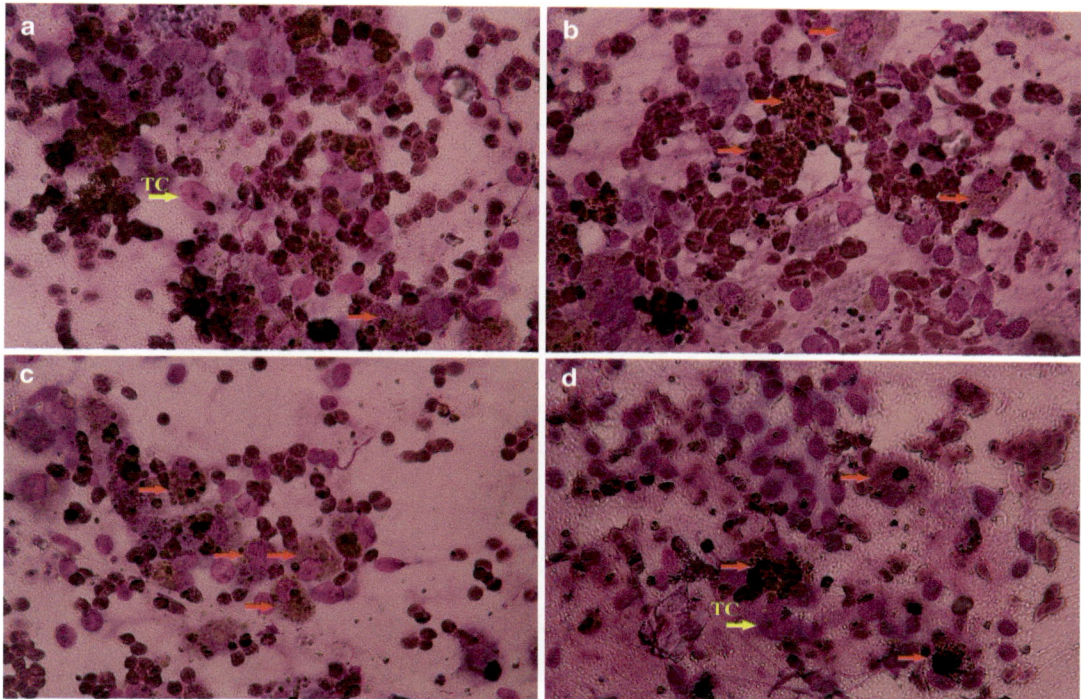

Fig. 12.9 (**a–d**) Abnormally proliferated smooth muscle cells (tumor cells, TC) (yellow arrow) and hemosiderin cells (red arrow)

12.3   Tracheal and Bronchial Amyloidosis

Brief history: Male, 77 years old, coughing for several months with mild shortness of breath.

Technology to obtain the target lesions: Biopsy under direct vision.

The preparation of cytological slides for ROSE: Imprinting (rolling).

Clustering (categorizing) analysis in ROSE interpretation:

There are visible pathogens, characteristic manifestations, or foreign objects.

Fig. 12.10 (a, b) Diffuse tracheal and bronchial wall thickening and atelectasis at some segments of the right lower lobe

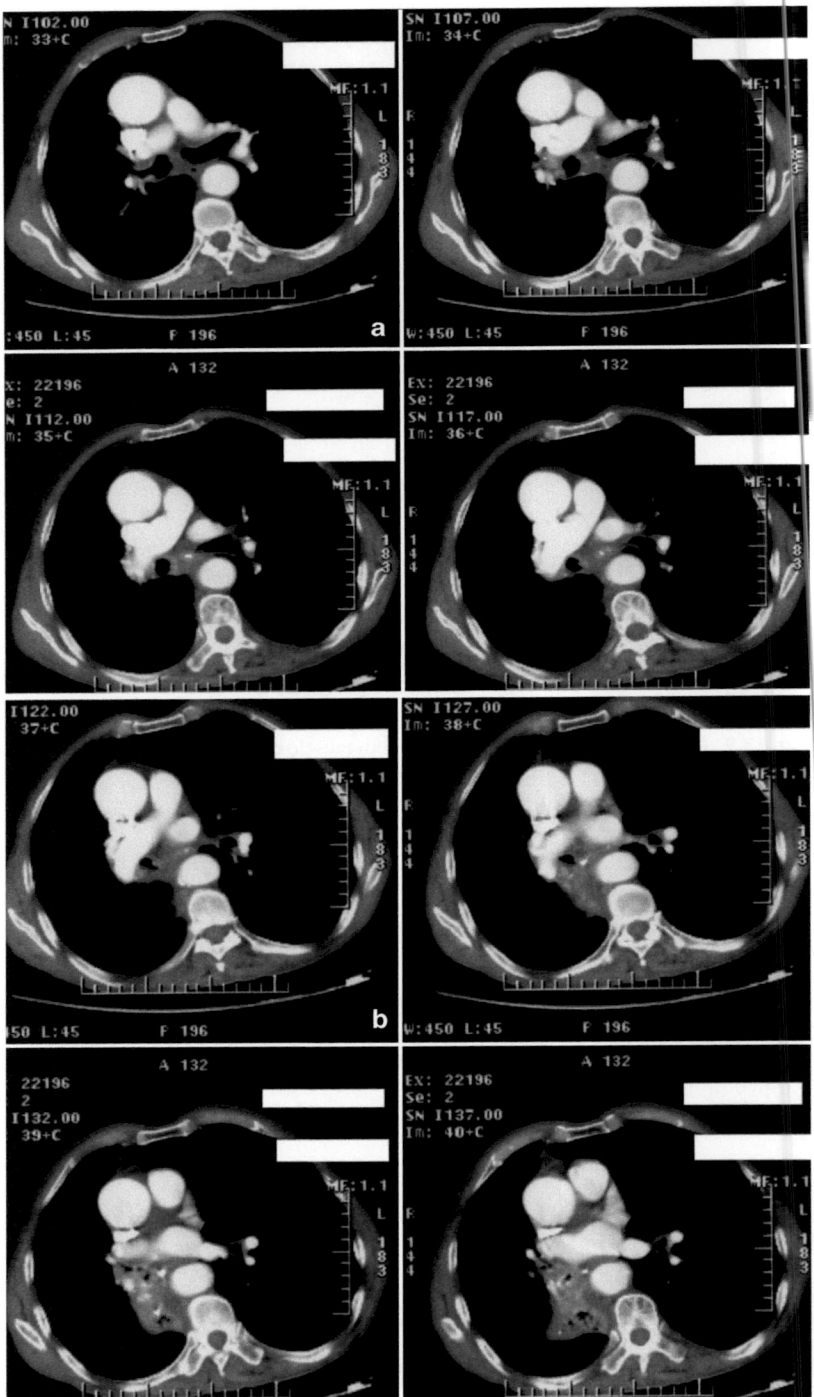

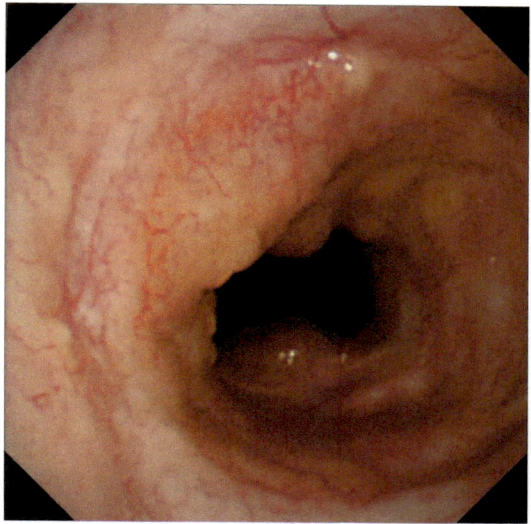

Fig. 12.11 Diffuse tracheal wall thickening

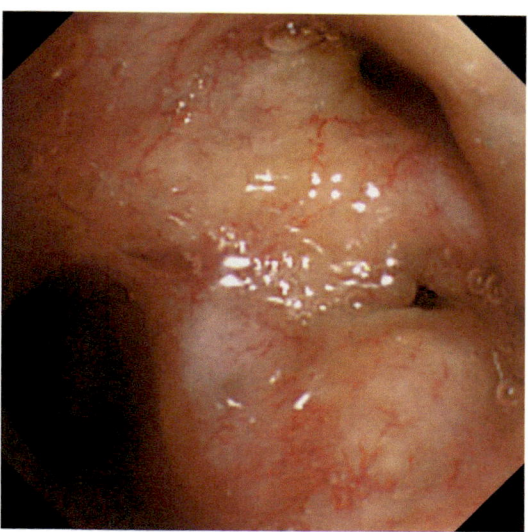

Fig. 12.13 The illustration showing the opening of the right upper lobe and mucosa thickening

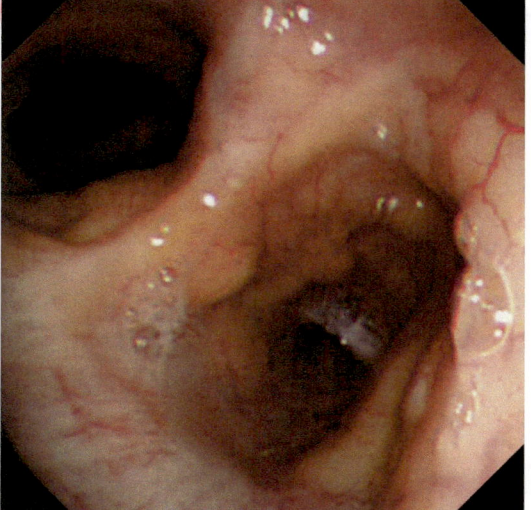

Fig. 12.12 Mucosal surface of carina unsmooth

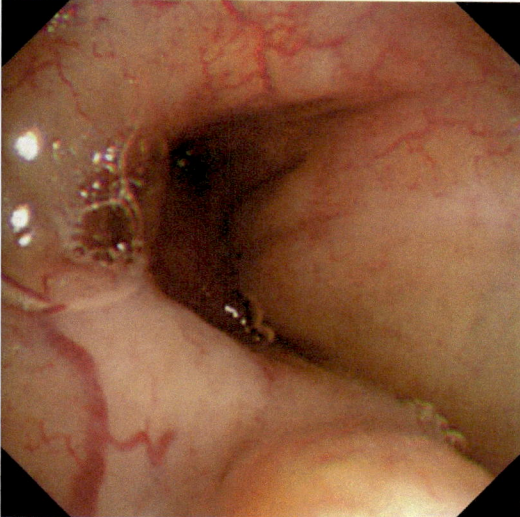

Fig. 12.14 The illustration showing the opening of the right bronchus intermedius and mucosa thickening, unsmooth

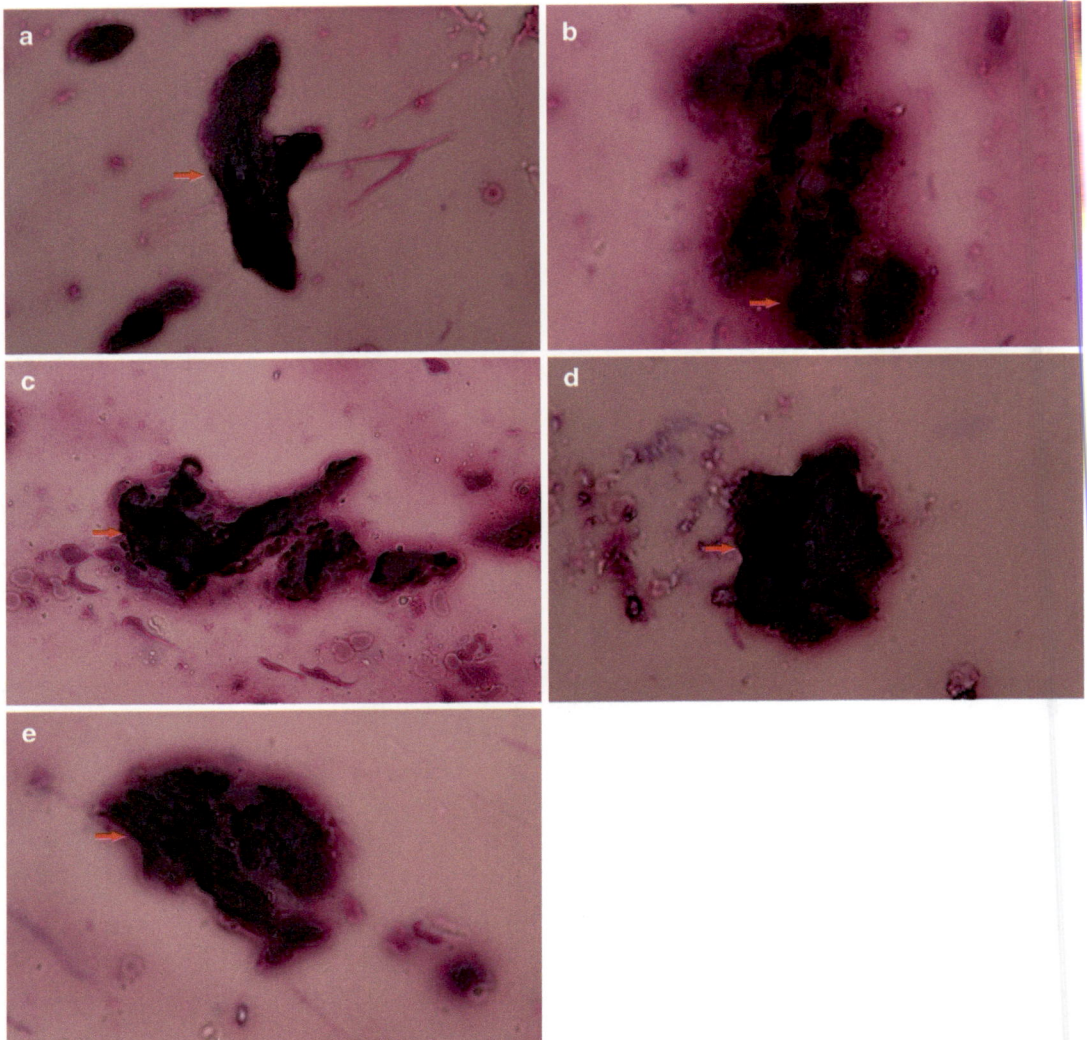

Fig. 12.15 (**a**–**e**) Cyanophilic amorphous substance (red arrow)

12.4　Primary Tracheobronchial Amyloidosis

Brief history: Female, 61 years old, persistent coughing with shortness of breath for 2 months, clinically diagnosed as primary tracheobronchial amyloidosis.

　　Technology to obtain the target lesions: Biopsy under direct vision.

The preparation of cytological slides for ROSE: Imprinting (rolling).

Clustering (categorizing) analysis in ROSE interpretation:

- "Inflammatory changes".
- There are visible pathogens, characteristic manifestations, or foreign objects.
- Necrotic "inflammatory changes".

Fig. 12.16 (a, b)
Enlargement of hilar and
mediastinal lymph nodes
and diffuse tracheal and
bronchial wall
thickening

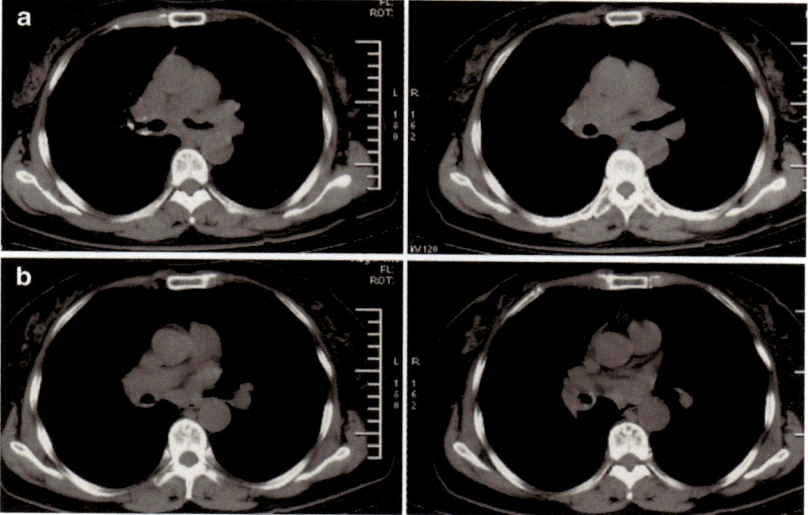

Fig. 12.17 (a, b)
Diffuse tracheal wall
thickening and rough
mucosal surface

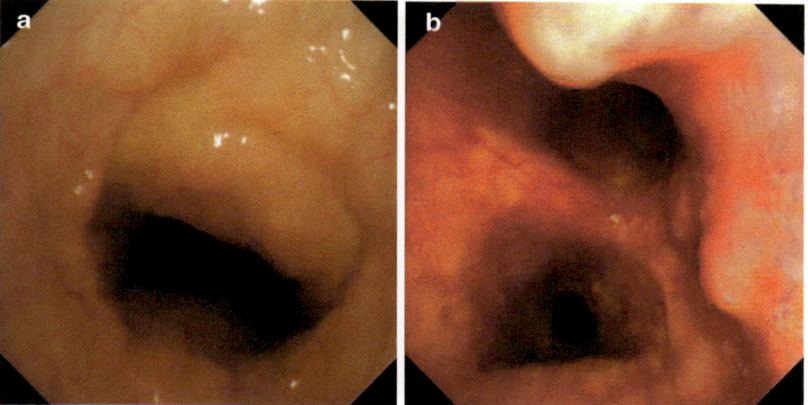

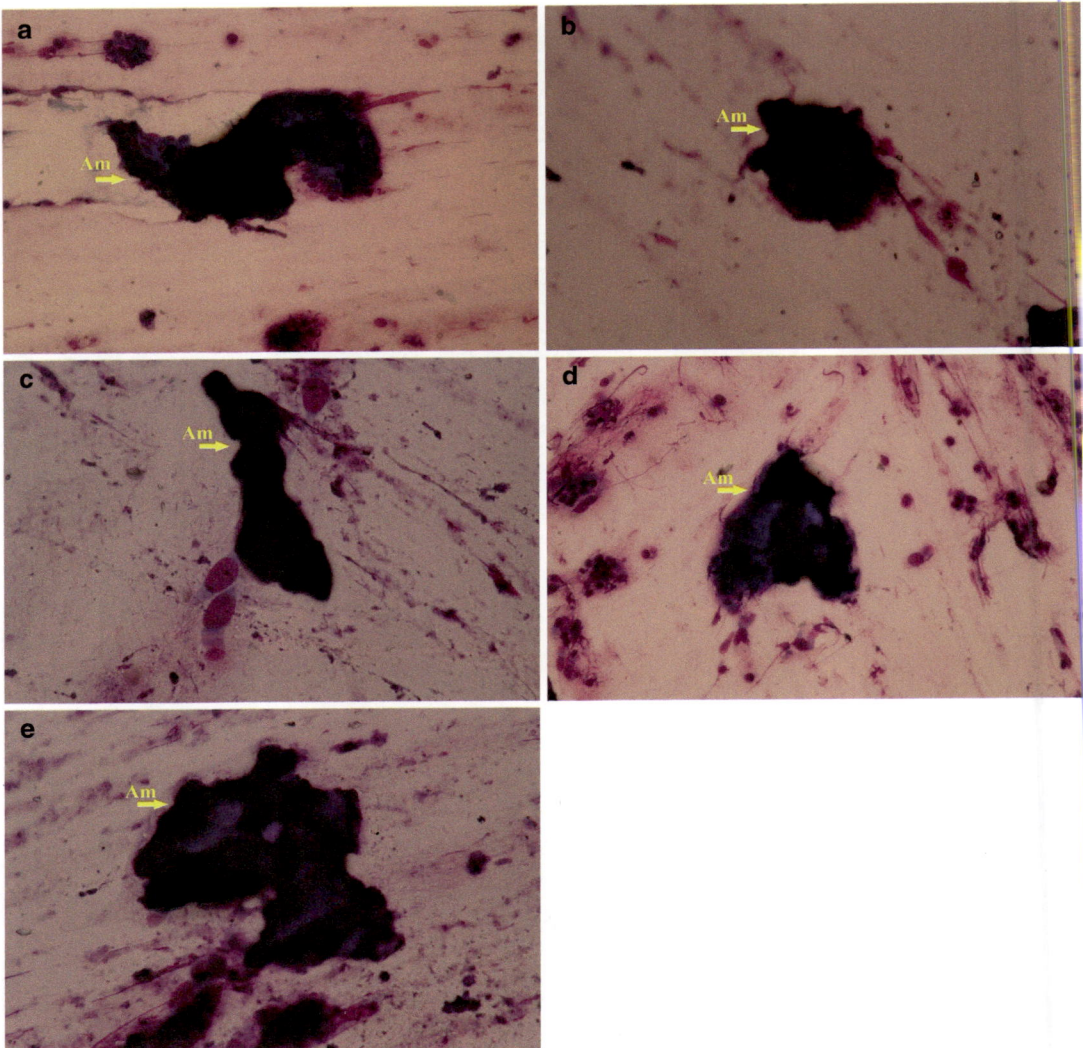

Fig. 12.18 (a–e) Annotated at the figure (yellow arrow)

12.5 Primary Tracheobronchial and Pulmonary Amyloidosis

Brief history: Female, 68 years old, persistent coughing with mild shortness of breath, clinically diagnosed as primary tracheobronchial and pulmonary amyloidosis.

Technology to obtain the target lesions: Biopsy under direct vision.

The preparation of cytological slides for ROSE: Imprinting (rolling).

Clustering (categorizing) analysis in ROSE interpretation:

- "Inflammatory changes".
- Granulomatous inflammation.
- Lymphocyte-based immune inflammatory response.
- There are visible pathogens, characteristic manifestations, or foreign objects.
- Necrotic "inflammatory changes".

Fig. 12.19 (a, b)
Diffuse tracheal and
bronchial wall
thickening and
reticulonodular
abnormalities involving
both lungs, resulting
from thickening of
interlobular septa and
intralobular irregular
lines

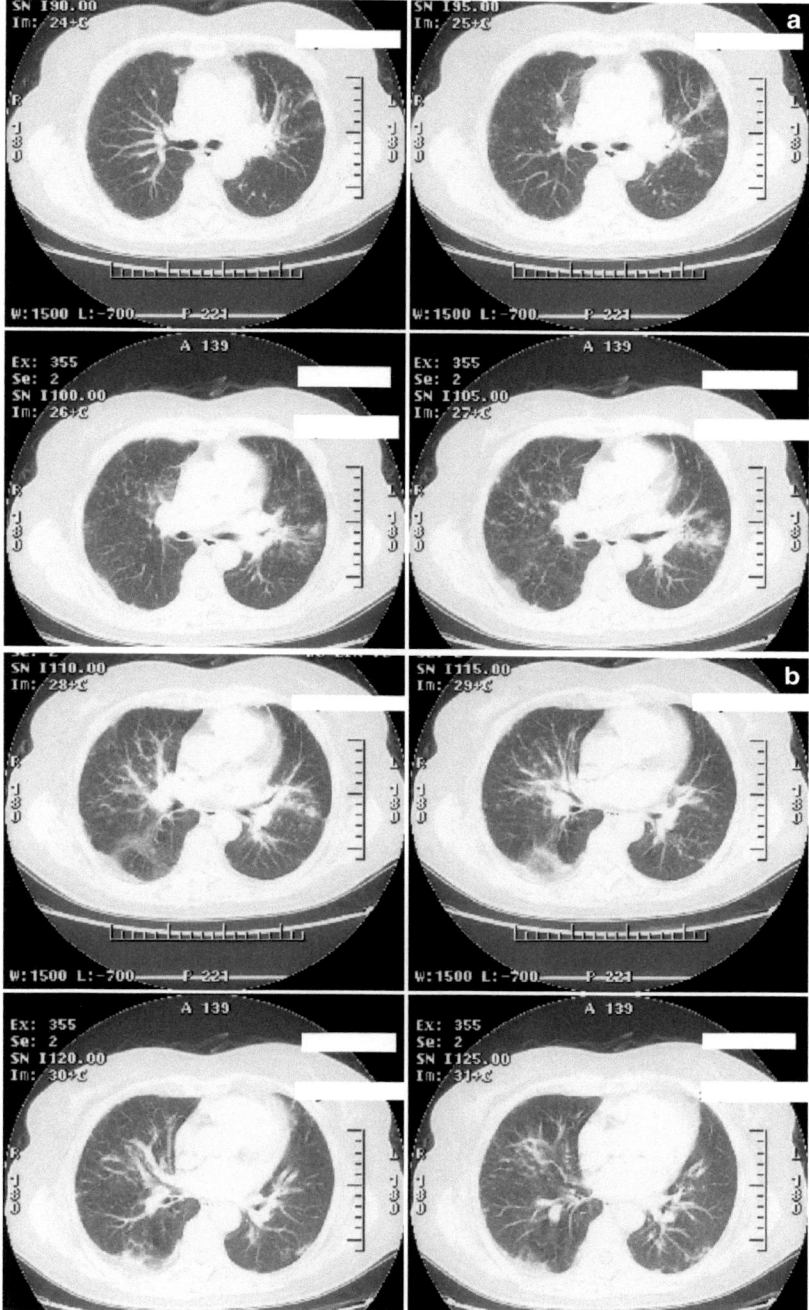

Fig. 12.20 (**a, b**)
Diffuse tracheal wall
thickening and rough
mucosal surface

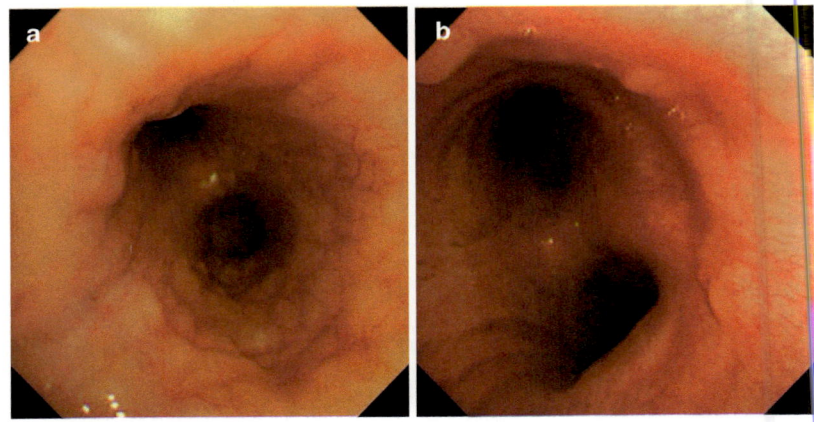

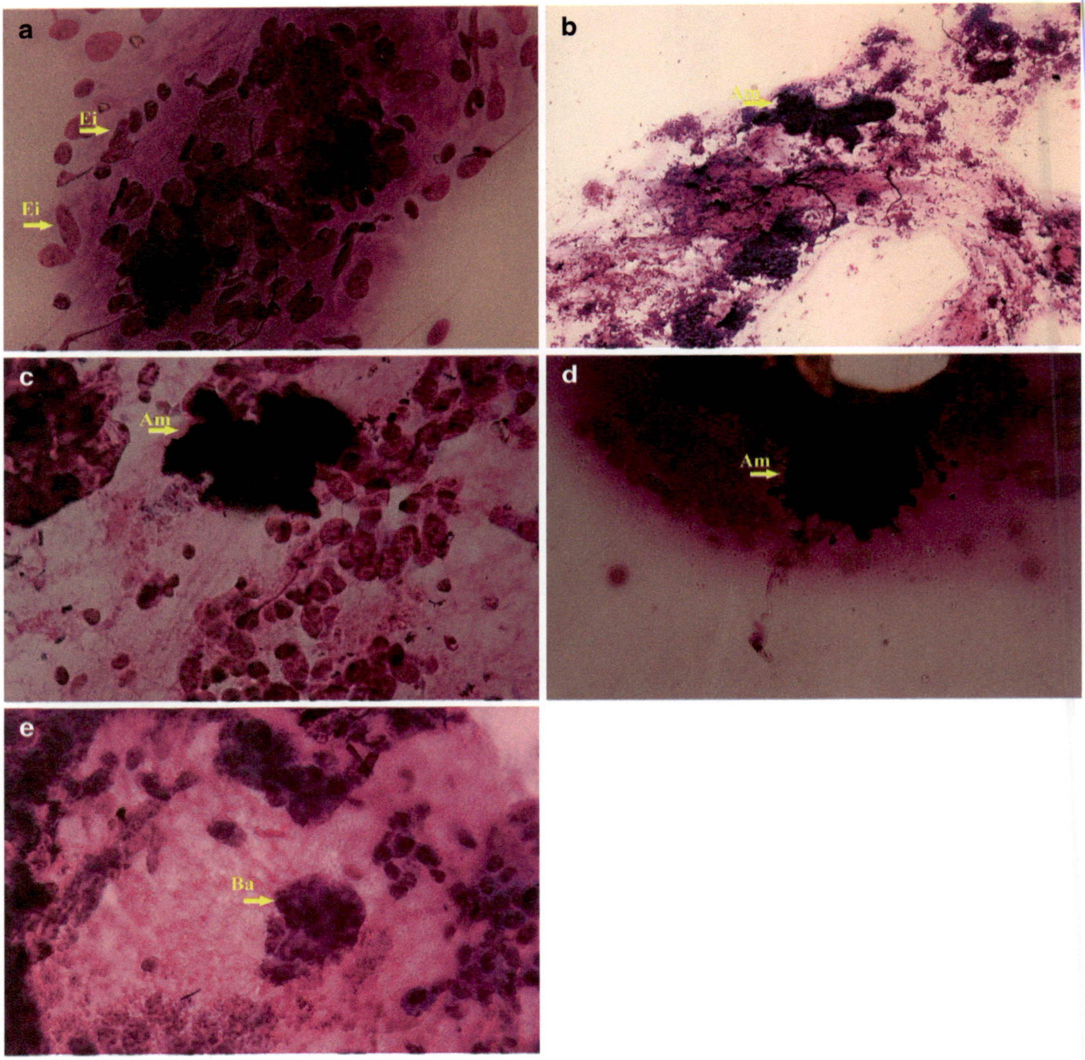

Fig. 12.21 (**a–e**) Annotated at the figure (yellow arrow)

12.6 Delayed Pulmonary Toxicity Syndrome (DPTS) Due to Cyclophosphamide

Brief history: Treated with a cyclophosphamide-containing regimen for lymphoma, after five cycles of chemotherapy.

Technology to obtain the target lesions: Transbronchial lung biopsy (TBLB).

The preparation of cytological slides for ROSE: Imprinting (rolling).

Clustering (categorizing) analysis in ROSE interpretation:

- "Inflammatory changes".
- Granulomatous inflammation.
- Lymphocyte-based immune inflammatory response.

Fig. 12.22 (**a, b**) Extensive ground-glass opacities and patches in both lungs non-contrast-enhanced CT

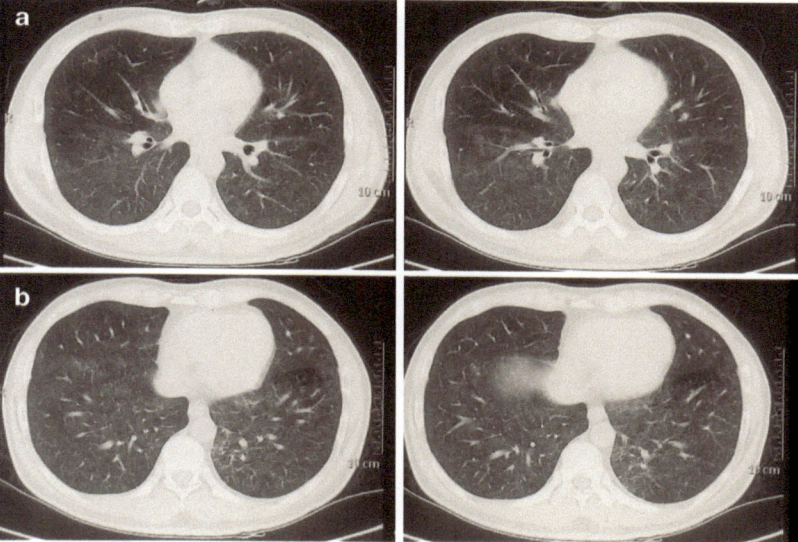

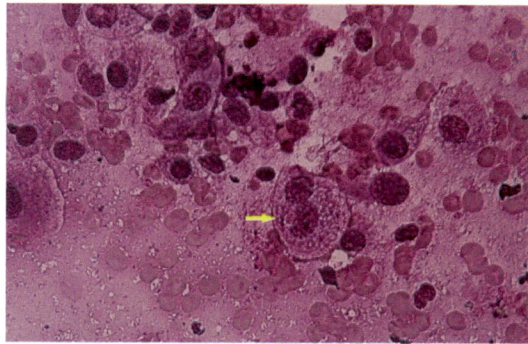

Fig. 12.23 Foamy macrophages (yellow arrow)

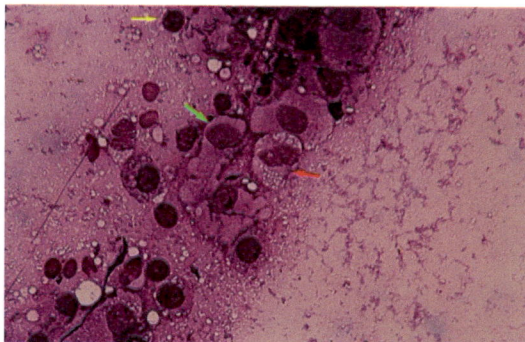

Fig. 12.24 Reactive lymphocytes (yellow arrow), lots of histiocytes (red arrow), and hyperplastic type 2 alveolar epithelial cells (green arrow)

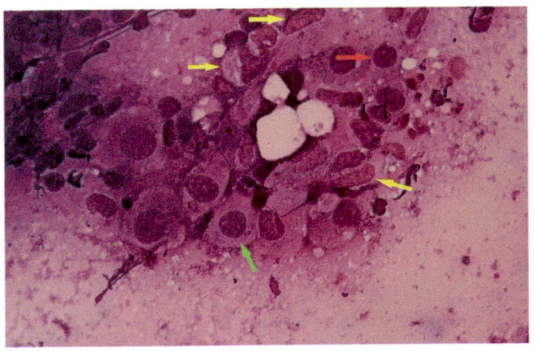

Fig. 12.25 Histiocytes and epithelioid cells (yellow arrow), reactive lymphocytes (red arrow), and hyperplastic type 2 alveolar epithelial cells (green arrow)

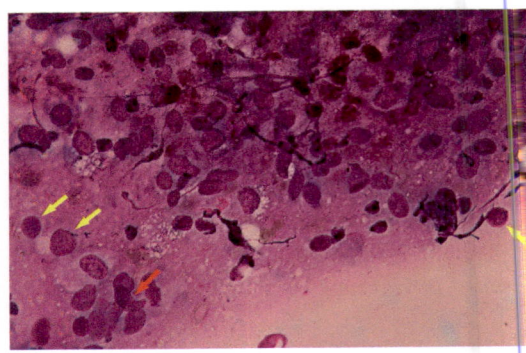

Fig. 12.28 Reactive lymphocytes (yellow arrow) and epithelioid cells (red arrow)

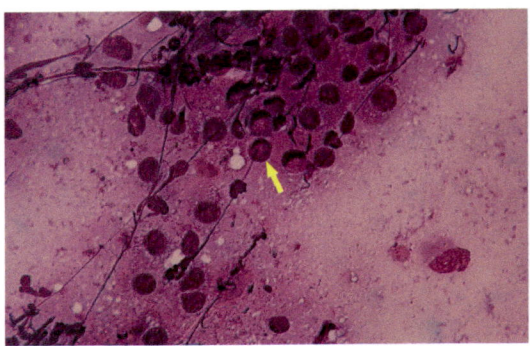

Fig. 12.26 Reactive lymphocytes (yellow arrow)

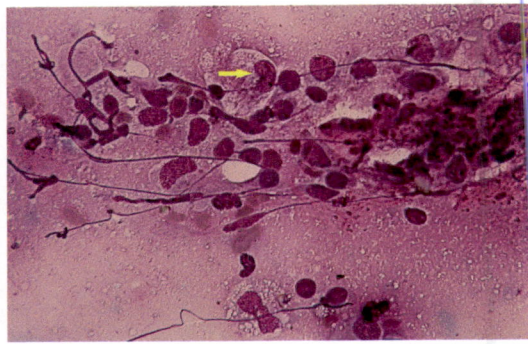

Fig. 12.29 Histiocytes (yellow arrow)

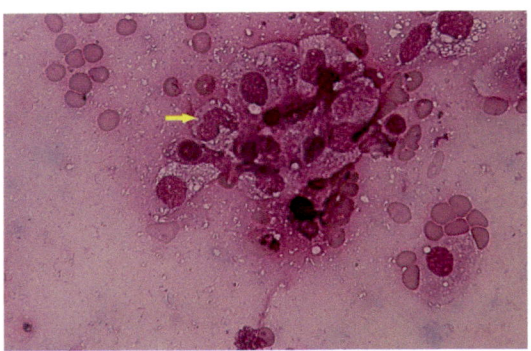

Fig. 12.27 Lots of foamy macrophages, histiocytes (yellow arrow)

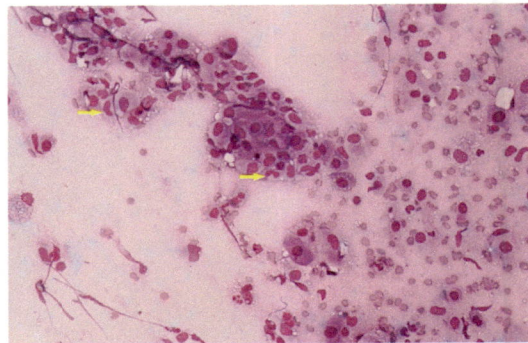

Fig. 12.30 Lots of foamy macrophages, histiocytes (yellow arrow)

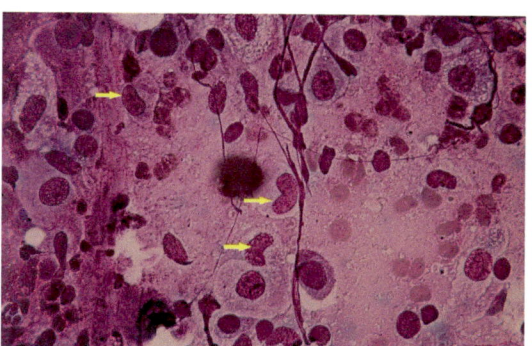

Fig. 12.31   Histiocytes (yellow arrow)

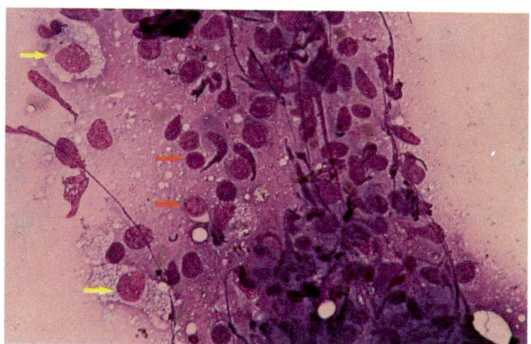

Fig. 12.34   Histiocytes (yellow arrow) and reactive lymphocytes (red arrow)

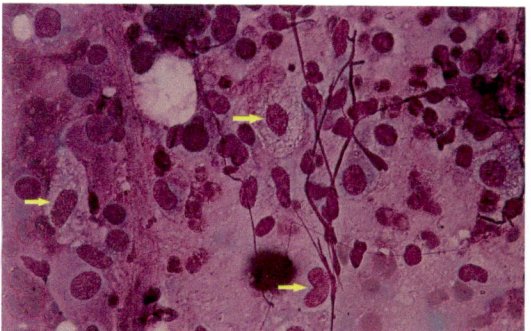

Fig. 12.32   Histiocytes (yellow arrow)

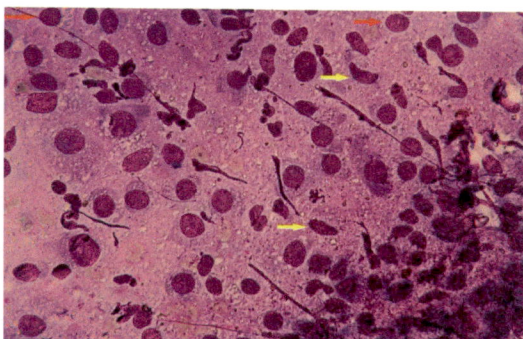

Fig. 12.35   Epithelioid cells (yellow arrow) and reactive lymphocytes (red arrow)

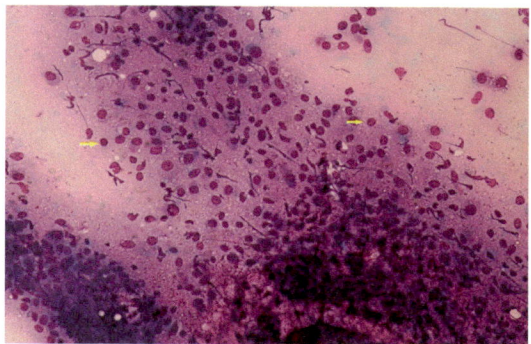

Fig. 12.33   Reactive lymphocytes (yellow arrow)

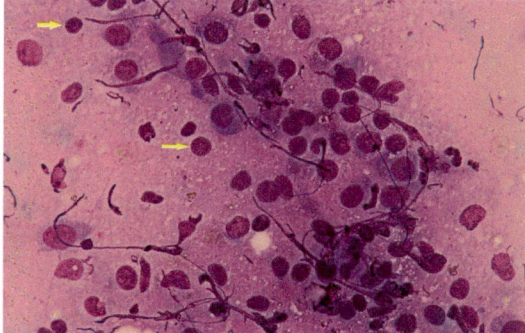

Fig. 12.36   Reactive lymphocytes (yellow arrow)

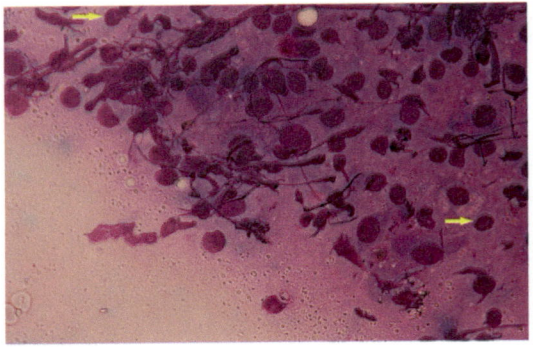

Fig. 12.37 Reactive lymphocytes (yellow arrow)

12.7   Acute Pulmonary Edema (Acute Left Cardiac Insufficiency)

Brief history: Male, 67 years old, wheezing, non-productive cough and progressive exertional dyspnea, clinically diagnosed as acute pulmonary edema (acute left cardiac insufficiency) finally.

Technology to obtain the target lesions: Transbronchial lung biopsy (TBLB).

The preparation of cytological slides for ROSE: Imprinting (rolling).

Fig. 12.38 (**a, b, c**) Extensive confluent consolidation and exudation in both lungs; smooth interstitial thickening distributed along the bronchial vascular bundles, especially at dependent areas; and pleural effusion at both sides

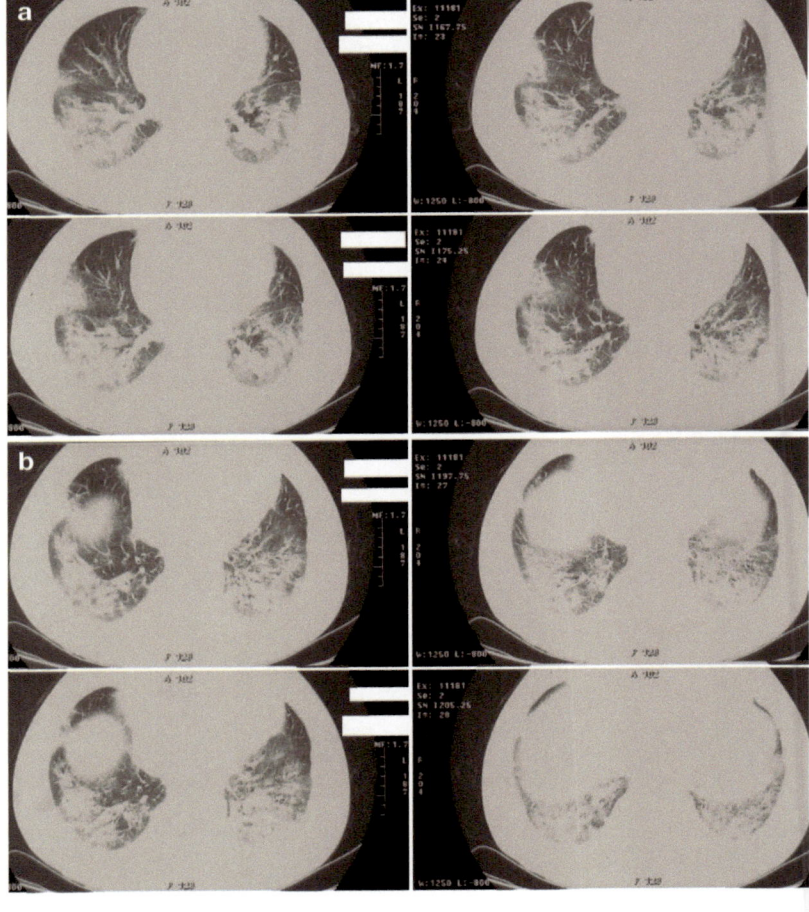

Fig. 12.38 (continued)

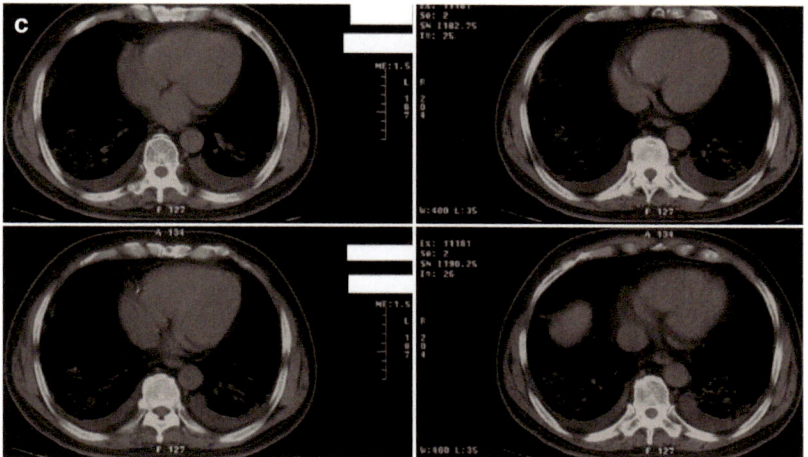

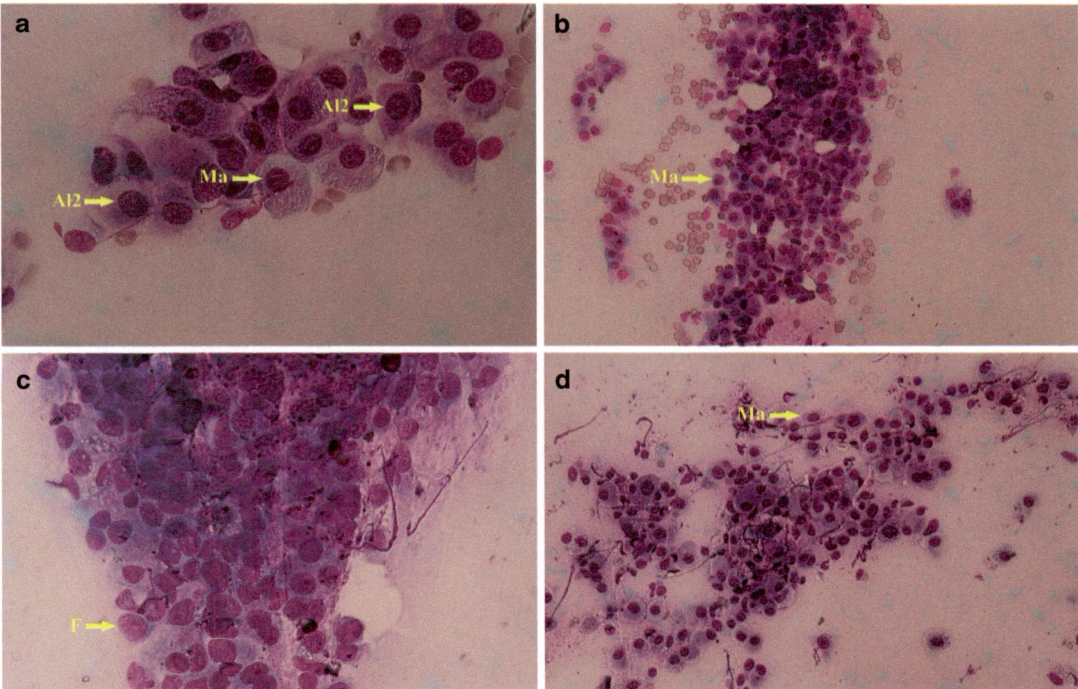

Fig. 12.39 (**a–e**) Annotated at the figure (yellow arrow)

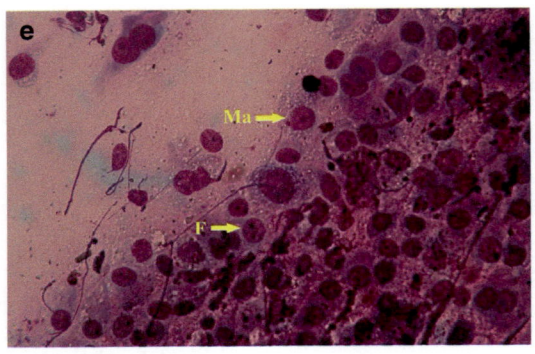

Clustering (categorizing) analysis in ROSE interpretation:

- Approximately normal/mild nonspecific inflammatory response.
- May conform to organization.

Fig. 12.39 (continued)